The Captured Womb

A history of the medical care of pregnant women

The Captured Womb

A history of the medical care of pregnant women

ANN OAKLEY

© 1984 Ann Oakley
except for text of Appendix I © Alison Macfarlane

First published 1984

Basil Blackwell Publisher Ltd
108 Cowley Road, Oxford OX4 1JF, UK

Basil Blackwell Inc.
432 Park Avenue South, Suite 1505,
New York, NY 10016, USA

British Library Cataloguing in Publication Data

Oakley, Ann
    The captured womb.

    Bibliography: p.
    Includes index.
    1. Prenatal care — Great Britain — History — 20th century.
    I. Title
    RG516.02   1984   362.1'982'00941   84–8856
    ISBN 0–631–14152–9

Typeset by Oxford Publishing Services, Oxford
Printed in Great Britain by Bell and Bain Ltd., Glasgow

FOR L

'It seems remarkable that a clinic designed for the routine supervision of all pregnant women, normal as well as abnormal, which is such a commonplace feature of obstetric practice today, has so short a history.'

(Forster, 1967, p. 85.)

'Until recently the gravid human uterus has been regarded as a sanctuary, its contained conceptus equally inaccessible to direct diagnostic manipulations and to therapeutic attack. . . .'

(Gruenwald, 1975, p. 98.)

'In a word, this is no ordinary medical issue by and of itself; it is an issue of civilization in origin and in solution.'

(Departmental Committee, 1930, p. 104.)

Contents

List of Figures

List of Plates

List of Tables

Introduction

This book is an attempt to write the history of the care pregnant women receive in preparation for childbirth and motherhood. More specifically, it is concerned with that type of care which has been deemed 'medical' because it is (has become) pre-eminently the province of the medical profession. Thus, the first and last question with which the book deals is one about the process whereby a particular area of social behaviour (pregnancy) comes to be separated off from social behaviour in general and reconstituted as a specialist, technical subject under the external jurisdiction of some expert authority. Why did this happen? How did it happen? What consequences did it have? The rise of medical antenatal care is an instance of the medicalization of health and human welfare, and of life itself. But while this is true, it does not itself serve to explain the incorporation of pregnancy in the medical domain.

Michel Foucault, in his *Discipline and Punish: the birth of the prison*, begins by saying that the study of punishment with which he is concerned must depend upon the concept of 'a political technology of the body'. Foucault's major objective in *Discipline and Punish* is to provide a history of the prison as an institution which organizes a field of objectivity: in such a field punishment is able to function openly as treatment, and penal sentences are inscribed among the accepted discourses of knowledge. Why, he asks himself, does he pursue such an objective? 'Simply because I am interested in the past? No, if one means by that writing a history of the past in terms of the present. Yes, if one means writing the history of the present' (Foucault, 1977, p. 31). To say that pregnancy is a medical activity because it is a biological one is to commit the error of 'writing a history of the past in terms of the present'. What is important is the development of the idea that any phenomenon belongs to this or that expert domain.

It could be argued that antenatal care is a subject of marginal relevance to most people's daily lives. Why, then, is it important to study antenatal care? In the first place, of course, since some 90 per cent of women in countries such as Britain bear at least one child, antenatal care is a process undergone at some time in their lives by almost half the population. This gives it some importance. But, secondly, as I shall argue later in this book, antenatal care is both an exemplar and a facilitator of the wider *social* control of women, and that is an even more significant matter. Antenatal care may be equated with other forms of social control over women on the basis of what is said by clinicians and policy-makers in Britain and other countries today. In some European languages (including Finnish, Danish, Norwegian, Swedish and Dutch), the term for antenatal care uses the word 'control': this can scarcely be irrelevant.

To appreciate antenatal care in all its aspects we need to step back into the past and examine its origins. We must do this because the phenomenon called antenatal care, as we know it today, cannot be explained in its own terms. According to the usual scientific–rational justifications, modern antenatal care is not justifiable (has not been shown effectively to prevent all 'avoidable' death and illness — however 'avoidable' is defined, and it is certainly subject to changing definition). It is, indeed, only justifiable in terms of its past, as the product and particular manifestation of a motivation to control the reproductive biology of women. The most characteristic aspect of modern antenatal care is the clinical insistence on the probability of pathology in all childbearing. In historical terms, the redefinition of pregnancy to abolish any idea of its essential normality was an obstetrical necessity, for, as William Arney, in a recent history, aptly puts it,

> The project of obstetrics as obstetricians originally defined it was the pathology of childbirth, but the continued existence of obstetricians depended on their ability to capture childbirth, all of it, treat it, and hold it firmly as part of their project. Until they could accomplish that, they would live with the threat . . . that someone would offer women an alternative approach to birth (Arney, 1982, p. 51).

With the definition of all pregnancies as potentially pathological, ante-natal care obtained its final mandate, a mandate written by the medical profession in alliance with the population-controlling interests of the state, and one giving an unprecedented degree of licence over the bodies and approved life-styles of women.

Most of the history of medicine has been written with an inclination towards positivism: there is a concern with the 'solid' facts of medico-scientific discovery and an energetic pursuit of truer and truer information via a scholarly documentation of these facts. Technical medical innovations are hailed as (mostly) unqualified benefits which automatically overrule the power of old ideas. Yet they are rarely totally free of hazard, and old ideas survive to challenge the new. In obstetrics, the fact that the last dwelling place of the old ideas tends to be 'the minds of uneducated women, a section of the population markedly unlikely to leave documentary record of its views' (Eccles, 1982, p. 119) in no way diminishes the vitality of the ideas themselves.

As Karl Figlio has pointed out, the positivist approach to medical history assumes that there are, indeed, solid facts to discover, and that their continuous discovery leads eventually (inexorably) to the present state of knowledge. The difficulty is that this assumption 'automatically isolates the endeavour called "scientific" or "medical" advancement from its social context. That is, it neither examines the non-intellectual contingencies which mould ideas, nor does it look at the use of scientific or medical concepts as cultural, social, religious or ideological tools' (Figlio, 1977, p. 265). Human societies are characterized both by the existence of a world of ideas about reality and by the social context in which such a world emerges. The 'mind–body' philosophical tradition of Western culture encourages us all to see a dislocation between the two — between minds and bodies — and in this respect a positivistic scientific medicine and a positivistic history of medicine are only particular examples of a general case. But of course the positivist case as applied to the medical field has always appeared to be strengthened by that very claim which is characteristic of medicine as a profession — the claim that medical knowledge, being highly esoteric, specialized and 'scientific' is, indeed, the exclusive property of medical practitioners. This means that the positivist formula is even more difficult, but no less important, to resist. We will obtain only a very limited (and self-legitimating) view of the history of medicine if we are not prepared to see so-called 'scientific' development as, at least partially, a culture of ideas influenced by the social relations of individuals and groups. As Saul Benison has remarked,

> The history and sociology of medicine and science . . . are not only important in themselves; they are of equal importance to the medical and scientific community. They are in a sense testimony that the development of modern medicine and science has reached a point in time when physicians and scientists, as well as social scientists, must stand back and reflect on the origin and meaning of medical and scientific ideas (Benison, 1971, p. 300).

Indeed, as chapter 12 shows, such a reflective activity as applied to antenatal care is currently going on within the medical field itself. But the interrelationships of sociology and history as applied to medicine are not easy: history tends to make a little of a lot and sociology a lot of a little (Lewis and Davies, 1982).

As part of this resistance to a traditional positivist history of medicine, I have deliberately not included in this book a glossary of medical terminology. Such a glossary within such a text as this reinforces the notion that medicine cannot be understood except by those who practice it; it tends to confirm the status of medicine as an obscure scientific craft. Most of the medical terms used in the text are either explained within it, or are self-explanatory. Many, indeed, are to be found in an ordinary dictionary.

The main theme of *The Captured Womb* is, then, the gradual reconstitution over the last 80 years of pregnancy as a distinct type of social behaviour falling under the jurisdiction of the medical profession. The process of tracing this reconstitution itself involves a large number of questions, themes, methodologies, and disciplines. For example, the history of the rise of medical antenatal care embraces all of the following 'histories':

the profession of midwifery
the medical profession, especially the subspecialties of obstetrics, general practice and paediatrics
the profession of health visiting
the position of women as mothers and in general
the organization, financing, and administration of the medical care system
the relation between the state and the medical and allied professions
the management of childbirth
the management of unwanted pregnancy
contraceptive techniques
the epidemiology of pregnancy outcome
non-medical forms of antenatal care
the relation between users and providers of medical care
the growth and social control of technology

It is clearly not possible in one book to do anything like thorough justice to all these fields and I have not tried to do so. Instead, I have selected an approach which focuses on ten questions:

(1) Why, how, and by whom, did pregnancy come to be defined as a medical phenomenon in Britain and other countries in the early decades of the twentieth century?
(2) How did this redefinition give rise to the theory and practice of clinical antenatal care?
(3) How has the theory of antenatal care related to its practice over the whole period?
(4) What *has* the practice of antenatal care consisted of?
(5) Who has provided antenatal care, and how have the various professional groups providing antenatal care related to one another?
(6) What strategies have been used, and what difficulties encountered, in extending antenatal care to cover virtually all childbearing women?
(7) How has the practice of clinical antenatal care related to non-clinical forms of care for pregnant women (for instance, health education)?
(8) To what extent does the evolution of antenatal care mirror, incorporate, or help to bring about, changes in the position of women as mothers?
(9) What has, or can, antenatal care achieve in terms of preventing deaths and illness in mothers and babies?
(10) Is antenatal care a separate case, or does its history merely run in parallel with that of other phenomena increasingly incorporated under medical jurisdiction during the twentieth century?

Some of these questions are taken in chronological order, whilst others are treated thematically. Hence, for instance, the way in which pregnancy has been ideologically transformed from a *social*, first into a *biological*, and, secondly, into a *medical* phenomenon, is treated in the beginning chapters; while the relationship between what doctors have said antenatal care ought to consist of, and what it actually has consisted of, is thematic to the whole book.

One difficulty with such research concerns the area it is intended to cover. Inevitably, this is to be defined by the researcher in relation to the data he or she finds available. But how far can one reasonably expect a researcher to go in determining the availability of data? For example, in my search for pre National Health Service antenatal records, I wrote to a sample of 15 maternity hospitals. I received the following by way of reply: none — eight; records damaged/destroyed — three; no records traceable — four. Fortunately, I was able to find some data eventually, but they were very limited. Historical series of GP case-records are even more difficult.

Most GPs have had no particular reason to preserve their confidential patient information, and only the unusually farsighted or the occasional historical accident has made available pre-NHS general practice case-material. The general question of sources for the writing of such histories as this one is not often discussed by their writers. I have used an eclectic mixture, mostly of secondary sources, though sometimes — as in the pursuit of case-note material — primary ones too. I have not attempted a systematic listing of these sources, but have referenced them in the bibliography, and appended a short list of the main hospital and other archives consulted (pp. 336–7). I am quite sure there are important sources I have missed, or some that I would have found had I continued researching for a longer period of time. Another problem in the compilation of such a history is that we may protest about the positivist bias in much existing medical history, but our ability to replace it with a more soundly-based social history is limited by the historical materials available to us. Women and patients are not the social groups most likely to leave a record of their views and experiences. We cannot ever know, for example, what 'most' women in the eighteenth century believed about pregnancy — whether they understood that 38 weeks was the normal period of gestation, or whether the curious notions of some of the 'professional' literature had injected women's beliefs with a dose of the scientific irrationality of the time.

In other words, I do not offer this volume as a comprehensive history of that exercise called antenatal care: I offer it as one approach to such a history, a beginning rather than an end.

Whatever its shortcomings, I could not have researched or written this book without invaluable help of various kinds. I am indebted to the Wellcome Trust for the financial support of a three-year Research Fellowship which enabled me to undertake the work. Also in the first place I am grateful to Murray Enkin and Iain Chalmers for setting me out on the road to finding out what I wanted to find out. They, and my other colleagues at the National Perinatal Epidemiology Unit in Oxford, have been important sources of advice and support. Alison Macfarlane in particular has contributed much in the way of essential statistical expertise in the form of Appendix I, and also throughout the book. Her support was provided by the Department of Health and Social Security. I should like to thank Lesley Mierh for typing, and Chris Catton for help in completing the bibliography. Other people who have commented at various stages of the work's gestation (or who have drawn my attention to relevant material or themes) are: Ms Gail Barlow, Professor Geoffrey Chamberlain, Dr Celia Davies, Ms Judith Emanuel, Dr Frank Honigsbaum, Dr Ludi Jordanova, Dr Gilliam McIlwaine, Dr Karl-Erik

Larssen, Dr Jane Lewis, Dr Irving Loudon, Ms Diana Palmer, Mrs Leonora Pitcairn, Dr Martin Richards, Professor Margaret Stacey, Dr Charles Webster, and Dr Louis Wood. Mrs Felicity Cave kindly translated from the Russian the paper on maternal impressions mentioned in chapter 1. I owe a special debt of gratitude to Dr Edgar Hope-Simpson and Miss Joyce Dawson for providing information on antenatal care in rural general practice during the period from 1946 to 1980, and to Dr Ivor Cookson for the same service relating to the 1940s and 1950s. Since much of my work has had to be done in libraries and medical record departments, I must also thank many library and medical records staff for their assistance, particularly Patricia Want of the library of the Royal College of Obstetricians and Gynaecologists, Miss Curtis of the medical records department at Queen Charlotte's Maternity Hospital, Mr Peskett, Miss Strous and Miss Gillon at the London Hospital, Miss Henderson and Miss Bone of the Glasgow Royal Maternity Hospital, Miss Williams of the Bristol City Archives Department, and the late Mrs Eaves-Walton and Dr Stephanie Blackden at the Edinburgh Medical Archives Centre. A number of individuals very kindly agreed to provide me with their own authentic autobiographical observations on the development of antenatal care, without which this book would have been the poorer: Professor Dugald Baird, Dr Ivor Cookson, Professor Ian Donald, Miss G. Humphreys, Dr Robin Mole, the late Dr Hugh Porter, Dr Hope Simpson, Dr John Sturrock and Professor James Walker, were all subjected to that process known as 'interviewing', and I hope did not find it too uncomfortable.[1]

I am very grateful indeed to all these people, but I do, of course, take responsibility for the final form of this work; any errors of omission or commission are all mine. Finally, I would like to thank Robin, and my three personal experiences of antenatal care, Adam, Emily, and Laura, for their continuing intellectual encouragement and domestic support.

---

1. Material from these interviews quoted in the text is referred to by the initials of the interviewee, followed by 'I' (for interview) in parenthesis. Thus, an interview with Dugald Baird would be denoted: (D. B. I).

Part I

Great Expectations: antenatal care 1900–60

I

Pregnancy before 1900

The immediate agency by which one living being is rendered capable of
giving rise to another similar to itself is enveloped in the most profound
and most hopeless obscurity.

Encyclopaedia Britannica, 1842, Vol. 17, p. 684

'Women when pregnant', wrote Alexander Hamilton, Professor of Midwifery at the University of Edinburgh, in 1781, 'should lead a regular
and temperate life carefully avoiding whatever is observed to disagree
with the stomach; they should breathe a free open air; their company
should be agreeable and cheerful; their exercise should be moderate . . .
they should . . . avoid crowds . . . agitation of body from violent or
improper exercise, as jolting in a carriage, riding on horseback, dancing,
and whatever disturbs either the body or mind' (Hamilton, 1781, pp.
160–1). This advice appeared under the heading 'Rules and Cautions
for the Conduct of Pregnant Women' in the first edition of Hamilton's
Treatise of Midwifery, and well represented prevailing medical attitudes to
pregnancy in the era before the establishment of modern obstetric care.

In the eighteenth and nineteenth centuries, antenatal care as a concept did not exist. Neither the providers of health care, nor pregnant
women themselves considered routine medical supervision necessary.
There were no clinics or hospital departments set aside for that purpose.
No professional body had successfully claimed the care of pregnant
women as its expert territory. There was, furthermore, no systematic
body of knowledge or techniques applicable to pregnancy which could
provide a rationale for medical supervision.

To say this does not mean, of course, that some idea of taking care of
pregnant women has not been built into most societies' ways of managing childbirth throughout history. On the contrary, classic texts such as
Engelmann's *Labor Among Primitive Peoples* (1883) had already, in the
nineteenth century, exposed the various customs followed in different

parts of the world for protecting the health of the pregnant woman and her unborn child — from the weekly changing of pregnant women's shoes in Esthonia (to throw the devil off the scent), to the more reasonable-sounding external abdominal massage and altering of fetal position practised in ancient Japan. To say that antenatal care in the modern sense did not exist does not mean, either, that some physicians did not practise certain medical interventions on those pregnant women who presented themselves for professional care; they did — bloodletting being perhaps the most prominent and alarming example (see pp. 22–3). Nor would it be correct to conclude that no pregnant women prior to the twentieth century attended doctors or midwives for the purpose of seeking a successful outcome to pregnancy; a few did so, although these would have been only those who could afford it. But these exceptions served to prove the rule, and the rule was that pregnancy itself, and in general, did not constitute a medical phenomenon.

There are two main stages in what has been termed the 'medicalization' of pregnancy. The first stage consists of its incorporation into medical discourse in the seventeenth and eighteenth centuries as a 'natural' state; the second is its gradual redefinition as pathology — as a medical phenomenon akin to illness: this process has really only become marked in the period since 1950, although it has developed along with the clinical antenatal care movement itself.

The 'medicalization' of pregnancy as 'natural': the message of the textbooks

In the 1980s there is still a rather uncomfortable ambience about cultural attitudes to pregnancy: is pregnancy a natural phenomenon, or is it so potentially or actually abnormal that it constitutes a medical condition? Medical practitioners themselves may be rather surer on this issue, but their predecessors in the eighteenth century upheld a paradigm of pregnancy which decisively appealed to *nature* as the arbiter of its proper management.

By the end of the nineteenth century in Britain there was already in existence a substantial corpus of medical advice literature for pregnant women.[1] There was also a more narrow, but overlapping, corpus of

---

1. Some discussions of advice literature written by experts to a 'lay' audience make an assumption of passivity or gullibility in the audience. I do not assume this. We have, of course, no reliable historical evidence as to who may have read the nineteenth-century pregnancy advice literature, or what they may have thought of it. See Mechling, 1975, for a discussion of this issue.

professional literature dealing with pregnancy. In the former category came such books as Thomas Bull's *Hints to Mothers for the Management of Health During the Period of Pregnancy and in the Lying-in Room* (1837), and P. H. Chavasse's *Advice to a Wife on the Management of her own Health* (1832). Predating these, the 'English Trotula's' early fifteenth-century handbook of health care advice to women must be mentioned, as it contains many references to pregnancy. There is, for example, the advice that drinking mead before going to bed will prove a good indicator of pregnancy; if the mead-drinker is pregnant, she will have 'much discomfort in her belly' (Rowland, 1981, p. 121); and there are a number of nasty-sounding recipes for suppositories that will succeed in evacuating a dead child from the womb.

Both men and women wrote such manuals of information and advice, and from a variety of motives. By the eighteenth century the market for maternity care manuals was obviously expanding, and some authors clearly had commercial interests in putting together packages of prevailing wisdom (see Eccles, 1982, for more on the midwifery literature of Tudor and Stuart England).

Squarely in the tradition of male-authored motherhood advice manuals is Dr John Grigg's *Advice to the Female Sex in General, Particularly those in a State of Pregnancy and Lying-in*, published in 1789. Grigg described himself as a 'Practitioner in Midwifery' and 'Surgeon to the Pauper-Charity in Bath and late of his Majesty's Navy'. He had no compunction about declaring the superiority of his own expertise, writing that

It is much to be regretted, that there are yet many of the [female] sex, who are prejudiced in favour of ancient, erroneous opinions and customs, and thereby exclude themselves from the advantages they might reap by consulting those who are better acquainted with the human frame, and have acquired a much greater share of this species of knowledge, than others can with any reason be supposed to be in possession of (Grigg, 1789, p. 144).

Perhaps wisely, he also noted (p. 103) that 'Nothing contributes more to the enjoyment of health, both of body and mind during this state [of pregnancy], than a firm reliance in the providence of God.'

Chavasse, some four decades later (1832, p. 172) provided a much-needed link: 'Nature', he states, 'is perfectly competent to bring without the assistance of man, a child into the world . . . Assist Nature! Can anything be more absurd? As though God in his wisdom . . . required the assistance of man.' But God did, for if there was one function these advice manuals had, it was that of telling women what kind of condition pregnancy was, and of informing them as to how 'nature' decreed they should conduct themselves when pregnant. Such manuals, and indeed their counterparts in the twentieth century, were also intended to *reassure*. Were pregnant women anxious? Were they more anxious in 1781 than in 1881 or 1981? We have no way of telling. We cannot merely assume that women were more anxious because the dangers of childbearing were greater; none of the early advisors on pregnancy cite the risk of death (of mother or child) as a rational basis for the worries they set out to dissipate, even though obstetric death rates at the time were a great deal higher than they are today.

The early literature on pregnancy made no separation between obstetric texts and the 'advice' literature. Thus, Augustus Granville's *A Report of the Practice of Midwifery at the Westminster General Dispensary During 1818* was, at the same time, a detailed account of Dispensary practice and proferred comfort for worried females. Surgeon Douglas Fox's *The Signs, Disorders and Management of Pregnancy* is both a textbook and an information source for women: 'it is essential', says Fox, 'that females should possess a work containing the information they require with a view to add to their mental comfort', and to this end he prided himself on producing a work 'free from all technical expressions' (Fox, 1834, p. iv).

The authors of these books did not simply view pregnancy as a normal physiological function. To do that would have been to defeat their purpose, which was to provide information. What they did was a good deal more complex; essentially, they constructed a schema of pregnancy which systematized what was taken to be the everyday experience of pregnant women. Thus systematized, this experience then came to be represented as technical–medical knowledge.

The first and most fundamental notion was that pregnancy itself was not a disease. 'Neither was it my intention to represent pregnancy as a state of disease,' wrote Montgomery in 1856 (p. 41), 'but as one in which a great temporary alteration takes place in the condition of particular functions'. Because of this alteration, pregnant women experienced many troublesome symptoms. But it was the troublesome character of these symptoms to their owners, not any medically-perceived danger *per se*, that gave rise to the 'need' for medical treatment.

A typical Contents list for the 'pregnancy' section of an advice manual ran as follows:

Part I The Signs, Disorders and Management of Pregnancy

The signs of pregnancy
The disorders of pregnancy
Indigestion and the management of the digestive organs
Feverishness
Nausea and vomiting
Fastidiousness and capricious appetite
Heartburn
Flatulence
Spasm, or cramp of the stomach and bowels
Costiveness [constipation]
Purging
Piles
Descent of a portion of the lower intestine
Distension of the bladder
Irritable bladder
Palpitations of the heart
Fainting
Headach [sic]
Toothach [sic]
Salivation
Tenderness and irritability of the external parts of the passage
Discharge from the passage
Pain from distension of the abdomen
Enlargement of the veins of the lower limbs
Swelling immediately underneath the skin
Cramp, or spasm of the lower extremities
Despondency
Miscarriage

(Fox, 1834)

Part II was devoted to 'The Treatment to be Adopted during and after Confinement', and Part III to 'The Management and Disorders of Children'.

This approach stands in marked contrast to that found in obstetrical writings or advice manuals today. In the first place, before the modern era, the whole period of pregnancy, childbirth and motherhood is viewed as a continuous entity. There is no parcelling out of childbearing and childrearing as the divided responsibility of different medical specialties. Secondly, the texts make no separation between what, nowadays, would be called *major* symptoms of *clinical* importance on the one hand, and *minor* symptoms of *nonclinical* importance on the other. Both were seen as 'natural' i.e. as the commonly occurring manifestations of the dramatically altered physiology of the pregnant woman's body. Related to this, there was no conceptual differentiation of 'normal' from 'abnormal' pregnancy of the kind that has become central to obstetrical discourse in the second half of the twentieth century.

The main remedies proposed for all disorders of pregnancy in the eighteenth and nineteenth centuries were based on the principle of adjusting the pregnant woman's bodily fluids and functions so as to bring them into a more balanced state. To this end, Dr Chavasse admonished that 'a lady who is *enceinte* ought to live half her time in the open air. Fresh air and exercise prevent many of the unpleasant symptoms attendant on that state; they keep her in health; they tend to open her bowels; and they relieve that sensation of faintness or depression' (Chavasse, 1911 (eighth edition, p. 203)). To ensure an adequate supply of fresh air, Chavasse advised ladies to check their chimneys and skylights (an act that would probably, also, he felt, abolish puerperal fever). He said a pregnant woman should be in bed by ten o'clock — with the windows open, of course.

Diet was most important. It was advisable to adjust this, not only in accord with the dictates of nature, but also according to the temperament of the pregnant woman. Water was the best drink, while tea and coffee caused heartburn and vomiting: meat was good for 'hardy and laborious' women, but bad for those who are 'indolent and sedentary' (Grigg, 1789, p. 90). (See pp. 290–1 for a return to the emphasis on diet in twentieth-century antenatal care.) The need to treat pregnancy nausea and vomiting, and the constipation that commonly afflicts pregnant women, are frequent themes. Dr Grigg recommended cold infusions of spearmint for severe vomiting or, if this failed to work, 'fifteen or more drops of tincture of opium' at bed time 'in a draught of mint, rose, or cinnamon water'. Grigg believed that keeping the feet warm was also very important, and that some vomiting might actually be a good thing. In another text, Dr Tyler Smith went so far as to say that patients who do not vomit in pregnancy 'should be puked occasionally with warm water, camomile tea, or a mustard emetic' (Tyler Smith, 1858, p. 116). Other remedies for pregnancy vomiting included leeches, ice, bismuth, enemas and belladonna.

But if vomiting wasn't entirely an unmitigated evil, constipation certainly was. 'The keeping of the intestinal canal open is an article of great importance', wrote Charles White (without saying why): 'for this purpose vegetables and ripe fruit in large quantities may be allowed, bitter antiseptic purges in small doses should be given every day, or every night . . . The use of these will prevent the intestine from being plugged up by accumulation of hardened faeces, whereby putrid flatulencies are generated' (White, 1773, p. 72). A careful diet and regular purging were the means recommended to avoid the dreadful fate of these 'putrid flatulencies'.

Most of the ordinary middle-class social entertainments of the day and passion, or anything resembling passion, were also contraindicated. Dr Chavasse counselled against the practice of 'gadding out night after night — one evening to a dinner party, the next night to private theatricals, the third to an evening party, the fourth to the theatre, the fifth to a ball, the sixth to a concert', and demanded to know 'How many miscarriages, premature births and stillborn children have resulted therefrom' (Chavasse, 1911, pp. 6–7). The tight corsetry of the time came in for some criticism, as did a mode of exercise hardly ever referred to directly, but coyly termed by Montgomery 'conjugal enjoyments'.

The problem of diagnosis

The pregnancy symptoms discussed in eighteenth- and nineteenth-century manuals had an essential significance to the obstetrician which they lack today: they served as guarantees of the very existence of the condition which could otherwise scarcely be diagnosed. Prior to the development of reliable and speedy laboratory pregnancy tests in the 1920s, the first obstacle to the development of clinical pregnancy care was the accurate diagnosis of the condition of pregnancy. Unless pregnancy could be diagnosed relatively accurately and early, antenatal care could be little more than a last-minute preparation for labour. Professional confirmation of pregnancy did not even begin to be a custom in Britain until the eighteenth century, and then only among the upper social classes. 'The most certain mode of knowing whether a woman be in a state of gestation or not', wrote Professor James Blundell of Guy's Hospital in 1834 (p. 153), pessimistically, but with some degree of accuracy, 'is by waiting till the term of nine months is complete.' The medical practitioner's claim to expertise rested on a somewhat shaky foundation: 'We can conceive no subject in regard to which a mistake might so utterly ruin a young man's hopes', cautioned William Leishman in 1873 (p. 154), 'than the determination, in delicate or doubtful cases, of this question of pregnancy. An obvious pregnancy overlooked, because the idea has never crossed the mind, is bad enough; and we have known a practitioner of thirty years' standing blister the abdomen in the ninth month under the idea that he was treating a morbid growth.'

A large part of the early texts is devoted to an elaborate classification of the signs and symptoms of pregnancy. W. F. Montgomery's classic text on this topic, *An Exposition of the Signs and Symptoms of Pregnancy* (first edition, 1838) took 492 pages to describe the means whereby a medical practitioner could reliably make a diagnosis of pregnancy. In so doing, Montgomery acquired for himself a place in the history of obstetrical nomenclature by describing the glandular follicles on the breast — 'Montgomery's tubercles' — which constitute an indication of pregnancy. (However, as an aside it should be pointed out that he was not the first to focus attention on them and he misunderstood their significance; he mistakenly thought that they produce a secretion which would stain the woman's clothing).

The basic problem was, as Leishman despondently remarked in the section on 'early signs of pregnancy' in his *A System of Midwifery* (1873, p. 155), that 'The earliest of all the symptoms have their seat in the generative organs but are of little value from a practical point of view, inasmuch as they consist in physiological and anatomical manifestations which are almost entirely beyond our ken.' Not knowing what was really going on, medical authors provided, instead, intensely detailed descriptions of what they thought *might* be happening. The usual approach was to divide signs of pregnancy into three classes — 'positive', 'probable' and 'presumptive'. Under the first heading came the detection by the medical practitioner of fetal heart sounds or movements; under the second, changes in the shape or consistency of the uterus or cervix; under the third, such occurrences as the cessation of menstruation, morning sickness and 'mental disturbances' (Williams, 1903). The descriptions provided of the signs of pregnancy reached an almost lyrical pitch at times, as poetic colours and textures were imaginatively ascribed to the participating tissues, which were endowed with an immense power of activity as a result of what was tendentiously termed the 'prodigious power of fecundation' proceeding from 'the male in coitu' (Montgomery, 1856, p. 3).

Easy, quick and early methods of diagnosing pregnancy had been energetically sought since at least 1350 BC (Cianfrani, 1960). The *Medieval Woman's Guide to Health* (Rowland, 1981) records some of them. One involved watering wheat and spelt daily with the woman's urine; if the wheat grew the woman was pregnant with a boy, and if the spelt grew she was having a girl. (Sex prediction tests were, seemingly just as important as tests for the diagnosis of pregnancy.) The wheat and spelt strategy was based on the recognition that a pregnant woman's urine contains hormones capable of germinating seeds — an observation made scientific by modern botany (Hon, 1961). Erle Henriksen tried the Egyptian germination test in 1941 and found it yielded a 75% correct positive and an 85% correct negative result (Henriksen, 1941).

Because of its easy availability, urine was intensively studied for centuries as holding the key to the mystery of pregnancy. Aristotle put it in a glass for three days and then strained it through a fine cloth: he declared if there were 'small living creatures' in the resulting deposit, then the woman was most certainly pregnant. Savonarola, in the fifteenth century, studied the colour particularly, and identified a pale lemon hue and cloudy deposit like 'carded wool' as characteristic of pregnant urine from conception until the sixth month. Magnus, in the thirteenth century, tried mixing it with milk and found that a gravid woman's urine caused the milk to float — but he did not find out why. Rueff in 1553 stuck an iron needle in urine overnight and said that if the needle was covered in black spots the following morning the woman was pregnant (see Henriksen, 1941, on the history of pregnancy tests). There was an enormous preoccupation for a long time, indeed, from at least the tenth until the close of the nineteenth century, with a substance that came to be known as kiestein. If a pregnant woman's urine was collected and allowed to stand exposed to the air for some days, it apparently produced 'a peculiar floculent sediment, like fine cotton wool . . . [which] rises to the surface and forms a pellicle which has been compared to the fat of cold mutton broth' (Playfair, 1898, p. 158). By the time of Playfair's 1898 text, widespread disappointment with the reliability of the kiestein test was noted.

Not surprisingly, in view of the state of the art, medical practitioners in the eighteenth and nineteenth centuries had to place some reliance on women's own opinions as to whether or not they were pregnant. 'If a patient apply to me anxious to know whether she is in a state of gestation or not', wrote James Blundell (1834, p. 154), 'one of the first questions I propose is — have you any feeling of bearing?' Some practitioners thought they could tell merely by looking: 'The countenance . . . becomes much altered from absorption of fat' declared Dr Tyler Smith (1858, p. 113), a little unpleasantly, 'the eyes look somewhat sunken, and surrounded with a dark areola; the alae of the nose are pinched; and the corners of the mouth dragged down, so that the mouth looks larger.' Vaginal examinations were not much employed — either to diagnose pregnancy or for any other purpose. As a matter of fact, even abdominal examinations in pregnancy were considered highly improper. When an abdominal examination was done, it was normally conducted under the bedclothes and with the examiner's eyes on the ceiling. In Britain,

Victorian morality dictated the choice of the absolutely non-confrontational left lateral position. Upper-class women who sought pre-delivery care might be given a vaginal examination at about seven months; for this they were sedated with opiates and had their labia rubbed with opium tincture and softened with linseed or starch fomentations (Smith, 1979). Two fingers of the physician's hand, well rubbed with lard and with nails trimmed, were inserted into the vagina (the rubber gloves available at the time were too thick to be practical and were not generally used for this purpose). Montgomery recommended using chloroform to render a vaginal examination possible in those few cases in which it was needed. But unless the woman was unconscious, the condition of her genitals and cervix would not be visually examined by the doctor, for this was regarded as far too embarrassing for both doctor and patient.

Theories about pregnancy

If medical practitioners were forced to rely somewhat on women's own information as to whether or not pregnancy had occurred, they were not in an enlightened position with respect to the *dating* of pregnancy, either. 'Wherefore women are most prone to conceive either just before or just subsequent to the menstrual flux', wrote William Harvey (1578–1657), (cited in Thoms, 1935, p. 9), the so-called 'father' of British midwifery, thus voicing an opinion that became accepted medical wisdom for some 300 years. J. W. Ballantyne (1861–1923), the so-called 'founding father' of antenatal care (see chapter 2), believed that conception occurs just after menstruation (Ballantyne, 1904), while others believed that 'the ovule is discharged at the height of menstrual congestion' (Hirst, 1900, p. 63), or just prior to the 'proper epoch' for the occurrence of a period (Playfair, 1898, p. 183). Even as late as 1913, R. W. Johnstone wrote (1913, p. 98) 'we have no certain knowledge as to when ovulation occurs, nor can we ever hope to know the exact time for fertilization. Coitus just before or after a menstrual period is more frequently fertile than at other times.'

There was a widespread belief in a phenomenon known as 'superfoetation', according to which the uterus did not 'close up' until the third or fourth month, so that multiple conceptions were possible, this feat being proved by the birth of differently sized twins, and even more definitely by the birth of black and white twins. J. Matthews Duncan, a most energetic defender of the superfoetation idea, in his 1868 *Researches in*

Obstetrics reproduced from William Hunter a drawing of a third-month pregnancy. In this, the fetus is shown sheltering tidily on the right hand side of the uterus while a 'free passage' like a motorway is sketched out between the cervix and the left-hand fallopian tube. One prevailing theory about the cause of this wonderful phenomenon was that it was due to the woman's specially receptive response to the 'Fervour of a very Libidinous Tickling Congress' (quoted in Eccles, 1982, p. 40).

Another area of ignorance was the question of where menstrual blood came from (an issue eventually settled by the examination in 1908 by Hitschmann and Adler of uteruses from women who died menstruating). Evidence about the timing of human fertility such as the habits of Jewish women, who regularly became pregnant whilst observing the Levitical ban on intercourse during, or for seven days after, a period, remained intensely puzzling. In view of the puzzle about when pregnancy began, it was logical that the matter of how long pregnancy lasted was also hotly disputed. 'With regard to this point,' wrote Montgomery humbly (1856, p. 495), 'it must be confessed, that our knowledge is by no means either so extensive, or precise, as might be, at first sight, expected in a matter apparently capable of being made the subject of daily observation.' He thought the natural period of gestation 280 days, and cited several cases of the only kind that could at the time furnish firm evidence for this being so, namely those in which the date of conception could be fixed with some certainty. A woman whose husband left the country on 5 April told her doctor she would require his services on 10 January, which she duly did; and when her husband came home he assured the doctor that the same regularity had also marked her previous pregnancy and labour. Other writers were more doubtful of their ability ever to determine the truth, citing Avicenna to the effect that 'at the appointed time, labour comes on by command of God' (Tyler Smith, 1858, p. 218).

Although medical writers of the eighteenth and nineteenth centuries were basically describing what they had observed from empirical experience to be the symptoms of pregnancy, they were also at pains to provide an *explanation* as to why these should occur. The principal theory about the physiology of pregnancy was that of 'plethora'. The theory of plethora rested on the old Hippocratean and later Galenic philosophy of disease, according to which health represented a condition of balance between the four 'humours' — black bile, yellow bile, blood and phlegm. The model was a fundamentally chemical one of disease as produced by disturbances of body fluids. The term 'plethora' was applied to a wide range of diseases, and it meant an excess of blood in the body, symptoms of which included a flushed face and strong pulse. Plethora was the main chemical disequilibrium of pregnancy, and was said to be due to the retention of menstrual blood which, in turn, was thought capable of causing a whole range of pregnancy disorders, from miscarriage and premature labour and convulsions to constipation, fever, and maternal depression.

The remedy was obvious. 'It is scarcely ever proper (except in the weakest constitutions) to omit taking away blood from the system' commented Dr John Clarke in 1806. 'Bleeding from a large vein . . . will often be found extremely useful, and has much more effect in appeasing the sickness and vomiting of pregnant women, than any medicines taken into the stomach' (Clarke, 1806, p. 111). Bloodletting was not only a treatment applied to pregnancy, but it was, prior to the twentieth century, thought by most practitioners of medicine to be the most powerful remedy in the treatment of all disease, and had possessed this status since the time of Hippocrates. W. S. Playfair remarked in his 1898 text that earlier in the century, 'it was by no means rare for women to be bled six or eight times during the latter months, even when no definite symptoms of disease existed', and noted that there were many recorded cases 'when depleting was practised every fortnight as a matter of routine, and when the symptoms were well-marked, even from fifty to ninety times in the course of a single pregnancy' (p. 153). In Thomas Denman's *An Introduction to the Practice of Midwifery* (last edition, 1821), there is a case of threatened abortion at four months treated by bleeding the patient 17 times in ten days, and withdrawing a total of 110 ounces of blood — the patient eventually, miraculously, achieved a safe delivery. The apparently paradoxical use of bloodletting to treat haemorrhage was based on the hypothesis that, by causing the patient to faint through removing blood, the force of the circulation was reduced, clotting could take place, and thus the haemorrhage would be checked. In Britain William Smellie (1697–1763) and William Hunter (1718–83) extended the therapy of bloodletting to the treatment of almost every pregnancy complaint. In America in the early part of the nineteenth century, physicians normally took 8–10 ounces of blood from every pregnant patient they could get their hands on, a practice that was carried out in order to relax a rigid cervix and prevent postpartum haemorrhage, infection and convulsions (Siddall, 1980).

The beginning of the end of bloodletting therapy came in 1843, when the laboratory studies of Gabriel Audral in France revealed that the blood of pregnant women contained a diminished number of red blood cells, rather than an increased number. By the mid-century, many practitioners had begun to reduce their use of venesection, although a new competing theory that puerperal convulsions were caused by a poison, a toxin in the system, led to a temporary revival of the practice, according to the logic that if you removed part of the blood, you also removed part of the poison (Allbutt, 1897; Williams, 1903); this logic held sway for almost another half-century in some places.

Theories and explanations relating to eclampsia and toxaemia (and later pre-eclamptic toxaemia — the terminology changes), conditions which were a major cause of mortality in childbearing, have a long and complex intellectual history. It was in 1827 that Richard Bright boiled a teaspoonful of urine to make the discovery of 'albuminous urine' in patients with oedema. Some years later, in 1843, his obstetric colleague, John Lever, thought to examine the urine of women with puerperal convulsions, and was forced to the conclusion, independently reached in the same year by Simpson, that albuminous urine in pregnancy was not always 'simply' a manifestation of nephritis, but indicated the presence of a condition peculiar to pregnancy itself. By the mid-century, the dangerous association of severe oedema, albuminuria, and headache or visual disturbances on the one hand with convulsions on the other was well known. But the aetiology of the syndrome was obscure — and still is, to a great extent (Redman, 1982).

Another key theory about pregnancy commonly held prior to the modern obstetric era was that of 'maternal impressions'. This theory stated that the condition and viability of the fetus was profoundly influenced by the mother's mental and emotional state — a view that, of course, fitted well with the prevailing model of successful pregnancy as guaranteed only by a life-style properly balanced in accordance with natural dictate. In 1727 Dr James Blondel provided the following clear and uncompromising definition of the maternal impression theory:

the child may receive some Hurt by Means of its Mother this being laid down as a general Rule, that the Prosperity of the Foetus does depend on the welfare of the Mother; and that, whatever is detrimental to her is directly, or indirectly, prejudicial to the other.

It suffers, not only by the Distempers of the Parents, but also by several Accidents, as great Falls, Bruises and Blows the Mother receives, by her laborious Work, by odd and constrained Positions of her Body; by the Irregularity of her Diet, and of her Actions; by immoderate Dancing, Running, Jumping, Riding, Excess of Laughing, frequent and violent Sneezing, and all other Agitations of the body.

The Child may also suffer by the Affections of the Mother's Mind. For the Disappointment of what she desires is sufficient to make her uneasy, and pine away; deprive her of sleep and Quiet, and even of Food, and consequently the Child runs the Risk, for Want of due and wholesome Nourishment, to grow feeble and weak, and at last to lose its life (Blondell 1727, pp. 2–3).

In this form, the theory of maternal impressions seems no more than a somewhat old-fashioned statement of the modern 'stress' or 'life-events' theory of disease, as applied to pregnancy outcome (Oakley, Macfarlane and Chalmers, 1982). Yet Blondell's definition was, in fact, a radical protest against the most widely held opinion of the time, which was that in maternal impressions lay the cause of all congenital malformations in the fetus. Until well into the nineteenth century, the question for most medical men who contended this matter was not *whether* maternal impressions could cause deformed fetuses, but *how* they did so. This was the main topic of an international congress held in 1755 at the Academy for the Sciences in St Petersburg ('Towards a history of the problem of the effect of the mother's organism on the fetus', Kopelevich, n.d.). By the early decades of the nineteenth century, the embryonic science of embryology was beginning to sound an isolated note of caution. In France, Geoffrey Saint-Hilaire analysed the statistics of legitimate and illegitimate births in Paris for the years 1817–21 and did not find an excess of malformed fetuses among unmarried mothers, the group presumably under most stress (Saint-Hilaire, 1822; see also Oppenheimer, 1968).

Blondell himself had noted that maternal emotions could not be 'so malignant to the Foetus as 'tis commonly reported, or else the Race of Men should insensibly degenerate into a Generation of Monsters' (p. 14), but the strength of the maternal impressions theory continued unabated in the philosophy of many medical practitioners. In 1834, for example, a Dr James Blundell (no relation), under the 'Causes of Monstrosity' in his *The Principles and Practice of Obstetricy* (1834, p. 137), cited the following case, typical of many discussed by eighteenth- and nineteenth-century medical authors under that heading:

There was a child . . . lately born at Plymouth, with excrescences pushing from the mouth, and which certainly resembled a large bunch of grapes . . . Before she was aware of this faulty formation, the mother was closely questioned by the accoucheur, and she certainly did state distinctly enough, that in the early period of her pregnancy . . . in passing along a street, she chanced to see a boy who had got a bunch of grapes, which he was eating very greedily, as boys will do . . .

As if this were not enough, 'Growing from the region of the sternum, too, there was an excrescence which might remind one of the wattle of the turkey cock, an animal by which she had been frightened a little earlier in her pregnancy.'

Babies without limbs, with heads of cats, with two heads, with all kinds of tumours — all these owed their origin to something the mother had seen, or experienced, during pregnancy.

Monitoring and intervening in pregnancy

As we have seen, antenatal care in the nineteenth century, and before, was mostly limited to advice on life-style, though a few therapies, for example bloodletting, were practised, and a few monitoring techniques were used, for example abdominal palpation, on the few women who presented themselves for clinical care during pregnancy.

The discovery of new therapies and monitoring techniques is an important part of the history of medicine, and thus of the history of antenatal care. It is rarely, however, a question of uniform progress towards greater and greater therapeutic effectiveness or towards increasingly effective techniques for monitoring health and preventing illness. At the same time, there is no doubt that the creation of a specific body of knowledge and relevant technical resources is intrinsic to the process of professional growth.

In this sense, many components of twentieth-century antenatal care have their origins in the nineteenth century. For example, it was in 1872 that John Braxton-Hicks (1823–97) described the now famous Braxton-Hicks contractions in his 'On the Contractions of the Uterus Throughout Pregnancy' (he used them to diagnose pregnancy). The change in the colour of the vaginal mucosa in early pregnancy (Chadwick's sign) was described by Jacquemier in 1838, and Hegar's sign — the softened lower part of the uterus in early pregnancy felt with a bimanual vaginal examination — was described by Reinl in 1884. The fetal heart was first heard through a corset and by means of an ear only by a surgeon, Francois Mayor (1779–1826) of Geneva, in 1818: he was listening for fetal movements at the time, and the discovery of the fetal heart sound was accidental. (Mayor never realized the significance for obstetrical practice of his discovery.) Fetal heart sounds were reported independently, and also accidentally discovered in 1821 by Jean Alexandre Lejumeau Vicomte de Kegaradec (1787–1877), a pupil of Laënnec, inventor of the stethescope proper. According to Montgomery, de Kegaradec

> wished to ascertain whether it were possible to hear the wave sound produced by the liquor amnii by the motions of the fetus: this he altogether failed to detect but, while making his investigation near the end of pregnancy, he one day heard a sound which he compared to the movement of a watch, being composed of two distinct sounds like those of the heart, which were repeated from 143 to 148 times in a minute, the mother's pulse beating at the time only 70 (Montgomery, 1856, p. 202).

By the time Montgomery wrote, it was acknowledged that the fetal heart could probably be heard sometime in the fifth month, but regular monitoring of the condition of the fetus by this means did not become accepted practice for many decades. Indeed, many authoritative medical men argued against it, including Professor James Hamilton, the son of the Hamilton whose admonitions to pregnant women began this chapter. In a fierce debate with the Master of the Rotunda Hospital, Robert Collins, in the 1830s, Hamilton asked if Collins would 'propose to apply the stethescope to the naked belly of a woman, for if so, he may be assured that in this part of the world at least, such a proposal would be indignantly rejected by every . . . practitioner of reputed respectability' (cited in Radcliffe, 1967, p. 71). Similarly, the technique of testing urine for albumin and sugar was learnt by medical students by the 1890s, but its practice as applied to medicine was confined to teaching hospitals for many decades.

Abdominal palpation, a technique still central to the practice of antenatal care in the 1980s, was pioneered by Adolphe Pinard (1844–1934) of the Paris Maternité Hospital in a work published in 1889: *Traité du palper abdominal au point de vue obstétrical, et de la version par manoevres externes*. Before Pinard, an Englishman, Gustavus P. Murray, had noted in the *Lancet* in 1858 the fact that farmers manipulated the abdomens of their ewes in order to predict the number of lambs that would be born, and that the practice might usefully be extended to humans, although he didn't see it being much help before the eighth or ninth month, and made various extravagant claims which strained his credibility within the obstetrical community, for example that the fetal vertebrae could actually be counted through the mother's abdominal wall. Pinard himself recommended the examination of pregnant women before the beginning of labour, and described a technique of using both the examiner's hands to determine the presenting part of the fetus. His method of estimating disproportion, by pressing the fetal head into the pelvic brim with one hand and judging the overlap over the pubis with the other, is the basic technique still in use today. In a similar manner, Pinard's method of external version (converting a breech into a vertex presentation) which he said should be undertaken on all breech presentations at the eighth month, came to be accepted practice world-wide — but slowly. When H. R. Spencer (1860–1941) published his famous article on external version of breech presentations in 1901, describing the method he himself was using at University College Hospital, London, he noted that the usual time of diagnosing a breech was still when labour began. 'The operation [of external version] of course, involves the necessity of the patient's being examined during pregnancy, a necessity which is not recognised by all doctors or patients' (p. 1196).

Two kinds of strategies have been especially important in establishing the rationale of modern antenatal care. One relates to the medical–professional claim to know what is going on inside the uterus better than the mother herself, and the other refers to the matter of controlling the termination of pregnancy — the onset of labour. In neither respect was nineteenth-century practice at all advanced. A number of different methods of inducing labour had been practised for centuries, with mechanical methods by far the most popular until, in 1872, the discovery that quinine possesses the power of intensifying uterine contractions seems to have turned the tide in favour of the pharmacological methods that have come to dominate modern obstetric practice (see chapter 8).

As to seeing inside the uterus, the modern era really begins with the discovery by the German experimental physicist William Conrad Röntgen (1845–1923) of a form of radiation which came eventually to be known as X-rays ('X' standing for the unknown).

At a late hour on Friday, November 8 (1895), when there were no assistants in the laboratory, Röntgen was testing the density of the black cover fitted over a Hittorf–Crookes (vacuum) tube . . . The shield was impervious to any light known. He noted a bright fluorescence in a screen of barium platino-cyanide which lay on a bench nearby. It seemed improbable that the effect could have been produced by cathode rays as their nature was then understood; but in order to exclude them he experimented with a screen at a greater distance than the known range of cathode rays. The fluorescence persisted. The next step was to interrupt the rays by various bodies which would have been quite opaque to cathode rays . . . In this way he deduced that he was dealing with a new kind of radiation . . . (Underwood 1957, p. 229).

Röntgen was lucky, in that dusk had fallen, making visible the tell-tale gleam from the screen on the bench. Several other physicists were on the verge of making the same discovery. One, Crookes, had earlier returned some photographic plates to the makers complaining that they were fogged (by X-rays, had he only realized) (Shanks, 1950).

The first X-ray in 1895 was of Mrs Röntgen's hand, and was produced so Röntgen could explain to his wife the nature of the important work that was making him late home every night. The first X-ray of a pregnant woman (with a dead fetus) was performed by E. P. Darts and W. W. Keen of Philadelphia, in 1896. Pelvimetry with X-rays was first described by Pierre Budin in France in 1897, who showed his colleagues at a Moscow Congress of that year an X-ray photograph 'prise sur la Femme Vivante' demonstrating that, as he put it, 'les rayons pourront donner des resultats tres utiles' (Budin, 1897). From 1899 came X-rays of living fetuses, and, in the early years of this century, a mounting enthusiasm for the use of X-rays in the diagnosis of pregnancy (see chapters 4 and 7 for further discussion of X-rays).

The institutional provision of antenatal care: beginnings

Since women in the eighteenth and nineteenth centuries did not usually visit doctors for medical care in pregnancy, the novels of the time give no glimpse of the antenatal consultation. The wise and well-off heroine of Defoe's *Fortunate Mistress* (1724), for example, took elaborate precautions for her confinement, hiring a midwife, a nurse, a female nurse-assistant, and a man-midwife; but she did not obtain any professional care during her pregnancy (Riley, 1968). In the second half of the nineteenth century, the practice of consulting a physician–accoucheur was becoming a little more popular among the wealthy classes. Yet even in these cases there would usually only be one or two antenatal examinations. It was not the obstetrician but the midwife whose hands conducted the bulk of the nation's deliveries — the Registrar-General's *Annual Report* for 1876 stated that midwives attended 70 per cent of all births in England and Wales, the proportion being above 90 per cent in some rural areas. Midwives did not, apparently, do any antenatal care, though they might do a cursory examination on 'booking' at the seventh or eighth month. Both midwives and medical men charged for their services, which meant that most British mothers could afford midwifery care only — if that, for many used untrained, experienced women in the community who, for an even more modest charge, would not only deliver the baby but provide all-round domestic help.

In the first half of the nineteenth century a delivery conducted by a male accoucheur would have cost from one guinea plus 5s–7s 6d (mileage extra) for women in 'moderate circumstances' — but the wealthier could expect to pay upwards of 100 guineas for the confinement alone (Smith, 1979). The midwife's charge, even for experienced midwives, was not more than a few guineas — a few shillings for the poor (Donnison, 1977).

Pregnant women who could not pay the cost of an accoucheur, but wanted one, could use the services of a Dispensary or Lying-in Hospital. Dispensaries pre-dated hospitals, and were set up from the late seventeenth century on to provide free advice and cheap medicines to the sick poor. By the nineteenth century, many provided a range of cheap or free treatments as well, including midwifery. Most towns had at least one dispensary; in 1890, there were no less than 44 in London (Abel-Smith, 1964). Those that did midwifery were readier than the hospitals to employ midwives for 'normal' cases, reserving the male accoucheur for more awkward ones.

The Lying-in Hospitals began as charities in the eighteenth century. The first in England was the British Lying-in Hospital (later the British Hospital for Mothers and Babies, Woolwich) founded in 1747; between 1739 and 1800, ten separate lying-in hospitals were founded. (Table A.1, p. 303, shows total numbers of maternity beds over the period from 1861 to 1938.) Given that the management of the acutely ill was the central function of the eighteenth century hospital, 'it is necessary to ask why this new type of institutional care was thought appropriate for healthy young parturient women' (Versluysen, 1981, p. 20). The answer is that the significance of the hospital lay in the service it could do to the emergent profession of obstetrics. It facilitated the restriction of competition from female midwives, established the principle of doctor control over client preferences, enabled clinical expertise to be taught to others, and set the stage for the later depiction of childbirth as potentially pathological. In order to gain the services of a hospital, a pregnant woman needed to prove the onset of labour, poverty, and residence in the right parish, and also to hold a letter of recommendation from a hospital subscriber. Some lying-in institutions only admitted married women, and for these proof of marriage was required. (Others only admitted unmarried women if it was their first pregnancy, so as not unduly to encourage vice.)

Institutional provision for maternity was more firmly established earlier on the continent than in Britain. Pinard, of abdominal palpation fame, wrote of the work of a Madame Becquet of Vienne (France) in the Avenue de Maine, Paris, where, in 1892, the first refuge for 'les femmes enceintes abandonnes' had been set up. Pinard claimed that delivery in this establishment (presumably with admission in late pregnancy) produced bigger and healthier babies. Between 1892 and 1904, some 10,000 women received the attention of such French 'receiving' institutions; 3,902 were married, but had husbands who were away or ill, 922 were widowed, and 4,442 were unmarried.

Although the maternal and infant welfare work initiated in France in 1890s is usually hailed as the proper beginning of the antenatal care movement in this country, there were several antecedents. In 1788 a professor of pathology at the College of Surgeons in Paris, Tenon, surveyed hospital provision in Paris at the time and noted that the famous Parisien hospital, Hôtel Dieu, a world centre for midwifery work, admitted pregnant women at the end of pregnancy. If they required a 'secret refuge' they were transferred to the Hôpital de la Salpétrière, where a special ward was reserved for them. The Hôtel Dieu's rules for admission allowed pregnant women who were ill to enter the hospital earlier in pregnancy; those who had heavy work or a long journey could come in at seven months 'especially when they have pains, when the womb is very low, and when at the same time the cervix is dilated' (Browne, 1935, p. 5). Two large wards were provided, comprising 67 beds. Forty-three of these were four and a half feet wide, and so accommodated between two and four patients each. According to François Mauriceau (1637–1709), pupil at the Hôtel Dieu, 'one of the duties of the assistant surgeon was to examine all those who applied and convince himself that they were so near term', an act achieved, apparently, by examining the condition of the cervix (Radcliffe, 1967, p. 27).

In Britain a similar institution to those in France, the Lauriston Prematernity Home, was founded in 1899 in Edinburgh, adjacent to the Royal Maternity Hospital, and with the purpose of providing care for unmarried pregnant women (see chapter 2). Until this time British hospital practice seems to have varied a good deal. The Lying-in Charity in Manchester (later the St Mary's group of hospitals), founded in 1790, admitted 'properly recommended' patients at any time during the last month of pregnancy. This appears from the annual reports to have been something of an abused privilege, some of the women lying about their dates in order to get into hospital for a rest (Young, 1964). The same fate befell the policy of the City of London Maternity Hospital which, in October 1753, changed its practice and only admitted patients in labour

(Cannings, 1922). Over a hundred years later, E. A. Barton, Outdoor Obstetric Assistant to University College Hospital in 1887–88, observed that 'there was no antenatal examination of patients, they were seen for the first time when labour started' (Merrington, 1976). The case-book of Queen Charlotte's Maternity Hospital for 1877–78 records only a desultory interest, shown at the time of admission in labour, in the patient's 'history of pregnancy'. This is usually described simply as 'ordinary', viz.

Ordinary — sick three months
Ordinary — nine months sick
Ordinary — sick all the time.

Thus, in the nineteenth century, hospital provision for maternity rarely included antenatal admission, and even more rarely any form of antenatal care. The Manchester Lying-In Charity appears to have been something of an exception to this rule. An out-patient service was started by the Charity in August 1791 for pregnant women, women suffering from 'disorders which are the consequence of childbirth' and for children under two. In 1793–94, 70 women and children attended as outpatients. By the time of the Charity's move to Quay Street in 1856, there was in existence an embryonic antenatal clinic to which putative patients applied with their form of recommendation. In the case of a first pregnancy or if the woman had a previous history of difficult labour, she was examined. Every patient had her urine tested antenatally (Young, 1964).

In 1819, Augustus Bozzi Granville, Physician–Accoucheur to the Westminster General Dispensary, wrote an interesting account of midwifery practice at the Dispensary during 1818. The catchment area of the Westminster General Dispensary formed a third of the total metropolis, and during 1818, 640 pregnant women were received there. The average age of the women was thirty; one woman, giving birth at fifty-two, was having her sixteenth child after an eleven-year gap. Twenty of the babies were stillborn, and the maternal mortality rate was one in 160. (Granville notes in defence of this figure that Dispensary patients were poorer, came later in labour and were not so carefully surveyed by doctors as patients attending lying-in hospitals.)

Granville also compared the cost of Dispensary care with that provided by the Lying-In Hospitals. For the latter he estimated the cost of each labour at £3. 12s. 10d. 'a sum sufficient to relieve sixteen poor married women . . . by the timely assistance of medicines, a midwife, and a physician, from the Westminster General Dispensary' (Granville, 1819, p. 17).

The 'deep, dark and continuous stream of mortality'

Granville reported a high maternal mortality rate: apart from noting the stillbirths, he gave no figure for infant mortality. At that time no national figures were available for deaths associated with childbirth. The production of such figures is a complex matter, depending on the definitions adopted of what constitutes (in women) a death due to, or associated with, childbirth, and what constitutes (in fetuses) a death rather than a failed gestation; and depending, also, of course, on the accuracy and completeness of the death and birth certification systems employed on the basis of these definitions. (See Appendix I; and also Macfarlane and Mugford 1981.) Some index of the deficiencies due to inadequacies in the production of obstetric mortality statistics is the estimate of the Registrar-General in 1872 that around 38,000 births in the period from 1841 to 1850 were probably not registered.

Without a comprehensive system of data collection, based on an appropriate classification, the dangers of childbearing in the nineteenth century, and before, can only be guessed at. There is no doubt that they were substantial. Infant mortality (deaths within one year of birth) — the only available measure of the danger to the child — probably averaged around 150 per 1,000 live births throughout the nineteenth century (Dyhouse, 1978). Figure A.2, p. 296, shows infant mortality from 1840 to 1980, and a decline that begins only in the late 1890s. William Farr (1837–1880), 'Compiler of Abstracts' to Britain's first Registrar-General, concluded in his *Vital Statistics* (1885) that insanitary conditions in the large towns meant that infant mortality was actually increasing in the latter part of the nineteenth century. When Farr came to consider in detail the topic of maternal deaths, he justified his interest thus: 'I have every year specially dwelt on the causes of death in childbirth for two reasons; firstly because the lives themselves are at the most precious age, and secondly because skill can do more here in averting danger and death than in other operations' (Farr, 1885, p. 278). Farr's analysis showed that maternal mortality was about one per 200 live births in the period 1847–76. During these years a total of 106,565 women died within a month of giving birth. In a most memorable phrase, he termed these fatalities 'a deep, dark and continuous stream of mortality' (p. 279).

Other commentators shared Farr's concern, but produced different figures. A considerably higher estimate was given by Dr J. Matthews Duncan in a book published in 1870 *On the Mortality of Childbed and Maternity Hospitals*. In Duncan's view, 'Not fewer than one in every 120 women delivered at or near the full time die within the four weeks of childbed' (p. 24). Puerperal fever was common, accounting for around 40 per cent of maternal deaths in the mid-nineteenth century (Farr, 1885, p. 271). Taking into account birth-rate changes, the Registrar-General's Decennial Supplement for 1901–10 concluded that there were actually more deaths from that cause than in 1861–70. Though these statistical debates cannot be decisively settled, Figure A.4, p. 298, collects together the available data for all-cause maternal mortality from 1840 to 1980, and also specifically for puerperal sepsis deaths.

The high rate of puerperal sepsis deaths was partly responsible for a debate that raged in the latter part of the nineteenth century about the merits of institutional confinement, or, as Duncan put it: 'To be, or not to be? — that is the question. It is now supposed by many to be settled that they ought not to be . . . The mortality of maternity hospitals is said to be so great that it is expedient, indeed absolutely necessary, to close them entirely' (Duncan, 1870, p. 110). Conditions in many maternity hospitals were scarcely salubrious, and must have been conducive to infection. 'It would be difficult to imagine any public institution more disgusting' said physician Charles Bell of the Edinburgh Royal Maternity Hospital in 1871; 'The wards were filthy in the extreme, the beds were not fit for human beings to occupy' (cited in Sturrock, 1958, p. 129).

This argument about the relative safety of domiciliary and institutional confinement still flourishes in the 1980s. Just as important as the actual statistics of mortality themselves is the matter of what people make of them. At the close of the nineteenth century, the importance of the high infant and maternal mortality rates hardly lay in their originality — since the deaths of mothers and infants had stood at about the same level since statistics first began to be collected. Their importance lay, rather, in the fact that other influences were leading people to define obstetrical deaths as a problem which it was the responsibility of the state, in alliance with the medical and midwifery professions, to solve. It was in this redefinition of obstetric mortality as a social problem, charted in the next chapter, that the movement for clinical antenatal care had its roots.

2

Children of the nation: the beginnings of antenatal care 1900–18

The future of our race and of the Empire depends on the subject with which we are now dealing . . . Let us remember that all men once lay in cradles, and were carried thither from cradles not made with hands, temples holier still, the Sancta Sanctorum of life.

C. W. Saleeby MD 'The Problem of the Future', 1915, p. 14

When the social costs of the industrial revolution began to be weighed against its benefits, sometime in the first half of the nineteenth century, health and illness were at first seen as rooted in the environment rather than the individual. The individual was the victim of the environment. Hence the painstaking topography of a survey such as the 1842 *General Report on the Sanitary Condition of the Labouring Population of Great Britain*. The battle against disease would be won when the country attended to its drains, cleared its public and private places of 'noxious filth', and let the fresh air blow through them.

Treat the environment and all will be well. Such a philosophy could hardly breed the idea and practice of personal antenatal care. For this to happen, two developments in thinking about health had to take place. First, a *personal* concept of health had to replace the environmental one. Secondly, childbearing needed to be singled out as an activity of proper concern to the state — one in which it was essential for the state to intervene in the interests of maintaining and improving the quantity and quality of the population. As George Newman (1870–1948) put it in his Annual Report to the Board of Education for 1913, the two basic truths are (1) 'that the health of the adult is dependent upon the health of the child'; and (2) 'that the health of the child is dependent upon the health of the infant and its mother' (Board of Education, 1914, p. 16).

Both these developments, necessary to the evolution of antenatal care, began at about the same time, in the last years of the nineteenth century. However, while the second — the state's proper interest in reproduction

— quickly became firmly established, the first — an individualized concept of health — took somewhat longer to take root.

The ruling of the world, and the hand that rocks the cradle

It might seem strange that the impetus for these changes in the philosophy and policy of health care in this country should come from an altogether different exercise — war — in an altogether different place — South Africa. The Boer War (1899–1902) disturbed the heedless imperialism of the nineteenth century, by revealing what appeared to be a shockingly low standard of health among the male population recruited to fight in that war. This revelation forced political attention on the actual condition of the Empire's citizens.

In January 1902 General John Frederick Maurice, writing under the pseudonym 'Miles', published an article entitled 'Where to Get Men' in the *Contemporary Review*. In this he argued that the general shortage of recruits reported by British military authorities was due to the fact that few were able to meet the physical requirements necessary for war service. The article provoked a frightened and angry popular discussion 'that linked together in men's [sic] minds, *so they could not again be separated*, the questions of public health and national welfare' (Gilbert, 1966, p. 85, my italics).

The maladies listed as inimical to Army service centred on anaemia, flat feet and bad teeth. The basic cause of these was stated to be poor feeding in infancy and childhood. To substantiate his argument, Maurice cited several colourful and pathetic anecdotes, including one in which a 'most respectable woman in a good situation . . . used habitually to give her six month old baby cold cabbage for supper' (Maurice, 1903, p. 45). The *underlying* cause of Britain's impending failure to be great and free was thus unequivocally identified as maternal ignorance and inadequate devotion to duty.

Maurice's writings are part of the standard story of the beginning of the British maternal and child welfare movements, and they led directly to the setting up of the Interdepartmental Committee on the Physical Deterioration of the Population. The Committee, which sat for 26 days and took evidence from 68 witnesses (23 of whom held official positions, two of whom were 'noted anthropologists' and 34 of whom were doctors), published its Report in 1904. It was not at all coincidental, from the point of view of the emergence of antenatal care, that part of the

Committee's brief was to comment on the role of the medical profession in securing the physical efficiency of the nation.

The Report's first conclusion — that the British race was *not* deteriorating — was reached by discrediting the 'alarmist' statements of General Maurice. The Committee decided that they all personally had bad teeth, so bad teeth could not be a sign of physical degeneracy. They also established that Maurice's figure of three out of five army recruits unfit was based on mere guesswork, and their examination of him showed him to be a generally untrustworthy witness. When he said that on Mafeking night he walked from Charing Cross to Cannon Street, and did not see among the crowds a dozen men fit enough to be enlisted, the Committee retorted that surely the streets were not lit well enough for him to see?

Nevertheless, the Committee made various recommendations for the surveillance and improvement of the nation's health. These included measures to deal with overcrowding, urban slums and smoke pollution, and better statistics relating to pregnancy and birth: the registration of stillbirths, infant mortality rates by locality, and the collection of occupational data in relation to infant mortality, especially for *mothers*. There was also to be systematic instruction for girls in infant feeding and management, and education for mothers in childrearing in leaflet form.

The Report voiced a principle that was to become more and more dominant as the century wore on, and without which there could have been no concerted movement for the medical surveillance of pregnant women. 'The public health is obviously a question of the highest general concern' said the Committee, 'and to the extent that local independence militates against its security, the principle of local self-government must be subordinated to more important interests' (Interdepartmental Committee, p. 24).

This was the clarion call for centralized policy-making in the provision of health services. It represented a challenge to the philosophy of individualism which had hitherto dominated British political decisions, both in the medical and other realms.

Lloyd George's National Insurance Act of 1911 established compulsory medical insurance for all men earning less than £160 per annum, and for all manual labourers, and a maternity benefit to the wife of an insured man at the level of 30 shillings payable at childbirth — double that if the woman herself was also a contributor. The Act was the first legislative codification of the new principle that personal health was the concern of central government, and was the logical forebear of the National Health Service itself. But before the revolution of 1946 was possible, there needed to be a fuller development of the new philosophy in relation to children as the adult citizens of the future and in relation to mothers as the individuals whose wombs constituted the *sancta sanctorum* of life itself.

Educating the mothers

The medical care of pregnant women was not referred to in the 1904 Report as conducive to improved health. There was, however, a great deal of emphasis in it on the welfare of the infant and young child, and it was the translation of these proposals concerning child welfare into legislation — most immediately the Relief (School Children) Order of 1905, the Education (Provision of Meals) Act of 1906, and the Education (Administrative Provisions) Act of 1907 — which initially marked the state's advance into an area previously regarded as one of private responsibility — the home and the family.[1]

In 1900 the infant mortality rate stood at 154 per 1,000 live births. It had fluctuated around that level since the beginning of official statistics in 1838, the highest level — 163 — being recorded in 1899. Most strikingly, the rate had not fallen in parallel with the drop in general mortality rates (from 22.7 per 1,000 in 1875, to 16.9 in 1901). This message stands out clearly comparing figure A.2 for infant mortality from 1846 to 1982 and figure A.5 for mortality in women from 1838 to 1982 (p. 296, p. 298). Deaths among women in general began to fall around the mid-nineteenth century, some half a century before infant deaths. What made matters worse was the decline in the birth rate: there were 153.5 births per 1,000 women aged fifteen to forty-four in 1876–80, and 105.3 in 1906–10 (Office of Population Censuses and Surveys, 1982) (see Figure A.1, p. 296). Thus, infant mortality must be considered — as the title of George Newman's book published in 1906, suggests, *A Social Problem*. There were 120,000 deaths of children aged under one year annually. The chief causes of death in the first three

---

1. Even before these developments was another, less visible, but very important development: the Registrar-General's Annual Report for 1904 contained a letter to the Registrar General from John Tatham MD, in which Tatham pointed out that the 1904 Report had obtained for the subject of infant life-preservation in the public mind 'a degree of importance that had never previously been attained since the establishment of civil registration in this country' (p. i). As a result a new table had been introduced into the Registrar-General's Annual Report for 1904 which showed for the first time the breakdown of infant mortality by month in the first year after birth and by year up to five years.

months were prematurity and immaturity. Although Newman said that 'The explanation [of the early infant deaths] is clearly to be found in antenatal conditions' (p. 62), he did not, like most of those writing at the time, propose medical antenatal care as part of the answer. The answers were, rather, the education of mothers in infant care, provision of better food for infants and mothers, and attention to the working conditions of poor women.

This emphasis on maternal ignorance and the need for educating mothers was not confined to eugenicists or a handful of policy-makers, but was the common feature in most discussions of infant mortality, and in the programmes of all the voluntary and municipal associations concerned with maternity and child welfare. Educating mothers was, certainly, a cheaper solution than the provision of adequate free medical services or improved housing, but the zeal with which it was promoted probably had more to do with perceptions of women's social function, than with a strictly cost-benefit analysis of different strategies for preserving children's health.

Why did mothers need educating? Why were they feckless? In the first place, they had little understanding of how to feed or care for their children hygienically. This could be seen, said the experts, most clearly from the diarrhoea death-rate which in 1911 still accounted for 28 per cent of total infant deaths, and had a strong seasonal component, being highest during a hot summer. Moreover, while sanitation had improved during the last quarter of the nineteenth century, deaths from diarrhoea had risen, suggesting that the cause could lie in maternal behaviour. Mothers were also deemed irresponsible in not consulting doctors often enough for advice on infant care, and, of course, in going out to work, a factor that was held by John Burns, MP, President of the Local Government Board, in his inaugural address to the 1906 National Conference on Infantile Mortality, to double 'the whole death rate of the neighbourhood' (p. 15). Not only did the babies die, he contended, but the surviving children were turned into gangs of 'anaemic, saucy, vulgar, ignorant, cigarette-smoking hooligans' (p. 16). (He himself had a good mother — she had 18 children and did not go out to work.) Others stated the case less strongly, seeing married women's employment as a product of those poor social conditions which would themselves be conducive to high infant mortality. The main point was, as Jane Lewis acknowledges in her *The Politics of Motherhood* (1980, p. 78), that the anti-women's employment lobby stemmed more from the belief that woman's place was in the home than from any convincing evidence connecting maternal employment with infant mortality. These were the years of the suffragettes; in 1905, with the imprisonment of Annie Kenney and Christabel Pankhurst, votes for women had just become a vital public issue. The following year saw large public meetings and the disassociation from orthodox political activity of the militant suffragette movement. The spectre of women publicly asserting their rights provoked, as it always seems to, the backlash ideology of shutting the kitchen door in their face.

In France, Britain and other countries the turn of the century saw the establishment of new municipal institutions known in this country as milk depots. The first was in St Helen's in 1899. (Seebohm Rowntree founded the first private one in York in 1903.) Plate 2.1 shows the Liverpool Milk Depot, founded in 1901. The main principle of the milk depot was municipal control over the quality of milk from before it left the cow until the mother opened the municipally-supplied bottle to feed it to her infant. The milk depots thus aimed to cure one cause of maternal fecklessness, namely contaminated milk. The origin of the milk depot lay in France where the first 'Consultation de Nourrisons' was set up by a Professor Herrgott in 1890 and the first 'Goutte de Lait' in 1892 by Pierre Budin (1846–1907), 'father' of the French infant welfare movement. Mothers who attended the former institution were encouraged to bring their one-month old babies back to the hospital where they were born, for weighing and medical examination, and were paid on a sliding scale according to the infant's progress (McCleary, 1933, p. 43). (Plate 2.2 captures all three activities of the Goutte de Lait.) Similar arrangements for the monitoring of infant nutrition and the provision of safe milk were made in other countries. In the USA the pioneer of the movement for compulsory milk pasteurization was a gentleman called Nathan Straus, later celebrated as the Jew who had done most to serve America. He began a milk depot in 1903 in New York on a pier at the foot of East Third Street where fresh milk was made available to a large tenement population. 'Awnings and seats were put up on the pier so that the babies and their mothers could . . . inhale the fresh air of the river' (McCleary, 1933, p. 57). By 1913, there were 77 milk depots in New York, most of them operated by the City Health Department.

In Britain in 1907 there were 15 milk depots administered by public health authorities. G. F. McCleary, at the time Medical Officer of Health for Battersea, and throughout his life closely identified with the infant welfare movement, described the *modus operandi* of the Battersea Depot in 1904:

The homes of the children fed on the milk are visited by the lady sanitary

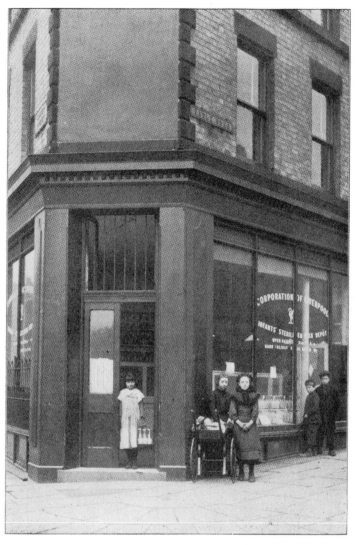

Plate 2.1 Infants' milk depot, Earle Road, Liverpool
source: McCleary, 1905

inspectors, who endeavour to secure that the instructions are properly carried out. If the child does not appear to be progressing favourably the mothers are strongly advised to seek medical advice, and if the child has been using the milk for more than two or three weeks and is not under medical supervision the mother is advised to give a little gravy or raw meat juice in addition to the milk, and written instructions for the preparation of raw meat juice are given to her (McCleary, 1904, p. 338).

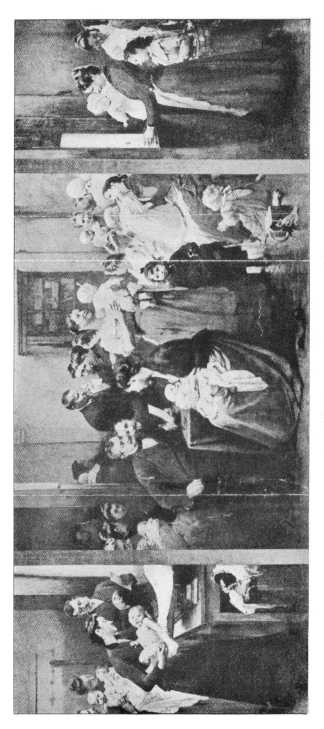

Plate 2.2 'L'Œuvre de la goutte de lait' (Dr Variot's consultation at the Belleville Dispensary, Paris).
From the painting by M. Jean Geoffroy, exhibited in the Salon in 1903, now the property of the Municipality of Paris. This picture illustrates the three main features of the work of the Goutte de Lait: (1) weighing the babies, (2) medical consultation, (3) distribution of sterilized milk

source: McCleary, 1905

Mothers were charged 1s 6d a week for a supply of properly sterilized 'Humanized Milk' (more if they lived outside the Borough) (Metropolitan Borough of Battersea, Annual Report, 1904–05, p. 211).

The principle of home visiting had been established, and mothers had begun to open their front doors to the designated experts of the state — or, rather, they had begun to do so back in the 1860s, when the Ladies' Health Society of Manchester and Salford started home instruction in domestic hygiene. By the turn of the century, there were a few municipally-appointed health visitors, and in 1910 when Sidney and Beatrice Webb wrote their treatise on the need for preventive medicine, *The State and the Doctor*, there were at least 3,000 voluntary visitors, plus between 200 and 300 municipally-salaried health visitors in the UK, some of whom were actually qualified medical practitioners. It was in the early years of this century that health visiting was formed as a separate profession, although the overlap with the medical profession remained until the 1920s (Owen, 1982).

Schools for Mothers

Home visiting was both a symbol and manifestation of the state's newly-designated right to determine what happened in the homes of its people. What the mothers thought of it we do not know. The Webbs said the poverty-stricken mother could only view the visitor as an unmixed blessing. In Somerset Maugham's *Of Human Bondage*, a novel recalling Maugham's own domiciliary midwifery practice in Lambeth in the 1890s, it is suggested that visiting was often perceived as unwelcome intrusion by women whose own backgrounds rendered them incapable of knowing what motherhood on or below the poverty line was all about.

The safe milk movement was, then, never merely a collection of milk shops, but from the start a systematic investment in the monitoring of maternal behaviour. Once networks of lady health visitors and sanitary inspectors had been established for the purpose of ensuring hygienic infant feeding, it was easy for their duties to extend beyond nutritional advice into every crevice of the whole realm of housewifery and motherhood. By 1906, when the first National Conference on Infantile Mortality was held in London, it had become a general assumption among medical professionals, health care administrators, and policy-makers, that the correct education of mothers was an integral part of the struggle to lower infant mortality. As Herbert Samuel, MP, put it in his preface to that invaluable document *Maternity: letters from working women*, in

1915: 'The infant cannot, indeed, be saved by the State. It can only be saved by the mother. But the mother can be helped and can be taught by the State' (Davies, 1915, reprinted, 1978). The ostensible curriculum was the correction of methods of childrearing (and childbearing), but this could be used to justify a much more broadly-based curriculum, which included almost every facet of women's behaviour.

In Hughes Fields Girls' Council School in Greenwich in 1913, girls in the top two classes had two half-hour periods weekly on domestic hygiene. These did not consist merely of talks

> or question and answer, but always contain something in the nature of a practical demonstration in which the girls can take part. Conditions likely to arise in their own daily lives are reproduced as far as possible, and such a subject as the care of the home during the absence of the mother gives opportunity for washing and dressing a doll, arranging a cot, preparing a baby's food, cleaning the house, treating an imaginary burn previous to the doctor's arrival, making a linseed poultice for a sick father, etc. (Board of Education, 1914, p. 237).

Both in, and outside, schools, class teaching was added to individual instruction as a strategy for improving mothers. Indeed a whole new category of schools, namely Schools for Mothers, came into being during these years as vehicles of instruction for adult women in house-wifery and motherhood. A School for Mothers was defined by the Board of Education in 1915 as 'primarily an educational institution providing training and instruction for the mother in the care and management of infants and little children' (Board of Education, 1915, p. 27). It could include classes, home visiting, and infant consultations, but medical treatment would be only 'incidental'. The first School for Mothers was set up in St Pancras in 1907 and was modelled along the lines of one in Ghent started in 1901. The School opened on 4 June 1907; it offered weighing machines (for mothers and babies) 'demonstrations by ladies' in the making of baby clothes; 'lantern lectures on baby culture and social gatherings to talk over experiences with ladies'; cheap dinners for expectant and nursing mothers (an experiment begun in 1906 in Chelsea and before that in 1904 in Paris); medical consultations; and 'a bureau for fathers' (principally for advice, it seems, but fathers' 'evening conferences' were held at which men could hear about their duties 'to the mother, the baby, the children, and the home' (McCleary, 1933, p. 131).)

The founder of the St Pancras School, Dr Sykes, Medical Officer of Health for the Borough, designed a card containing 'Advice to

Mothers', and packets of the cards were sent to the various hospitals, dispensaries, maternity nursing associations, etc., and also to midwives with the request that whoever was booked to attend the confinement should be responsible for giving the card to the mother. Leaflets on infant care were the most common mode of instruction in the early days, and were produced by many voluntary associations. It was, in fact, a voluntary association, the National League for Health, Maternity and Child Welfare, that set up the first non-hospital based antenatal clinics in London in 1915 (see p. 56). Voluntary organizations also performed a significant function as pressure groups. The Women's Co-operative Guild, known today for its powerful documentation of women's experiences as mothers at the outbreak of the war in 1914, put a great deal of pressure during the war years and afterwards on local authorities to initiate schemes for helping mothers. The Guild's Congress Report for 1915–16 notes resolutions sent to 33 separate local authorities (Davies 1915).

Before this, the Guild had carried out a survey of their members asking how women provided for the costs of childbirth. Finding that the doctor or midwife's fee invariably came out of the general housekeeping money, the Guild then sent deputations to the Attorney General and Lloyd George asking for maternity benefit provision to be included in the forthcoming National Insurance Bill. When the Act was passed giving this benefit to the husband, the Guild campaigned to have the money paid to mothers instead, a change duly effected in 1913.

Another large organization that has maintained its impetus and is alive and relatively well in 1982 is the National Association for Maternal and Child Welfare which started out as the National League for Health, Maternity and Child Welfare in 1905 (as one of the many organizational responses to the 1904 Report on the Physical Deterioration of the Population). It was in 1915 that the League added to its agenda the objective of establishing maternity centres 'with a view to supervising the antenatal as well as the postnatal care of infants and the education of the mothers' (NLHMCW Annual Report, 1915, p. 8).

The structure of the League and its affiliated organizations illustrated an important element in the voluntary work for maternal and infant welfare, which was that the membership of voluntary and local authority organizations often overlapped. For example, the Executive Committee of the National Association for the Prevention of Infant Mortality and for the Welfare of Infancy, one of the League's affiliated organizations, consisted of 48 members, divided into one quarter representatives of Statutory Administrative authorities, one quarter practising medical professionals, one quarter medical officers of health, and one quarter 'others'.

In 1908 the St Pancras School for Mothers received a grant from the Board of Education to help fund its classes in infant care and housewifery. The grant was for £5 13s 5d rising to £15 12s in 1909, and was given under the Regulations for Technical Schools which provided grants for organized class teaching. By 1912, 27 institutions were in receipt of grants of this kind — 150 in 1913; and in 1914 the Government determined that the importance of maternal and child welfare work merited greater investment. Consequently, the Board of Education and the Local Government Board (LGB) issued circulars explaining that such grants (to 50 per cent of approved actual expenditure) would in future be payable to voluntary associations as well as local authorities. By this date, 1914, the emphasis in maternal and child welfare work was beginning to shift from work that was primarily educational to that which included a medical component. Indeed, the LGB circular of 30 July 1914 specifically drew attention to the limited character of much infant welfare work, which concentrated on the first year after birth, stating: 'it is clearly desirable that there should be continuity in dealing with the whole period from before birth until the time when the child is entered upon a school register' (p. 9). The scheme for maternal and child welfare outlined in the circular placed the local supervision of midwives first, the provision of antenatal care second, skilled assistance with the confinement third, and postnatal care of mothers and children fourth in order of priority. So far as antenatal care was concerned, listed under that heading were outpatient or clinical antenatal care, home visiting of expectant mothers, and inpatient care, in that order. But most significantly the circular, in its own words, 'contemplates that medical advice and, where necessary, treatment should be *continuously* and *systematically* available for expectant mothers (LGB circular, 30 July 1914, p. 9; my italics).

The LGB's words enshrined two important principles that have governed work in this field ever since: the principle that the state's interest in motherhood begins at conception[2] and ends with the onset of fulltime schooling (when the child is passed to the supervision of the school medical service), and the principle of the *continuous* and *systematic* provision of antenatal care.

2. Or before; see chapter 11 on pre-conceptional care.

Ballantyne and 'antenatal therapeutics'

The years immediately following the publication in 1904 of the Report on the Physical Deterioration of the Population were also the years in which, within the medical profession itself, the idea of antenatal care was gestated and born.

The official story of the birth of antenatal care begins with an article entitled 'A Plea for a Pro-Maternity Hospital' published in the *British Medical Journal* on 6 April 1901. Its author was a forty year-old lecturer at the University of Edinburgh, Dr John William Ballantyne (1861–1923). The son of a seedsman and nursery-garden-owner, the great-grandson of a botanist who re-afforested Scotland with Canadian trees, and the great-great-grandson of the man who introduced Himalayan azaleas to Britain, Ballantyne qualified at the University of Edinburgh in 1883 and went to work first in the Edinburgh Royal Infirmary and next in the Royal Maternity Hospital, where he published in 1885 a study of sphygmographic tracings in eclamptic women. His first interest was paediatrics, but his family background in botany had bequeathed him a fascination with teratology (the study of malformations). His MD thesis in 1889 was entitled, 'Some Anatomical and Pathological Conditions of the New-Born Infant in Relation to Obstetrics', and consisted of 700 handwritten pages detailing the anatomy of several fetuses which Ballantyne had examined in complete transverse frozen sections. Described as a 'colossal worker' (McCleary, 1935, p. 50) Ballantyne wrote some 10 books and 500 medical articles, and personally edited 18 volumes of the *Encyclopaedia Medica*. A 'little dapper man', renowned for being 'courteous and fastidious' (Russell, 1971, p. 23), who championed the cause of female medical education, opened the first VD clinic in Edinburgh, could lecture in Latin to foreign students, and was very much part of the international academic medical community, Ballantyne established for posterity his reputation in this area when he published in 1902 and 1904 two learned volumes on the subject of antenatal pathology and therapeutics. (Volume I weighed 3½ lbs and volume 2, 4 lbs.) In these he expounded the view that 'Preventive medicine would not progress until the laws governing antenatal health were known.'

In his prolific writings, Ballantyne did not use the term 'antenatal care', but talked interchangeably about antenatal therapeutics, antenatal hygiene and antenatal prevention, by which terms he intended to refer to the 'prevention, cure or amelioration of morbid states arising in ante-natal life' (Ballantyne, 1902, p. 465). Defining the practical implications of this, he said that 'The first step . . . in the direction of successful treatment of the unborn infant must be successful treatment of the pregnant mother.' But, 'Here, on the very threshold of the subject, we meet with a check; for, when we come to consider it, we realize that about the physiology of pregnancy . . . our knowledge is very imperfect . . . As a matter of fact, the profession does not understand the physiological changes of pregnancy' (Ballantyne, 1902, p. 465, p. 471). The medical profession was willing, he went on to observe, to endorse such popular 'fog-shrouded' notions about pregnancy as the importance of diet and the powerful effect on the fetus of maternal emotions.

The 1901 article, ('A Plea for a Pro-Maternity Hospital'), for which Ballantyne is remembered, is not, in itself, one of his most striking contributions, but is remarkable rather for its repercussions in medical circles. (The prefix 'pro', was intended in the Greek sense of 'before', not in the Latin one of 'in favour of'. But some found it misleading and in his later writings, Ballantyne reverted to the prefix 'pre' as used in his original 1900 lecture on the topic (Ballantyne, 1907–08).) In the article Ballantyne suggested an annex of the Maternity Hospital 'for the reception of women who are pregnant but who are not yet in labour'. He anticipated the women who would occupy these beds as being initially those with a poor obstetric history or present complications of pregnancy, and later on for poor working women who needed to rest during pregnancy. He pointed out that there was, at the time he wrote, no official hospital in-patient provision for pregnant women. A case of 'morbid pregnancy' might be treated in a general hospital, but with reluctance — in case a birth should occur. It would be only by the admission of complicated pregnancies to hospital that clinicians could hope to learn more about the aetiology of antenatal disease. Finally, he observed that a pre-maternity ward could also be expected to justify itself on economic grounds: providing working women with rest might well result in healthier babies.

Ballantyne's ideas were not especially novel. As a rejoinder published in the *British Medical Journal* on 13 April 1901, from a Professor Kynoch observed, they had been practised in some places for Centuries. But there was no doubt that Ballantyne's notion of a pre-maternity ward was new in some important ways. The arrangement he proposed differed from existing institutional provision for pregnant women in that women would not have to be either married or unmarried to qualify for it, but solely 'ill and pregnant . . . The permission to enter would be always *medical*' (Ballantyne, 1907–08, pp. 28–9). Moreover, his concept of pre-maternity care was all-embracing: what he did *not* think could be cured or prevented by antenatal care was not worth mentioning. His amusing description of an international prototype — 'A Visit to the Wards of the Pro-Maternity Hospital?' — ends with a Dr Geburtsmal saying 'In this twentieth century, Mein Herr, we prevent everything, war, disease, hurricanes — everything, except the doing of good to others' (Ballantyne 1901b, p. 597). The hospital was situated in Germany, supported by the French, and funded by an American from Chicago. Its characters included a Frenchman, Dr Leoufmalade, a Russian, Dr Embryonowsky, a Greek, Dr Teras Teratos, and a Dr Anthony Nathan Patholog of mixed blood. There were wards for the treatment of syphilis, for the cure of chronically alcoholic women, and for the prevention of abortion and prematurity, and one ward inscribed simply and hopefully with the word 'Heredity'. There were also laboratories for the microscopic investigations of urine and excreta, not to mention 'the Röntgen [X ray] Room, where the art of antenatal diagnosis was being perfected' (Ballantyne, 1901b, p. 597).

Ballantyne's dream, was then, intrinsically a technical–scientific one. A new scientific understanding would combine with new medical technologies to endow the physician with virtually complete power to extract every fetus from the womb live and healthy. The purest demonstration of this is to be found in another piece of Ballantyne's wry science fiction, the inaugural address on the future of obstetrics which he gave to the Edinburgh Obstetrical Society in 1906. In this, the President of 1906 is telephoned by an unknown voice who claims to be the President of 1940. The voice asks Ballantyne if there is anything he would like to know about obstetrics in 1940. Ballantyne enquires first about obstetrics teaching and learns that this has been vastly simplified by an instrument called the 'electric phantom'. The electric phantom is a model of the female pelvis containing a full-term uterus and fetus: the fetus is delivered by electric means at a rate selected by the teacher, and there are various buttons to press to narrow or widen the pelvic inlet or outlet, thereby presenting the student with a practical case to solve, like the student pilot in a practice cockpit. There are also machines which show for teaching purposes, on closed circuit television, the real deliveries of real fetuses, and reproduce accurately fetal heart sounds.

Moving on to obstetric practice, Ballantyne is then told of the discovery which revolutionized twentieth-century practice — a 'tocophoric serum' obtained from the blood of pregnant animals, which effected the safe and speedy induction of labour. 'In this way', explained the President of 1940, 'a labour could be brought on and a child born with almost the same degree of certainty with which it used to be possible to perform a surgical operation' (Ballantyne, 1906–07, p. 14). Improvements in vital statistics were anticipated and 'the hygiene of pregnancy began to be studied in detail and with an enthusiasm and thoroughness never before arrived at'. It was anticipated that pregnant women regularly consult the doctor 'early enough for his [sic] remedial measures to avail both the maternal and the infant lives' — in fact in the first weeks of pregnancy (Ballantyne, 1906–07, pp. 23–5). Eclampsia, stillbirth, and habitual abortion had become rare. 'New and more effective means of keeping prematurely born infants alive' had been introduced, and destructive delivery operations 'yielded to methods which gave a chance of survival to the child'. The majority of complications were detected antenatally, so that even caesarean sections were infrequently done on anything other than an elective basis. In this way Ballantyne anticipated many of the advances in obstetrics that were to be achieved in the coming few decades: systematic antenatal care, hormonal methods of inducing labour (see chapter 8), electronic fetal heart monitoring and obstetric ultrasound (see chapter 7), and neonatal intensive care (chapter 9) included.

Visionary as Ballantyne's conception of antenatal care was, he did not see it as especially of benefit to the mother, and he did not anticipate routine out-patient antenatal care as we know it today. His interest was above all in pathology, in understanding and treating 'morbid' pregnancies. His notion of routine antenatal care was limited to the suggestion (1906–07, p. 150) that pregnant women needed a 'medical man's eye' kept on them and 'the medical man ought to pay an occasional visit to his pregnant patients, even if it be only to relieve them of some of the minor ailments of pregnancy, to keep their minds at rest, and to secure a regularly-sent sample of urine for analysis.'

Three months after the publication of Ballantyne's 'Plea' in 1901, the first bed for the in-patient treatment of pregnant women was endowed in the Edinburgh Royal Maternity and Simpson Memorial Hospital. Officially the endowment was anonymous, but the endower was in fact a Dr Freeland Barbour, who was himself a wealthy member of the staff of the hospital, a friend of Ballantyne's and the author of a pioneering work on pelvic anatomy. The offer was made by Dr Barbour in a letter of 15 July 1901 to the Board of Directors of the Hospital. Barbour wrote:

> At present patients who are suffering from the diseases incident to Pregnancy are admitted to the Hospital only on sufferance. If the Board will authorize one case of this nature (at a time) to be treated in the Hospital, I shall be glad to give a sum of £1,000, the interest of which will I understand cover the cost of maintenance.

The Board unanimously agreed to accept Dr Barbour's offer and the details were subsequently worked out. In a letter of 22 October 1901, Dr Barbour requested that the bed be used only for patients suffering from 'a non-infectious disease complicating pregnancy, e.g. cardiac disease, chorea, albuminuria'. He suggested that, in order to extend the benefit to as many patients as possible, no case be allowed to remain more than one month. To commemorate the founder of the hospital (Alexander Hamilton) he wanted the bed known as the 'Hamilton bed'.

The first patient to occupy the Hamilton bed was recalled by Dr Caleeb Saleeby at a Conference on Infant Welfare held in London in July 1924 as 'a little Englishwoman from smoky Leeds with a rickety pelvis'. The patient did not survive caesarean section, and soon afterwards her infant died in the arms of Dr Saleeby, then resident physician at the Edinburgh Royal Maternity Hospital. 'It was a tragic beginning', commented Saleeby, 'for one of the greatest and happiest ideas of any age' (National Association for Maternal and Child Welfare Annual Conference Reports 1924–31, p. 215). Ballantyne's own memory of the first case was different. With customary modesty he described the first case as a thirty-seven year-old multipara with hydramnios in whom he diagnosed a malformed infant; the woman gave birth easily and unexpectedly to twins: 'Such was the almost ludicrous termination', commented Ballantyne, 'of our first attempt to forecast the future of antenatal affairs' (Ballantyne, 1907–08, p. 36).

The first outpatient clinic

Like the first patient to occupy the Hamilton bed (and many such historical 'firsts'), there is some dispute about the first out-patient antenatal clinic. At the same time as Ballantyne was developing antenatal therapeutics in Scotland, and other hospital physicians were beginning to think along similar lines, the sphere of municipal provision was independently enlarging. But the apocryphal first out-patient clinic in the authorized version of the birth of antenatal care was the one opened in Edinburgh in 1915, and also associated with Ballantyne's name — though erroneously, as it turns out.

The Minutes of the Board of Directors of the Hospital refer on 11 December 1914 to a letter suggesting the supervision of expectant mothers. The letter was from a Dr Haig Ferguson (1862–1934) a family doctor for 20 years, who later moved into hospital practice, qualifying as a Fellow of the Edinburgh Royal College of Surgeons in 1902. Remembered by Dr John Sturrock, who was Ferguson's registrar in 1926–27, as a 'handsome and impressive' figure with a sartorial and persuasive manner and a habit of referring to patients by the name of the town from whence they came ('Kircaldy, you're on the mend'),[3] Ferguson was one of the founders of an institution located at 4 Lauriston Place, Edinburgh, known as the Lauriston Prematernity Home. He served as Chairman and Visiting Physician to the Home for many years, and was personally responsible for the medical supervision of the unmarried pregnant girls resident there, some 50 per cent of whom were under twenty, and most of whom were servants of the 'respectable working class' (Mackenzie, 1917, p. 119). The women could enter the home from six months of pregnancy, but most did so about two months before their due date. Becoming convinced of the value of medical supervision to preserve the health of mother and baby in such cases, Ferguson believed it should be made available to all mothers. In his Presidential Address to the Edinburgh Obstetrical Society in 1912, 'Some Twentieth century Problems in Relation to Marriage and Childbirth' Ferguson observed that what he termed 'intra-uterine puericulture' was the first duty of the obstetrician. Prenatal care would obtain a lower preterm delivery rate, higher average birthweight, and decreased neonatal mortality. Further, he went on, referring no doubt to his observations at 4 Lauriston Place, and echoing the precepts of the still-surviving nineteenth-century life-style paradigm of pregnancy, 'rest before confinement, good food, healthy surroundings and avoidance of excitement, seem to give the mother greater vitality, more perfect nutrition, full-term labours, and good recoveries' (p. 4). If such results can be achieved, argued Ferguson, for the mothers of illegitimate children 'how much more, then, should these advantages be obtainable for all married women' (p. 5). The eugenicist streak was strong in Ferguson, who did not believe in birth control, was fond of terms such as 'racial duty', and advocated the restriction of girls' education on the ground that it injured their pelvic organs. But, unlike Ballantyne, Ferguson stressed that the preservation of the mother's life and health was a prime duty for obstetricians. Unlike Ballantyne, also, he considered the question of the financing of the maternity services, and much bemoaned the passing of the National Insurance Act which, he thought, would lead to the retrogressive development of women increasingly booking midwives for their confinements: this would have

---

3. For my information on Haig Ferguson's role in the development of antenatal care in Edinburgh, I am indebted to an interview with Dr John Sturrock.

the effect of depriving the hospitals of the normal cases necessary for the teaching of future doctors.

By June 1915 Ferguson's 1914 letter on the benefits of prenatal care had borne fruit, and 'infant and prematernity consultations' under his direction had begun in the Edinburgh Royal Maternity Hospital. Mr Paterson, the hospital secretary, provided a form of printed ticket for patients to bring back on subsequent visits. R. W. Johnstone recalls the difficulty of purveying to respectable married women (as opposed to unrespectable unmarried ones) the new ware of antenatal care. Since the moral association of medical surveillance with illegitimate pregnancy did not motivate take-up of care among married women,[4] for their convenience 'entrance to the clinic was arranged from an unfrequented side street, and I well remember the great consideration that had to be given to their modesty in putting up an unobtrusive and discreetly worded direction board' (Johnstone, 1950, p. 13).

A report on the health of Scottish mothers and children, sponsored by the Carnegie United Kingdom Trust in 1917, described Britain's 'first' antenatal clinic. It was not at all a grand place:

> The premises in which these clinics are held consist of one room, divided into two by means of a wooden partition, and lavatory accommodation in the basement of the hospital. There is a separate entrance from a side street, which is on a level with the basement. The patients wait in the outer half of the room, and are seen by the doctor in the inner half. Assisting the doctor there are one of the resident doctors and two nurses. The consulting room is rather noisy and not very well lighted, having one window of translucent glass. Artificial lighting is by means of gas; the floor is covered with linoleum; a coal-grate and a sink are fitted in the doctor's room (Mackenzie, 1917, p. 51).

According to some sources (Joint Committee, 1948, p. 22; Kerr, et al., 1954, p. 151), prior to Ferguson's suggestion for out-patient clinic antenatal care, Ballantyne had arranged for the home visiting by nurses of expectant mothers booked for delivery at the Hospital for the dual purpose of giving advice and testing urine. But aside from preparing a pamphlet for distribution to pregnant women on the benefits of the new clinic consultations, Ballantyne was not himself involved in the new venture. However, some time after the clinic started, when Ferguson's

---

4. The opposite is the case today, and the 'stigma' of illegitimate pregnancy may be a reason for late antenatal attendance.

other commitments had become too pressing, Ballantyne was (reluctantly) persuaded to take over its supervision. By 1919, the relevant memoranda in the Minutes of the Meetings of the Medical Board of the Hospital are signed by Ballantyne, not Ferguson. In June of that year, Ballantyne recorded that the antenatal clinic (thus called) was held in the hospital annex on Tuesday and Friday, and was staffed by one doctor, one trained sister, two probationary nurses, and a woman medical student 'who acted as clerk and also received clinical instruction'. From 1917 the clinic was in receipt of an annual grant from the local authority of £200. In addition to small fees from women students trained there, Ballantyne as Physician-in-Charge received an honorarium of £105 per annum.

This development in Edinburgh did not occur in isolation, but was part of a national and international movement. In Australia, T. G. Wilson received permission from the Board of management of the Adelaide Hospital to run an out-patient antenatal clinic one day a week in 1910, which he did, singlehanded, until 1914. J. C. Windeyer followed with a clinic at the Royal Hospital for Women in Sydney in 1912. Both Wilson and Windeyer had visited Edinburgh in 1908–09 and seen the developments there, but the Australian clinics were a natural evolution of work already in progress; 'prematernity work' was, before the establishment of a formal clinic, carried out in the gynaecological outpatient department. In Sydney, 29 per cent of the women delivered at the hospital attended the antenatal clinic during its first two years: by 1920–22 this had increased to 50 per cent (Windeyer, 1922).

In the USA the first move towards routine hospital antenatal care came from the work of the Instructive District Nursing Association which, in 1901, began making antenatal visits to some of the patients of the Boston Lying-In-Hospital. By 1906, all pregnant women received at least one visit from a nurse at some point between applying to the hospital for confinement and the actual confinement itself. A Mrs William Lowell Putnam of the Infant Social Service Department of the Women's Municipal League of Boston then began in 1909 an 'experiment' in intensive prenatal care.[5] This was described in 1913 by Dr James Huntington of the Boston Lying-In Hospital's Pregnancy Clinic as involving the home visiting of all pregnant patients by the nurse every

---

5. I have not been able to discover why the term 'prenatal' was adopted in the United States and the term 'antenatal' in Britain. In the early years of the 'antenatal' movement in Britain — at least until 1918 — the two terms were used interchangeably.

ten days. At each visit the patients were questioned not only as to the proper care of their bodies but were reassured and encouraged as well' (Huntington, 1913, p. 763). It was not, apparently, a controlled experiment, yet the results of the work were regarded as so good that in May 1911 Mrs Putnam's efforts blossomed into a full-blown clinic. The clinic, like the one in Edinburgh, does not seem to have been a particularly grand affair, being located in a four-roomed tenement apartment opposite the hospital's main entrance: rent $300 per annum.

Within Britain, recognition of the importance of antenatal care within the hospital system was uneven. There are references to antenatal departments before 1915 — the City of London Maternity Hospital acquired a new building which included an antenatal department in 1907 (Cannings, 1922) for example — but their exact function is not known. In 1866, the Annual Report of the Glasgow Royal Maternity Hospital described an outpatient dispensary system which offered free advice on 'diseases peculiar to women and children only' twice a week at 3 o'clock in the afternoon. By 1912, the Hospital's Reports were noting 'a marked increase' in consultations among patients referred by their doctors for such advice. 'Married women of the poorest class' formed 95 per cent of such patients (Annual Report of the Glasgow Royal Maternity Hospital, p. 29). Three years later this work was formally organized into an 'Ante-Natal Dispensary', which provided a two-day-a-week service, soon rising to four days a week. What transpired in Glasgow was almost certainly a general pattern: over the years it had been customary to treat pregnant patients with complications in the outpatient gynaecological dispensary, and as the gospel of antenatal care began to be spread, this service was reorganized to form a separate department of each hospital's work.

Municipal antenatal care

The 1918 Maternity and Child Welfare Act enabled the municipal authorities to aid the funding of maternity and child welfare work wherever this occurred. Grants could be paid to voluntary associations or to hospitals already carrying out such work. The Act was permissive rather than mandatory in its outlining of the comprehensive ideal maternity and child welfare service, which included salaried midwives, health visitors, antenatal clinics, day nurseries, and free or cheap food for mother and child. But the Act did require every local authority to set up a maternity and child welfare committee which had to have at least two women members, and this, together with the general ardour prevailing for official action, signified the beginning of the end of the period of intense voluntary activity. Although hospital-based antenatal care was the structure which eventually came to dominate antenatal care in Britain, for the first 40 years it was municipal antenatal care that ruled the field. The development of municipal antenatal care over the period from 1916 to 1944 is charted in figure A.8, p. 302.

The first problem in organizing a municipal antenatal service was knowing who was pregnant. The question of a system for the compulsory notification of pregnancy was frequently raised over the years in medical and administrative circles (see, e.g. Hope, 1917) and, although officially it was frowned on for ethical reasons (LGB, 1918), local initiatives tackled the problem in a variety of ways. In a lecture delivered to the Royal Society of Medicine in 1915, a Dr Cates described the method used in St Helens, Lancashire from 1914. Since 95 per cent of mothers in St Helens engaged a midwife for the delivery, the link-person was obviously the midwife; and as the Local Health Committee was also the local supervising authority for midwives, they instructed midwives to notify all their bookings immediately to the Medical Officer of Health. A form was provided for this notification which included questions about sanitary conditions in the home and the financial circumstances of the patient. A nurse then visited the patient to give advice and arrange a private medical referral where necessary. A somewhat different system was instituted in Huddersfield, in 1916, with *voluntary* notification of pregnancy. The doctor or midwife booked for the confinement gave the name and address of the patient, with her consent, to the local Public Health Department, and was paid a fee for so doing; by 1937 when the system was still operating, the fee was 2s 6d. In 1916 some 11 per cent of registered births in Huddersfield were notified antenatally; by 1934 this had risen to 77 per cent (Ministry of Health 1937). Dr Moore, Medical Officer of Health for Huddersfield, compared the Huddersfield system with results from six other towns in 1924 and found the proportion of pregnancies notified (and thus presumably examined) antenatally some 27 per cent higher in Huddersfield than elsewhere, with a maternal death rate among notified cases one third that resulting from unnotified pregnancy (Moore, 1928).

Despite the LGB's circular of 1914, no antenatal clinic as such was established by that time, or in that year. The Forty-Third Annual Report of the LGB for 1913–14 noted that questions had been asked in 1912 of all Medical Officers of Health for the county boroughs about provision in their localities, and that the answers demonstrated that 'a considerable amount of work among expectant mothers is carried out' (LGB, 1914, p. xxx). For the most part, this consisted of home visiting by voluntary agencies. The situation changed when, in 1915, a Captain and Mrs Beamish gave £500 to the National League for Health, Maternity and Child Welfare to set up six experimental antenatal clinics attached to existing municipal infant welfare centres in the vicinity of the Royal Free Hospital in London (so that the Hospital could be used as a consulting centre). By 1918, the League was responsible for ten such clinics and in its Annual Report said it aimed to start 30 more. The actual 'first' strictly local authority antenatal clinic is not known. McCleary records (1935, p. 57) the clinic at the Town Hall, Woolwich, in 1915, as 'one of the first'.

By 1918 there were some 120 local authority antenatal clinics. The *raison d'être* of the antenatal centre was 'medical supervision', as it was not of its sister institution, the School for Mothers. The new centres were not intended for middle-class women and those with obvious complications of pregnancy who were expected to go directly to a private doctor or hospital. The antenatal centre would therefore serve principally the 'normal' working-class community of women with midwife-booked deliveries, and would be important centres for midwifery work. By 1915 the Central Midwives' Board had made it a rule that midwives should enquire into their patient's general condition in pregnancy, and obviously the local authority antenatal centre was a good place for them to carry out such an enquiry.

In a Memorandum on Health Visiting and on Maternity and Child Welfare Centres, dispatched by the LGB to the local councils in 1915, Newsholme provided a description of an ideal centre. He recommended 25–30 cases per session, including no more than 8–12 new cases; 'Crowding, and protracted waiting of mothers and of their children, should be avoided, and the interview of the doctor with each mother and child should not be hurried' (Local Government Board, 1915b, p. 18). Three rooms were desirable, one for waiting and undressing, one for weighing, and one for medical consultations. Figure 2.1 shows the record cards for mothers and infants advised by Newsholme.

As Newsholme indicated, medical officers at the antenatal centres did not provide treatment, and this eventually proved to be a fatal weakness in the system. What the centres provided was some hope of alleviating the uncomfortable minor ailments of pregnancy. This task was supported by the dominant model of pregnancy at the time, which, continuously with that obtaining in the nineteenth century, stated its essential normality: 'The condition of pregnancy', said the LGB itself 'should

A. *Mother*
Name ....Age ....Address
Patient of..
Date of first attendance..
Date of expected birth...
Occupation { present...
           { before marriage..
Occupation of husband ....
Former pregnancies   { 1st............................... 4th ....
(including miscarriages). { 2nd .... 5th ....
                          { 3rd............................. 6th...............................
(State in each case whether the child is still living, and, if not, cause of death.)
Previous medical history of patient..
Present health (teeth, constipation,
   digestion, obstetrical, &c.)   ....
Adequacy of food ....
Arrangements for confinement —
   Present condition (doctor's note) ....
   Treatment recommended ....
   General notes...
   Dates and notes of subsequent attendances (on back page).

B. *Infant*
Name .... Date of first attendance ....
Address..
Date of birth..................................... Maturity.....................................
Weight at birth ....
Health prior to attendance ....
Method of feeding...
Digestion and bowels ....
Sleeping...
Clothing...
Bathing ....
Open air...
Present state and weight...
Doctor's notes (including nutrition)..
Dates and notes of subsequent attendances (on back page).

C. *Home Conditions.*
Occupants of house........................... Adults .... Under 15 ....
Number of rooms and size ....
Sanitary conditions...
   Ventilation..
   Light ....
   Repair ....
   Dampness, &c...
   Cleanliness...
   Refuse Receptacles ....
Social conditions and habits...
Dates and notes of revisits (on back page).

The back of the sheet should be reserved for further notes, especially for medical notes of reconsultations and for consecutive weighings.

Figure 2.1 Maternity and Child Welfare Record Card, 1915
source: LGB, 1915a, pp. 19–20

not ... be regarded as pathological, but attention should rather be devoted to the prevention and ... treatment of ... minor departures from the normal' (LGB, 1914). The wisdom of medical tomes on this topic was not far advanced over that conveyed in the nineteenth century (see e.g. Russell, 1912), although some authorities had begun to edge their way slowly towards a less optimistic view of pregnancy: 'Pregnancy is a natural physiological state' said R. W. Johnstone (1913, p. 10) 'but owing to the conditions of modern life it tends to border upon the pathological.'

The state of the art

There were few advances during these years in obstetric knowledge or monitoring or intervention techniques. Exceptions were the recognition of the different ABO blood groups by Jansky (1907), and the description of X-ray measurement of the pelvis by Riddell in the same year (although X-ray pelvimetry did not become a widely-used technique until the 1920s (Kerr et al., 1954)). In 1914 Ballantyne could still write that 'the great desideratum of the present time is an absolutely reliable test of the presence of a child in the womb' (Ballantyne, 1914, p. 51).

This, then, was the technical background to the persistence of the hygiene model of antenatal care in the early municipal clinics. But how general was municipal antenatal clinic provision, and what proportion of pregnant women attended?

Undoubtedly the bulk of the provision was urban — a survey carried out for the Carnegie United Kingdom Trust in 1917 showed that among large towns with a population of more than 50,000, 58 had no local authority antenatal consultations. None of the 47 counties provided local authority antenatal care. In the towns, the extent and pattern of provision was very variable: thus, in Bradford, an antenatal clinic in Horton Lane consisting of 'a waiting room and consulting room properly furnished and equipped' had been in operation since 1915 (Hope, 1917, p. 232), whereas, in Dewsbury, there was no antenatal clinic at all, and in Leicester the Medical Officer of Health simply noted that 'A number of expectant mothers consult the Medical Officer at the School for Mothers' (p. 309).[6] Figure 2.2 shows the system in operation in 1917 at the North Islington Maternity Centre and School for Mothers. The

---

6. This suggests that some strictly medical consultation may have taken place at these institutions.

centre was set up in 1913 by a voluntary committee and the antenatal clinic opened in 1914. By 1917 the staff consisted of three visiting women medical officers, five full-time nurses, a paid secretary, and 37 voluntary workers, 21 of whom worked as visitors. The antenatal consultations held once a week consisted of advice plus recommendations for hospital treatment where necessary — and, of course, the homes were visited by the voluntary workers.

No national figures are available for the proportion of expectant mothers in receipt of antenatal care at the close of the first world war. Judging by the frequent references in the medical press to 'reluctant antenatalism' throughout the 1920s, it could have been no more than a very small proportion. Although in theory midwives could attend the antenatal clinics with their patients, and some probably would have done so, the practice of booking one's midwife a couple of months in advance of the expected birth was, apparently, as much to ensure that one's relatives knew who to send for in the event of a premature delivery as to secure pre-confinement care (Lane-Claypon, 1920, p. 140). Figure A.9, p. 303, brings together a number of different available sources of data on use of antenatal care over the whole period to 1980, and is a testament as much to the lack of systematically collected information as to what *is* known about the proportion of pregnant women using different types of care in the various periods.

Monday	LCC Dental Clinic	9.30 to 12 a.m.
	alternate Mondays	2 to 4 p.m.
	LCC Lectures to Midwives,	
	alternate Mondays	2 to 4 p.m.
Tuesday	Babies under 2 years of age	2 to 4 p.m.
	Children 2 to 5 years of age	2 to 4 p.m.
Wednesday	Expectant Mothers	2 to 4 p.m.
	Sewing Class	2 to 4 p.m.
	LCC Dental Clinic	9.30 to 12 a.m.
Thursday	LCC Dental Clinic	9.30 to 12 a.m.
	Babies under 2 years of age	2 to 4 p.m.
Friday	Babies (with ailing mothers)	10 to 12 a.m.
	Babies under 2 years of age	2 to 4 p.m.

The Superintendent is on duty every morning, and is able to see mothers who desire her advice for urgent matters.

Figure 2.2 Service-provision at the North Islington Maternity Centre and School for Mothers *source*: Campbell, J *Report on the Physical Welfare of Mothers and Children Vol 2*, 1917, p. 87. Reproduced by permission of the publisher Carnegie United Kingdom Trust.

The First World War both hampered and hastened the growth of antenatal work. There was, of course, practical disruption of antenatal

services, but good antenatal care also meant the survival of infants —
male infants — to fight in the future for their country's survival; or, as
Dr Hope put it in his 1917 Report for the Carnegie Trust, if in the 50
years prior to 1917 infant mortality had occurred at the rate prevailing in
that year, 'five hundred thousand more men would have been available
for the defence of the country today' (p. 1).

Some years before the end of the war it had become clear that the first
objective of the maternity and child welfare movement was already in
process of being achieved: infant mortality had fallen from 151 per
1,000 births in 1901, to 110 per 1,000 births in 1915 (Medical Research
Committee, 1917, p. 27). Indeed, by 1904, the year of the publication of
the Report on the Physical Deterioration of the Population, the infant
mortality rate was well into a decline that has been sustained until the
present day. Although infant mortality had begun to fall, recognition of
the decline is not marked in public documents until at least 1910, by
which time a fashion for analysing regional variations in infant and child
mortality rates was deflecting attention away from the overall fall.

Why did infant mortality begin to fall? As the Medical Research
Committee (MRC) said in its discussion of the subject, the general habit
was to attribute the declining mortality to 'such measures as the Midwives' Act, the Notification of Births Act, and the establishment of
prenatal clinics, Schools for Mothers, infant consultation centres, etc.'
(MRC, 1917, p. 27). Yet this motherhood surveillance system was
unlikely to be the cause of the falling infant mortality. Looking at the
exact relationship between the new milk depots and infant mortality
rates, for example, the MRC found 'a wonderful uniformity in the
behaviour of different curves' — of infant mortality in widely separated
towns, some of which had milk depots and some of which did not (p.
38). Moreover, infant mortality was falling all over Europe. The Committee was forced to conclude that milk depots would not be demonstrated to have had any beneficial influence, and quoted the words of
one sagacious 'chief lady health visitor' who even thought there might be
too much 'visiting' going on (after finding herself the fifth visitor in one
house).

Dr Brend, writing in the 1917 MRC Report, was of the opinion that
the answer lay in the air — in atmospheric pollution; but the Medical
Officer of Health to the London County Councils the author of a
number of unusually challenging and argumentative reports, discredited
this explanation in his Annual Report for 1917, on the grounds that the
rate was excessively low in the London area (98 in 1911–14), over which
'no wind blows that has not passed over an air-polluting district' (LCC,

1918, p. 4). This was the beginning of a debate which we shall investigate further in the next chapter about the relative effect of social versus biological causes of obstetric mortality, a debate which was of more than academic importance. What was at issue was the question of *preventability*, for the proportion of obstetric deaths that could *theoretically* be prevented constituted the proper domain, and thus testing ground, of antenatal care.

3

Save the Mothers: antenatal care 1918–32

It has been calculated by competent authorities that 75 per cent of the diseases peculiar to women owe their origin to impregnantion.

Berkeley, 1929, p. 72

In chapter 2 we saw how the need for antenatal services tended to be referred back to the single index of infant mortality. By the end of the First World War, however, the focus of the new antenatalism had shifted to a new index — maternal mortality.

In 1925 the Women's Co-operative Guild petitioned infant welfare workers at the Annual Conference on Infant Welfare to put the welfare of the mother before that of the child. By that year it had become apparent that whatever social and medical engineering or natural evolutionary process had brought about the decline in infant deaths, it was not achieving the same results for mothers. In this sense, the interests of mother and child clearly could not be assumed to be coincidental.

Maternity equals eternity

At the close of the First World War in 1918, one mother died for every 264 babies born alive. By 1932 this figure had risen to one maternal death for every 238 live births (Registrar-General Statistical Review for 1932, p. 87; Figure A.4, p. 298) — not perhaps a highly significant increase, given the year-to-year fluctuations, but the essential point was that deaths of women from causes due to, or associated with, childbearing, were not falling, as, indeed, they had not done throughout the entire history of their coverage by official statistics. This meant that some 3,000 women a year in England and Wales had to learn the lesson that 'maternity is another word for eternity' (Porritt, 1934, p. 1) — a stream of mortality as nearly as deep, dark and continuous as when William

Farr wrote in 1885. 'If every year 3,000 people died in their sleep and because of sleeping' remarked F. J. Browne in 1931, 'or if a like number of men died every year because they had eaten an ordinary breakfast, one can imagine what an outcry there would be and the efforts that would be put forth and the money that would be expended to find a remedy' (p. 688).

The first Government Report devoted specifically to maternal mortality was published in 1924. It was written by Janet Campbell, Senior Medical Officer to the department dealing with maternity and child welfare within the newly created Ministry of Health. Her report described maternal mortality as a major problem confronting the public health service. As she pointed out, most of the women who died were in the prime of life, and busy 'rearing children for the nation'. Many maternal deaths were associated with the death of the infant too, and with impaired survival among the remaining children. When mothers did not die, they frequently endured long-term ill-health: all in all, a considerable 'burden of avoidable suffering' (Ministry of Health, 1924, p. 5).

'Avoidable' was a key word. The definition of death or illness as potentially avoidable establishes the rationale for trying to avoid it. By earmarking a specific proportion of deaths or illnesses in a certain category as avoidable, the health care administrator, policy-maker or provider is staking out new territory as the legitimate domain of medical care. In her 1924 report, Dr Campbell did not put a figure on the proportion of maternal deaths that could be considered avoidable, but she did the spadework for such a calculation by initiating the first national 'confidential enquiries' exercise.[1] She asked a sample of Medical Officers of Health in different parts of the country to investigate all cases of puerperal fever (fatal and nonfatal) and all maternal deaths occurring in their areas between October 1921 and December 1922. The result of this investigation covered a series of 380 deaths of which 256 were puerperal fever deaths. Running through a list of factors possibly implicated in these deaths, Campbell found that the occupation of the woman did not seem to be important, that the cleanliness or otherwise of the home was less influential than might be expected, that the use of gloves and of sterilized gowns and forceps was less usual than it should be, and that antenatal care in these cases was either entirely lacking or 'perfunctory in character'. Out of the total sample of 380

---

1. Confidential enquiries into all maternal deaths have been the subject of a special report in England and Wales from 1952 until the present time.

deaths, only 48 women were said to have received any clinical antenatal care.

The methodology of Campbell's exercise prevented any comparison with the pregnancy histories of women who did not die, so that the efficacy of antenatal care in preventing avoidable deaths could only be an assumption. But the main burden of the report did, indeed, suggest that the prevailing standard of antenatal care was low. In Breconshire, for instance, antenatal care consisted purely of the occasional testing of urine by midwives — there was no routine physical examination; in Westmoreland, no one even tested urine, although 'the District nurses visit their prospective patients pre-natally' (Ministry of Health, 1924, p. 23). Of likely causes of maternal mortality, Campbell singled out the following:

(1) the quality of professional attendance in pregnancy, at delivery and postnatally;
(2) abortion and miscarriage (the former especially leading to maternal deaths from sepsis);
(3) rickets (as a cause of contracted pelvis producing difficult or obstructed labour);
(4) the employment of women;
(5) general sanitation and housing.

Of these rather disparate causes, the first was the one to receive most emphasis. Campbell observed that if the quality of professional attendance were good then 'nearly all other conditions become of minor importance' (p. 30).

To remedy this unsatisfactory standard of practice, Campbell proposed improvements in medical education and the training of midwives — two of the subjects of her earlier reports (Ministry of Health, 1923a; Ministry of Health, 1923b). Such improvements would, she hoped, focus on the practical need for antenatal care. She was quite certain that in antenatal care lay the main solution to the problem.

> It is the key to success in any scheme of prevention and it must be insisted upon in and out of season until it is no longer ignored or looked upon as a luxury for the well-to-do woman . . . Until antenatal supervision is accepted by patients and their advisers as the *invariable* duty of the professional attendant . . . we shall never make substantial progress towards the reduction of maternal death and injury (Ministry of Health, 1924, p. 74; my italics).

One main goal of the 1924 Maternal Mortality Report, to focus the spotlight on *avoidable* maternal deaths, had already been established for infant and child mortality. In its 1917 Report, the Medical Research Committee had called 52 per cent of infant deaths avoidable (apparently on the basis of no evidence other than assuming that the rate, which was then 104 per 1,000 live births, ought to be 50). By 1922, when Eardley Holland came to publish his report on the slightly different subject of *The Causation of Foetal Death*, the proportion of deaths considered preventable still stood at the magic figure of around a half, but he located the causes of death much more decisively in the prenatal environment. Holland concluded that about 20 per cent of fetal deaths could be prevented by antenatal care alone; a further 12 per cent by 'combined antenatal and intranatal methods', and about 20 per cent by primarily intranatal methods (Ministry of Health, 1922).

Whereas the official reports on obstetric mortality over the period from 1917 to 1932 spoke with a united voice of the *avoidability* of death, and each in its own way spoke *to* the role of antenatal care in this, the 1920s and 1930s were not years in which the utterances of official medical/governmental reports were the only ones that could be heard. The pronouncements and conclusions of the official reports had, indeed, to be heard above a clamour of opinion, often dramatically phrased and frequently backed by appropriate political action, on the emotive subject of maternal mortality.

'A woman's issue'

The outrage of avoidable maternal death and its necessary solutions were topics on which an extremely wide range of voluntary organizations all felt qualified to comment — the Women's Co-operative Guild, the Women's Labour League, the National Council of Women, the People's League of Health, the Trades Union Congress the Fabian Women's Group and the National Union of Women's Suffrage Societies (NUWSS), all had opinions on the subject. Emmeline Pankhurst, working as a registrar of births and deaths in Manchester, was first inspired to militancy on the avoidable death issue by the many infant deaths from syphilis she had to register in her capacity as registrar. Apparently, in these cases, information on the cause of death came in sealed envelopes signalling a conspiracy between doctor and husband to prevent the woman knowing why her baby had died.

By taking up this issue as a women's cause, the early feminists colluded with the state to divest men of some of their patriarchal power over family life. 'Opening out' the family in this way, and welcoming the state in, was one means of diluting the traditional power of men to control women's lives. Another motive was the suffrage organizations' need to define their future political programme in view of the imminence of the vote and the general post-war gynaephobia. During the war these organizations had suspended their militancy for work which had embedded them firmly in the arena of maternal and child welfare. It was therefore a logical development that after the war the NUWSS should change its name to the National Union of Societies for Equal Citizenship, and under the appropriate presidency of Eleanor Rathbone, mother of the Family Allowance system, should outline a set of objectives that included all aspects of women's social function, especially motherhood. Even the militant Women's Social and Political Union changed its name to the Women's Party in 1917 and formulated a truly imperialist agenda which included medical care for mothers and children; funds left over from the militant feminist campaign were devoted to the suitably maternal act of purchasing and equipping a home for female children in London (Rosen, 1974; and see Lewis, 1975).

Although Mrs Pankhurst senior became a peripatetic lecturer on moral hygiene (another logical development), the valiant Christabel took to a new belief in the second coming of Christ. The other famous Pankhurst daughter, Sylvia, recalling the safety of her own son's birth and the traumatic stillbirth of the Pankhurst family servant Ellen, witnessed years earlier, wrote a book called *Save the Mothers* (1930). In this she remarked that the 'contemptuous neglect of the mother's needs and her all-important function' represented 'as grievous an injury to women as any they suffered in the dark period of their political and social subjection' (p. 46). What was needed, said Pankhurst, was a comprehensive 'national maternity service'. Central to this idea was antenatal care, and to this she devoted a chapter. But she was not only talking about medical care: what she envisaged for mothers was a broad programme of economic and social protection, including wages for mothers during pregnancy and for one year after childbirth, with a woman's job being kept open for her for the same length of time.

In 1927 an 'unofficial' maternal mortality committee had been formed at the instigation of May Tennant, an infant welfare campaigner and ex-Inspector of Factories, and Gertrude Tuckwell, a vigorous trade unionist, whose interest in maternal mortality developed when she was a member of the Royal Commission on National Health Insurance in the 1920s and was confronted with evidence of very high sickness rates among married women. The unofficial committee was a highly influential group, with representatives of all political persuasions, and from all the leading women's organizations. Much organizational involvement in maternal mortality issues was, however, on a local basis. Thus, in Manchester the case of Molly Taylor, a nineteen year-old woman who died within hours of giving birth to a son in the out-patient department of St Mary's Hospital in September 1934, achieved such notoriety in the hands of the local women's organizations that the local authority was forced to agree to a public inquiry. Molly Taylor had a problem-free first pregnancy; she paid her £2 voluntary subscription to St Mary's Hospital and attended for Hospital antenatal appointments. When she finally turned up at the hospital in labour, she was told by a doctor that her baby would not arrive for some time — but it started to do so on the hospital steps as she left. After the birth, and because there was no bed available in the hospital at the time, mother and baby were transferred to nearby Crumpsall Hospital, where Molly Taylor died early the following morning.

Manchester City Council eventually agreed to hold a public inquiry into Molly Taylor's death, and the last straw persuading them to do so was a petition with over 9,000 signatures gathered by local women's organizations. The Manchester Public Health Committee noted that about 200 people, mostly women, attended this enquiry 'and at intervals they either applauded or dissented from the answers given by witnesses. Although the conduct of the Enquiry was thus disturbed', continued the Committee philosophically, 'we considered it inadvisable to direct the removal from the room of persons who took part in the demonstrations, and so impair the public character of the proceedings' (Public Health Committee Minutes, Manchester, 31 October 1934).

Many issues were raised by the case, including the exclusive right to determine the shape of maternity care claimed by the hospital's medical staff: against this, the women of Manchester were not satisfied to delegate responsibility for their lives to what they saw as a self-interested medical profession. After the Molly Taylor inquiry (which was inconclusive) a maternal mortality committee was set up on the initiative of women from the local Communist Party. The aim of this committee was continuing surveillance of the maternity services in the area. An index of the widespread support it received from within the women's community was the fact that its 1938 conference, which gave rise to a comprehensive 'Mothers' Charter', was attended by women from over 60 local associations, including three trade unions and seven Conservative associations (Emanuel, 1982).

In identifying as a priority the issue of maternal health and survival, these women's organizations were making the point that the deaths of women in childbearing were the tip of the iceberg of women's health, and women's health was, by any civilized standard, poor in an age characterized, not only by depressed living conditions, but by no access to free medical care for working-class women.

The public debate about maternal mortality thus engendered another debate, the debate about maternal morbidity referred to in the quotation at the head of this chapter. Janet Campbell's reports drew attention to the disabling and uncounted sequelae of childbearing in women. W. Blair Bell, first president of the British College of Obstetricians and Gynaecologists, complained in 1931 that at least 60,000 women annually in England and Wales (10 per cent of all mothers) 'are more or less crippled as the result of childbearing' (p. 1171) — though he and other gynaecologists who attached a statistic to the complaint had to rely to some extent on guesswork, since they could not know the degree of morbidity among women who did not present themselves for medical care. Bell quoted a series of 2,275 women attending the gynaecology out-patient clinic of Liverpool's Royal Infirmary in which 34 per cent were found to have disabling lesions attributable to childbearing, and made reference to other studies showing rates of 40–70 per cent lesions due to childbearing (mostly trauma or infections) among women attending gynaecology out-patient clinics all over the country (Blair Bell, 1931).[2]

While it was important, therefore, to the nation that women survive the perils of childbearing in order to attend successfully to their existing children and have more, life rather than death — and a good quality of life, at that — was a fate energetically to be pursued on behalf of women themselves. This putative separation of women's interests from any of the various available conceptions of the national interest is evident in documents such as Margery Spring Rice's *Working Class Wives* (1939); or in the Women's Co-operative Guild's (WCG) *Maternity: letters from working women* (Davies, 1915), a book based on letters solicited by the WCG to substantiate their campaign for the improvement of maternal and child health care.

Maternity is one of the few sources of evidence we have available to us of how women in these years felt about motherhood. The women who

---

2. Maternal morbidity is still an issue today. For example, a recent study of women having babies in Berkshire revealed that three months after birth, 20 per cent of women were troubled with varying degrees of incontinence (Sleep, et al., 1983).

contributed to the book are, of course, the survivors, and the letters in which they record their experiences are remarkable for the absence of any reference to women's own fears (or statistical chances) of dying in pregnancy or childbirth. Allusions to maternal mortality are to be found in novels — death in childbirth was an important fictional means in the nineteenth century of portraying the victimization of women. But death, even the deaths of healthy young women, were in an important sense an accepted fact of life in the era before they had come so enticingly to be redefined as 'avoidable' by the medical profession.

The impression conveyed by the letters in *Maternity* is one of 'perpetual overwork, illness and suffering' (p. 3). Among the 348 women who gave information, the stillbirth and miscarriage rate was 215 per 1,000 live births, and the infant death-rate 87. As one writer, the mother of seven children and two miscarriages, on a weekly wage of 30s said: 'It is quite time this question of maternity was taken up and we must let the men know we are human beings' (*Maternity*, p. 68).

One manner in which 'this question of maternity' was taken up was in the creation of the Ministry of Health in 1919. Although there had been pressure for such a department before, the pressure had been almost entirely concerned with environmental reform — with sewers and drains rather than 'scientific' medicine, and doctors as a group had only been really interested when they had needed to strengthen their economic position. The new Ministry of Health immediately initiated a great deal of important work on maternal and child health, and it did not do so purely because this was the climate of the time; rather, it did so because its own creation represented a solution to the administrative problem of which national body should be responsible for this branch of the public health. Lloyd George may have reserved a place for maternal and child welfare in his 1914 Budget, but a dispute about which department should handle the grant was only settled when the Local Government Board and the Board of Education, the two main competing bodies (see the chart in figure 3.1), agreed to turn the whole matter over to a Ministry of Health as soon as one could be created. The Ministry of Health was, in this way, an administrative answer to the maternal and child welfare problem. It was also seen by women's organizations as the great hope for women's health, since it could finally resolve the conflict between a health service for women based on the insurance principle and one based on a freely provided municipal service (the alternative preferred by most such organizations). Pressure from women's groups was instrumental in getting the Bill for the new Ministry through Parliament on the eve of the 1918 Election, and though the women did

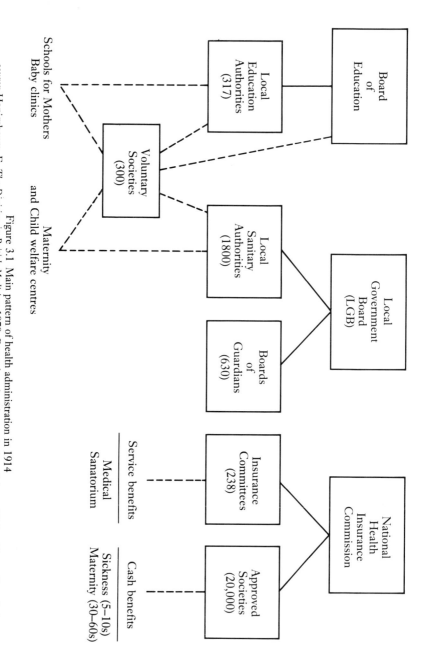

Figure 3.1 Main pattern of health administration in 1914

source: Honigsbaum, F. *The Division in British Medicine*, 1979. Reproduced with permission of the publisher Kogan Page Ltd.

not get their ultimate prize, a female Minister of Health, they did get Janet Campbell as Senior Medical Officer to the Maternity and Child Welfare section.

Janet Mary Campbell (1877–1954), later Dame Janet Campbell, was a remarkable woman. Born in Brighton, Sussex, the daughter of a banker, she graduated as a doctor in 1901 and entered the school medical service in its own infancy in 1905. Three years later she became the first whole-time woman medical officer at the Board of Education. She served on many committees, wrote many reports, and she took up many themes in women's health, from industrial medicine to liquor control, and from nursery education to the League of Nations. When she married the registrar of the General Medical Council in 1934 she was forced by the 'marriage bar' to leave the civil service. Thereafter she became a JP for Surrey, and attended the roses in her garden — at what a loss to the country's mothers and children no one will presumably ever know.

Apart from *Maternal Mortality* (1924), Janet Campbell wrote a report on *The Training of Midwives* (1923) and one, the same year, on *Obstetrics and Gynaecology Teaching*. These were followed by *The Protection of Motherhood* (1927), *Infant Mortality* (1929a) and (with Isabella Cameron and Dilys Jones) *High Maternal Mortality in Certain Areas* (1932). Campbell's work was influential in leading the Ministry to set up, in 1928, a Departmental Committee on Maternal Mortality and Morbidity. Campbell herself was a member of the Committee, chaired by George Newman. In its reports we can see an attempt to disentangle a profound argument which had developed between the providers of medical and midwifery care on the one hand, who, in the persona chiefly of the BMA, contended that the continuing high rate of maternal mortality was not due to poor clinical care, but to faults in the service-user and her environment, and, on the other hand, the lay organizations and a number of experts, including Janet Campbell, who argued that the crucial factor was, rather, the appallingly low standard of clinical care.

A unique commentary on the relevance to contemporary conditions of these two different interpretations is provided by the Rhondda experiments of the mid-1930s. The Rhondda area of Wales was one of the 'high mortality' blackspots, and the National Birthday Trust Fund in 1934 provided the money for a campaign to improve the situation. The campaign began by increasing the amount, and coverage, of specialist antenatal care in the area. Despite these changes, maternal mortality rose. In 1935, and the first six months of 1936, the tactic was changed to providing free food (2,910½ lbs of beef extract, 184 lbs of dried milk,

1,635¼ lbs of Marmite and 5,763 tins of Ovaltine) and the maternal death rate subsequently fell by more than a half (Rhys-Williams, 1936).

Blaming the victim?

In 1930 and 1932 two reports were published by the Departmental Committee on Maternal Mortality and Morbidity which expanded upon Janet Campbell's 1922 investigation of the causes of individual maternal deaths. A total of 4,655 deaths due to pregnancy and childbearing was reported, and a 'primary avoidable factor' located for almost half the deaths. Deficiencies in facilities, or judgements made by staff, were considered responsible for 50 per cent of the avoidable deaths, lack of antenatal care for 33 per cent, and negligence on the part of the patient for 17 per cent. Lack of antenatal care figured chiefly in deaths due to eclampsia (where it was implicated in 58 per cent of avoidable deaths), followed by shock (43 per cent) and sepsis contracted in cases of complicated labour (40 per cent). Negligence of the patient, on the other hand, was most implicated in deaths from embolism (42 per cent), other toxaemias (29 per cent) and postpartum haemorrhage (26 per cent).

The Committee also made suggestions for the improvement of the medical maternity services. Attention was drawn in both the 1930 and 1932 Reports to the need for all mothers to be cared for by registered midwives, for all to be examined antenatally and postnatally by doctors who would also be responsible for abnormal deliveries, and consultant referral where necessary. But if one single message emerged, it was that pregnant women were themselves deficient: they lacked the necessary intelligence, foresight, education or responsibility to see that the only proper pathway to successful motherhood was the one repeatedly surveyed by medical expertise. 'In the first place', said the 1930 Report (p. 92), 'it is necessary to draw attention to the responsibility of the expectant mother herself . . . a potent factor in maternal mortality is her neglect to make use of facilities already available.' This observation could scarcely be read into the statistics presented by the Committee, which did not show maternal neglect to be a 'potent' factor. 'In order to counteract this attitude', the Report nonetheless continued, 'it is necessary to educate the expectant mother, to provide free choice of doctor and midwife for her, and to devise a thorough and efficient system of following-up. It is felt that to ensure her co-operation it may also be found advisable to offer some financial inducement, e.g., to pay a portion of a cash maternity benefit in advance' (see pp. 272–3 on this repetitive formula of financial bribery). Yet, at the same time, not wanting to frighten women into anything beyond a simple medical care-seeking model of behaviour became an obsession among policy-makers in the 1930s. In 1935, the British Medical Association passed a resolution declaring that the publicity the topic of maternal mortality was receiving in the lay press caused terror to childbearing women — and even led to increased mortality (though the Association did not spell out the route whereby this effect was being achieved) (BMA, 1935, p. 245).

Good care and educational propaganda were the solutions recommended in the Departmental Committee's 1930 and 1932 Reports for a problem whose cause was assumed to lie in patient ignorance, and whose prime manifestation was the bogey of non-attendance. As the antenatal services developed, and as the claims made for their effectiveness expanded over the years, the spectre of non-attendance hovered with a deepening shadow over the visionary enthusiasm of the antenatalists. But the problem — so perceived — was there from the beginning. It could even be considered to be endemic to the process of imposing on women control of reproduction by means of a medical surveillance system:

[medical] supervision [during pregnancy] can only be effective when the mothers themselves appreciate the necessity of it and are prepared to make use of the facilities provided. Thus educating the mothers to look for antenatal care is no less important than securing opportunities for obtaining it (Ministry of Health, 1922, p. vii).

The problem to be solved is not to obtain theoretical assent to the value of ante-natal supervision . . . but to persuade the professional attendant to offer it and the patients to expect and welcome it . . . most women desire as little examination as possible and do not realize how great a safeguard it may be (Ministry of Health, 1927, p. 51).

There is still a large section of the population that does not realize the advantages of obtaining competent prenatal advice . . . The patient herself is often her own worst enemy, whether from ignorance or apathy, illhealth or prejudice, etc., and until she is able and willing to co-operate doctors' and nurses' attempts to assist her can never be fully effective (Departmental Committee, 1930, pp. 24–5, 39).

. . . many mothers who would benefit from existing facilities do not make full use of them (Royal Commission on Population, 1949, p. 198).
(See pp. 265–71 for the same theme in more recent reports.)

It was a simple knowledge–attitudes–practice model. Imparting the

knowledge would alter attitudes which would alter practice. But where
was the evidence that ignorance among mothers of the benefits of
medical care was the problem? Since antenatal care had not by the early
1930s reduced the rate at which mothers died in childbirth — and this
fact was well-publicized — a healthy scepticism on the part of potential
service-users was, perhaps, hardly remarkable. As Sylvia Pankhurst
sagely remarked in her *Save the Mothers*, since it was recognized by
government and medical professionals alike that antenatal care was not
yet as effective and efficient as everyone hoped, mothers could not be
expected to attend clinics in large numbers. If they did, they often met
the frustrating disincentive of waiting with young children for a long
time to be seen in uncomfortable conditions. (See chapter 11 for further
discussion of the 'maternal ignorance' issue.)

Although most emphasis (then and now) was placed on methods for
eradicating non-attendance, a few voices were heard in the 1930s
advising research into its causes. The Chief Medical Officer to the
Ministry of Health suggested in 1933 that in areas of low attendance the
responsible authority should 'examine the various causes which prevent
attendance and endeavour to locate and rectify the defects, whether in
personnel or conduct' (CMO, 1934, p. 76). It was also noted in some
quarters that, since non-attenders were more likely than attenders to be
poor, it was no use simply demanding that these women went to antenatal clinics. Attention geared to the individual woman's circumstances
needed to be 'paid to the social conditions and to the possible need for
nourishment, rest or domestic assistance during pregnancy as well as at
the time of confinement' (p. 36). But despite these qualifications, the
firm and unmistakable message was that, could the women only be got to
the clinics, antenatal care would be their one true salvation.

Working mothers

Those who denied the significance of poor medical care in maintaining
high levels of mortality and morbidity may have blamed social conditions. But what exactly was the contribution of social conditions to
mortality and morbidity? Given the anti-feminism of the 1920s, and the
economic recession of the 1930s, it is not surprising that in the attempt
to disentangle the influences of different social conditions, the evils
of women's employment should have received a great deal of attention. Many service-providers and policy-makers recommended the

abolition of women's paid work outside the home, but this was very often in contradiction to the statistical picture emerging from the analysis of obstetric deaths. Referring to the Reports of the Health of Munition Workers Committee, Janet Campbell noted in her 1924 *Maternal Mortality* Report that the evidence as to the effect of women's war work on maternity was that it was beneficial rather than harmful. The Medical Research Committee reporting on infant mortality in 1917 came to a similar conclusion — that industrial employment was not a direct cause of infant mortality or of low birthweight, and what had to be borne in mind was the heavy agricultural work traditionally carried out by women in areas with low mortality.

Campbell subdivided the potential effects of women's employment into direct and indirect. The indirect effects were the long-term ones adversely affecting the nutrition and development of girls, so as to render them biologically inefficient mothers in their turn. The direct effects, mainly those of heavy work, were compounded by discrimination against women which led them to be concentrated in 'the rougher kinds of factory work, charring, and relatively unskilled work, or worse still . . . some form of ill-paid home work . . . It is the women who work because they must, and who cannot always choose their occupations, who are most liable to suffer' p. 37.

In her later report on *The Protection of Motherhood*, Campbell made no bones about the fact that 'Outside employment is often less arduous than much of the household work ordinarily done by the mother of a family, and relief when necessary from heavy housework seems of greater practical importance than the restriction of paid employment' (Ministry of Health, 1927, p. 6).

The importance of looking elsewhere

The most persuasive evidence for the importance of social conditions came not from broad surveys of these in relation to maternal or infant survival, but from observation of striking regional and international differences in mortality rates. The 'league table' approach to evaluating birth and death had been important, as we saw in chapter 2, in the genesis of the early infant welfare movement. As the movement developed, and as antenatal care became one of its main canons, the comparison of the British record with that obtaining in other countries remained extremely important, and was indeed, purveyed with increasing

Table 3.1 Maternal mortality rate* 1911–13, selected countries

Scotland	5.70	Germany	3.48
Spain	5.27	Norway	2.90
Switzerland	5.21	Italy	2.44
France	4.78	Sweden	2.42
England and Wales	3.94	Holland	2.29

*per 1,000 live births
source: Ministry of Health, 1924, p.11

sophistication.[3] Campbell published a table of this type (Table 3.1) in her 1924 report (with appropriate reservations about the comparability of different statistical systems). So alluring had the low rates of obstetric mortality quoted for certain European countries become by the time of the Committee's Final Report in 1932, that a special delegation of experts was sent to Holland, Denmark and Sweden to investigate the truth behind these countries' enviable records.

The delegates saw large differences between England and Wales, on the one hand, and the three comparison countries on the other, which they thought had to be relevant to the discrepancies in death-rates. For a start, there were many smoke-polluted slums and much overcrowding in England's urban areas, but these problems did not exist in Holland, Denmark and Sweden. Diet in the comparison countries was also deemed superior, especially in terms of the consumption of milk by adolescent girls, producing a low incidence of pelvic deformity. Midwifery was said to be much better and earlier organized than in England and Wales; no general displacement of the midwife by the doctor as the supervisor of normal reproduction had occurred, and midwives enjoyed a higher professional status and an advanced standard of training. Most impressive was the fact that in Holland there existed groups of women who were trained as maternity nurses, as assistants to the midwife (whereas in England and Wales midwives were already in danger of becoming mere handmaidens to obstetricians). In all three countries the generally good health and development of the population was considered to be a basic cause of low mortality. The members of the delegation grew quite lyrical when describing the quality of the population in the countries visited. In Sweden, for example:

3. The question as to which countries are represented on such a table is, of course, important, and crucially affects the lessons capable of being drawn from the statistics. See Kerr, 1980.

The developing girls ride to their work on bicycles instead of in crowded buses and tubes, and after their day's work they resort to the parks, which even the smallest towns possess where they can listen to the orchestra and take a meal at the open air restaurant. The population is largely of the Nordic type, their bronzed faces, flaxen hair, and generally healthful appearance being in marked contrast to the sallow complexions and stunted growth which are only too common in our large industrial centres. Temperamentally the women are placid and self-controlled, and appear mentally as well as physically fit for childbearing (Department Committee, 1932, p. 76).

The British experts who examined other countries' maternity services for lessons applicable to Britain during this period were, doubtless, correct in drawing attention to the differing social conditions lying behind the different mortality figures. The low infant mortality rate in Norway, for example, was associated with a low level of urbanization, and, until 1940, infant mortality remained lower in the country than in the towns. Until the mid-1920s, at least, the efforts of Norwegian maternity care reformers were focused first on better living standards and conditions, and, second, on maternal education. Clinical antenatal care does not begin to predominate as an answer in Norway until the late 1920s; and, when it does, it is perhaps surprising to learn that Norwegian antenatalists were looking to England as their model for what should be done to 'control' mothers in pregnancy. The early birth control activists in Norway were also transplanting English ideas, and the first Norwegian birth control clinics were replicas of Marie Stopes's clinic in London (Blom, 1980).

The parallel observation to international differences — that mortality rates could exhibit gross differences by region *within* countries — provided a further route to the unravelling of the 'influence of social conditions' argument. William Farr had noted in 1885 that within Britain, there were healthy districts and unhealthy districts and 'mortality increases as the density of the population, or the nearness of the people to each other', or 'great cities are the graves of mankind' (pp. 147, 153).

Regional variations in maternal mortality were the subject of a special report, written by Janet Campbell and her collaborators in 1932. In the years 1923–29 there were three main areas located in the West Riding of Yorkshire, Lancashire and Wales, where the maternal death rate had been especially high at over 5 per 1,000 births. The excess of deaths was not attributable to a higher rate of puerperal sepsis, but to other complications of childbirth, and the high maternal mortality was accompanied by higher than average rates of stillbirth and neonatal deaths, indicating a concentration of reproductive problems in these areas. Poverty and unemployment, with the nutritional deficiencies probably associated with these conditions, were identified as the major culprits: attempted abortion was also singled out for its injurious prevalence among working-class married women, and freely available birth control instruction proposed as the remedy — a most radical suggestion for a Ministry of Health Report at the time.

Of the towns listed in the 1932 Report, Rochdale in Lancashire had the highest rate — 8.33 maternal deaths per 1,000 live births in 1925–29 (Oxley, et al., 1935).[4] In the 1930s, Rochdale was the focus of an experimental scheme designed to improve the mortality record, which was to serve as a model for others to come. In 1930 the newly-appointed Medical Officer of Health, a Dr Andrew Topping, instituted a propaganda campaign with the principal aim of telling women to use antenatal clinics. The apparent result was a fall in the maternal death-rate from 8.9 in 1929–31, to 2.99 in 1932–34 (Topping, 1936). Commenting on this apparent miracle, in the *British Medical Journal* (1935), obstetricians Oxley, Phillips and Young attributed the improvement in the later period to less fatal obstetric intervention, which was in turn due to the earlier hospital admission of women with complications of pregnancy and labour. They felt (an opinion which was not echoed especially strongly by outsiders who enthused about the Rochdale Scheme) that a raised standard of medical and midwifery practice had been the chief result of the propaganda campaign — they could not say with any certainty either that there had been widespread adoption of antenatal care by Rochdale mothers, or that this factor was of any importance in preventing death.

The message that environmental factors were important causes of maternal and other obstetric mortalities was not popular at the Ministry of Health. But neither was the Ministry especially keen to develop the argument that the low standard of clinical care was at fault. Behind both attitudes was the Ministry's inborn structural weakness — it lacked coercive powers over either the local authorities or over the medical profession — and its shortage of funds: the demand for maternal mortality to be decreased by almost any means had to struggle with the 1920s tightening up of expenditure on the public services (Palmer n.d.). The identification of women themselves as blameworthy — for being

---

4. Rochdale's early sinister significance in this field has been maintained until today. The media debate about perinatal mortality in the late 1970s and early 1980s tended to single out Rochdale as a 'black area'.

insufficiently enthusiastic antenatalists — neatly let both government and the medical profession off the hook, and was, in that sense, a convenient and understandable ideological response. The stress on the need for health education was prominent in official policy by the early 1920s — in 1925 the Public Health Act included a clause enabling local authorities to provide more in the way of health education.

A minimum standard

If women were to be educated to seek antenatal care it was necessary to secure consistency in the standard of antenatal care available throughout the country. One of the first tasks of the Departmental Committee on Maternal Mortality and Morbidity was to issue a Memorandum on minimum standards in antenatal care: 'Ante-natal Clinics: Their Conduct and Scope' (Ministry of Health, 1929, reprinted Departmental Committee, 1930). This is the Magna Carta of antenatal care: it laid down standards from which the practice of antenatal care, even in the 1980s, is directly derived.

The 'principles' of antenatal care as laid down in the Memorandum were:

(1) to predict 'difficult labour' from examination in pregnancy;
(2) to detect and treat toxaemia;
(3) to diagnose/treat/prevent infection (e.g. dental, cervical);
(4) to diagnose and treat VD;
(5) to ensure 'the closest co-operation' between the clinic and all persons in charge of pregnancy care;
(6) to recognize 'the educational effect of a well-organized clinic' (p. 140).

The ideal patient would attend first when 16 weeks pregnant, have a full medical and obstetric history taken, and 'if she is prepared' a physical examination including urinanalysis, blood pressure and external pelvic measurements (vaginal examinations being left to the Medical Officer's discretion). After this, the nurse should enquire into the patient's home conditions and advise her on hygiene, visiting the home if necessary. Following the first visit, said the Memorandum,

routine examinations should take place either at the clinic or the patient's home as follows: At the 24th and 28th weeks, from then every fortnight until the 36th week, and thence weekly until she is confined. The uterine height and girth should be taken, the foetal heart listened for, the urine tested, and general enquiries should be made, with special regard to the action of the excretory organs. The midwife should be able to do this examination in most cases at the patient's home, but any abnormality, however slight, must be brought to the notice of the Medical Officer of the clinic.

In place of, or supplementing, the routine examinations, special examinations should be made by the Medical Officer at the 32nd and 36th weeks. These will be directed mainly to ascertaining the presentation of the foetus, and the relation of head to pelvis.

It is advisable that, where possible, the blood pressure should be examined weekly during the last month, as a rise of pressure may be the first sign of a commencing toxaemia.

It is important that the expected date of confinement should be ascertained early in pregnancy, and be confirmed from time to time, and any patient going beyond the 40th week should be referred to the Medical Officer (Departmental Committee, 1930, pp. 142–3).

No justification was offered in the Memorandum for adoption of these particular guidelines, which were, it seems, derived from an *ad hoc* survey of antenatal care as practised by a number of public health departments at the time.

It was clear to the Departmental Committee, as it was to everyone else, that, even according to this somewhat arbitrary minimum standard, most British women in the late 1920s and early 1930s were escaping the antenatal care net. The *British Medical Journal* calculated the proportion of women attending for antenatal care per 100 births as 33.89 per cent in 1931, and 38.89 per cent in 1932 (*British Medical Journal*, 7 December 1935, p. 246). The growth in antenatal care is charted in Figures A.8–A.10 in Appendix I, and the gap in the 1930s between total births and use of municipal and voluntary antenatal clinic care can be clearly seen in figure A.9 (p. 303). As to the doctors who worked in maternity and child welfare, 'little credit and less cash' was the epithet attached to their seemingly unenviable status by the early 1930s. According to Davies's survey, the field was held about equally by men and by women. But the fact that maternity and child welfare work offered non-career posts made it specially attractive to married women doctors, thus slotting it in to an emerging sexual division of labour in medicine (Davies, n.d.).

Little could be assumed from the plain fact of attendance for antenatal care. Of the 18,828 women delivered at home by the district service of the Glasgow Royal Maternity Hospital in 1926–30, Kerr and MacLennan found that antenatal care had been limited to 27 per cent of the women, and, of these, 'only 10–15 per cent attended the antenatal clinic regularly' (Kerr and MacLennan, 1932, p. 177).

Among patients attending Glasgow Corporation antenatal clinics in 1929, most diagnoses were of the obstetrically unexciting diseases of poverty — carious teeth, 'alimentary' conditions, general debility: these accounted for half of all detected medical conditions (Report of the Medical Officer of Health for Glasgow for 1930). Writing of habits at University College Hospital in the mid-1920s, Norman White, at the time Outdoor Obstetric Assistant to the hospital, said there was only one antenatal clinic a week there, blood pressure was never taken and the patient's urine examined only once. A woman who had already had one baby without complications was not examined at all (Merrington, 1976). At St Mary's Hospital Manchester, during the same period, about 35 per cent of women attended at delivery by the hospital staff had received some antenatal care, but this did not start until the third trimester of pregnancy.

Dr Edgar Hope-Simpson who practised as a GP in Dorset in the 1930s recalls:

We were very lucky if we got them — they'd come if they weren't well, then we'd keep an eye on them until they'd had their baby. But there was nothing routine about it. We had a District Nurse, of course, but she didn't do much antenatally. When we got them we did blood pressure and urine for albumen and sugar . . . We had no feeling that we could do them very much good if we did get them early. Except for high blood pressure, that sort of thing, but even then, eclampsia, we'd been taught, came out of the blue. No, I think we had very little idea about what was likely to cause trouble except for the position of the baby (E. H. S. I).

Similar observations were made by Dr John Sturrock, who qualified in 1923. He remembered the practice of antenatal care at the Edinburgh Royal Maternity Hospital in the late 1920s:

There were four clinics on Monday, Tuesday, Thursday and Friday afternoons, and the women came up: you saw them initially and then it depended — in the middle trimester you would probably miss a month . . . They came at the 36th and then 38 weeks and these last two ones were particularly important, to see that the head would go in, and it wasn't too big . . . You wanted them to come as early as possible. Miss two periods and then come. But of course a great many just didn't (J. S. I).

Figure 3.2 shows the layout of the Edinburgh clinic at the time, and signals an important architectural and ideological link between the control of pregnancy and the control of venereal disease. Figure 3.3 reproduces the form used to record the patient's condition in the same clinic. On the other side of this sheet (not shown here) fifteen spaces were allowed for recording antenatal signs, though this must have been

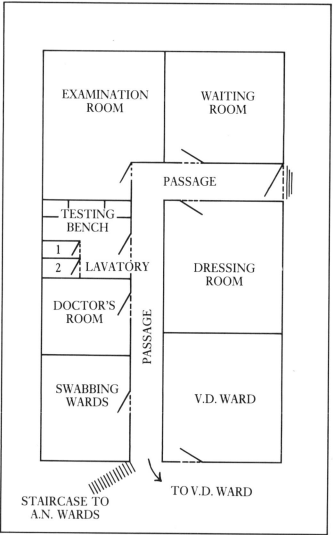

Figure 3.2 Plan of Ante-Natal Department Edinburgh Royal Maternity and Simpson Memorial Hospital, 1929

source: Haultain, W.F.T. and Chalmers Fahmy, E. *Antenatal Care: a practical handbook of antenatal care and the abnormalities associated with pregnancy*, 1929. E. & S. Livingstone. With permission of the publisher.

Recommended by Dr.………………

D.K.* No.

EDINBURGH ROYAL MATERNITY AND SIMPSON MEMORIAL HOSPITAL
ANTE-NATAL CLINIC

No.   Date

Name   M. S. or W.   Age   Ext. Version.………………

Address   †Pads.………………

GENERAL HEALTH

In Childhood

In Adult Life

General Notes on Health of Husband, Father and Mother; Family History as to Deformities, Twin-Bearing, Serious Illness, Etc.

HISTORY OF PREVIOUS PREGNANCIES, LABOURS, ETC.

Date of Birth Month and Year	Sex M.	Sex F.	Born Alive	Still-born	Miscar-riage	Duration of Pregnancy	ABNORMALITIES DURING PREGNANCY AND LABOUR	NATURE OF Spon.	NATURE OF Inst.	State of Health	CHILDREN Weight at Birth	CHILDREN Cause of and Age at Death
1.												
2.												
3.												
4.												
5.												
6.												

PRESENT CONDITION

PRESENT PREGNANCY: Date of Last Period

ARRANGEMENTS FOR CONFINEMENT: Own Home.   Hospital   Expected Date of Delivery

WASSERMANN: Date   Result

(1) SYMPTOMS: Pain.—

Discharge.—Red, Yellow, White. Micturition.—Frequent, Painful, Difficult, Impossible. Vomiting.—Duration

Digestion.—Heartburn, Constipation, Diarrhœa. Other Symptoms.—Headache, Blurred Vission, Twitchings, etc.

(2) PHYSICAL SIGNS:

General Conditions, as to Anæmia, Deformity, (Edema, etc …………………

Breasts and Nipples ……………………………………………

Heart ……………………………………………

Lungs ……………………………………………

Teeth ……………………………………………

(3) SPECIAL ADVICE OR TREATMENT: ……………………………………………

…………………………………………………………

…………………………………………………………

* D.K. refers to veneral cases.   † Refers to pads for Occipito-posterio cases.

Figure 3.3 Antenatal Clinic Record Card in use in Edinburgh Royal Maternity and Simpson Memorial Hospital in 1920s
source: Haultain and Fahmy, 1929, p. 7 with permission of the publisher.

more hopeful than practical. The patient was not weighed, and no space was provided for recording fundal height, the presence or absence of fetal heart sounds, movements, position or presentation.

Antenatal care, where it existed, took place in circumstances both primitive and sophisticated compared with the previous century. Some of the ecological limitations of maternity work included the fact that hospitals in the 1930s were still heated by means of coal fires, creating a lot of dust and work. Miss G. Humphreys, a midwife who qualified in the 1920s and did her midwifery at the General Lying-In Hospital in York Road, London, remembers having to walk up and down all the hospital stairs instead of using the lifts, which were reserved for the doctors and for the men who took the coal up to the wards. The hospital was divided into three districts and each district had a house where all the 'antenatals' were done. Antenatal care began at four or five months and consisted chiefly of advice plus urinanalysis — blood pressure was not taken unless there were adverse symptoms. The district midwifery staff did two visits to the homes 'which were poor, to see that they had a good pile of newspaper and a handywoman and a runner'. The handy-woman's job was to look after the woman and her other children after the birth. A 'runner' was the person who had to run to the nearest district house, or to the hospital, when the woman was in labour to fetch the midwife and carry one of the midwife's bags back to the house. The midwives went out with two bags:

And you were told, when you get there keep your hat on your head, roll your overcoat up as tight as you can and put it on some article of furniture away from the wall. The homes were all full of bugs and fleas. I remember bathing a baby on the district once and there were two plops and a voice from the bed said 'what is it nurse? Is it a mahogany flat or is it a blackhead?' Blackheads were fleas and mahogany flats were bugs (G. H. I).

Yet the times were changing, clinically if not socially. Dr G. F. Gibberd, a registrar at Guy's Hospital in London, published in 1929 a comparison of midwifery at Guy's in 1928 and 1870. He included some statistics on what he called obstetric interference, showing that the increased use of forceps delivery, caesarean section and instrumental induction of labour had raised the obstetric interference rate at the hospital from 1.35 per cent in 1863–75, to 8.86 per cent in 1928. Maternal mortality had apparently fallen considerably between these years, 'but it does not follow', cautioned Gibberd, 'that by doubling the present interference rate we should again halve the mortality rate. *We must find the amount of interference that will give the minimum mortality'* (Gibberd, 1929a, p. 536).

Proving the value of antenatal care in the more specific sense of effecting a drop in maternal mortality was, as we shall see in the next chapter, fast becoming an epidemiological exercise in which clinicians were forced to engage whether they liked it or not. And finding the degree of interference in pregnancy, labour and delivery that yielded the minimum mortality was, not coincidentally, emerging at the same time as the priority of the new obstetrics.

4

No Magic Answer: antenatal care 1932–39

Supervision at an antenatal clinic will not by itself save life.
Lancet, 24 November, 1934, p. 379

In the second decade of the twentieth century, antenatal care had been hailed almost as a universal panacea, the cure for all reproductive ills. Twenty years after the founding of the first antenatal clinic a more cautious, even cynical, attitude had set in. What had antenatal care achieved? Why had so much been hoped for, and so little apparently gained, from its practice? Was antenatal care simply not the magic answer it had been held out to be?

Disillusionment in difficult times

Throughout the 1920s and 1930s the overarching aim of maternity care, as we have seen, was to preserve the life of the mother. The influence on clinical practice of this struggle to reduce the risks of childbearing for women was still profound at the end of the 1930s, as Professor James Walker of Dundee recalls:

> I remember delivering a woman of a baby in the middle of the night and getting a baby with a broken collar bone, a breech. And the next morning my chief said to me, 'I hear you did a breech in the middle of the night, how is the mother?' I said, 'she's fine.' *Two hours later* he said 'oh, by the way, how did the baby do in that case?' (J. W. I)

This was the era before perinatal mortality, when babies did not count the way they do today. The primary aim was to get the mother safely through childbirth. Yet this was the very objective which had not been achieved after nearly one generation of antenatal care. In his preface to Janet Campbell's *The Protection of Motherhood* (1927), George Newman called the situation 'obscure and perplexing'. By 1934, the medical profession was prepared to admit to the perplexity of the situation more publicly, and in that year the *British Medical Journal* carried a series of contributions under the general heading, 'Are we satisfied with the results of antenatal care?' Professor F. J. Browne of University College Hospital in London who, the following year was to publish the first edition of his famous and long-lasting *Antenatal and Postnatal Care*, launched in with an examination of how antenatal care had fared in relation to trends in the various obstetric mortalities. The stillbirth rate appeared to have risen slightly between 1927 and 1932, but then notification had only been in progress since 1927. Infant mortality was falling, but neonatal mortality, which was chiefly due to 'prematurity, malformation, and obstetrical injuries' was not. As to maternal mortality, Browne thought he detected a fall in deaths from eclampsia from 1930, 'Yet, considering that eclampsia is almost entirely a preventable disease, the incidence and death rate are still far too high' (Browne, 1934, p. 195). Browne's comments are reflected in figures A.2–A.4 (pp. 296–298).

All in all, there was certainly no room for complacency, and a concerted effort was needed to find the reasons for the comparative failure of antenatal care. Browne himself identified three sets of reasons: (1) an increase in first births as a proportion of total births; (2) a higher level of intervention in labour and delivery; and (3) the inadequacy and ineffectiveness of much antenatal care. His observations on standards of antenatal care were that, although some 80 per cent of expectant mothers were by now receiving antenatal care (about half in municipal clinics), the quality of care left much to be desired. 'Examinations are too infrequent, perfunctory and unskilled to accomplish anything useful' (p. 96). Municipal clinics could not offer treatment. Many GPs were uninterested in antenatal work. More consultant care was needed. On intervention, Browne observed that antenatal care could sometimes simply transfer mortality from one column to another: from fetal death due to obstructed labour, for example, to maternal death due to caesarean section. Ammunition for this point of view was supplied by Mr A. J. Wrigley of Guy's Hospital in London, who analysed the induction of labour statistics for five hospitals in 1934, and showed that in about half of all cases, induction of labour was carried out for a mistaken diagnosis of disproportion. 'It is suggested', wrote Wrigley, 'that ... antenatal supervision, in its anxiety to find a possible abnormality, has tended to overlook the extreme difficulty of its diagnosis and to underrate the consequences of treatment. We must ask ourselves the question "Need we induce?" not "Can we induce?" ' (p. 89).

Wrigley was impressed, too, by the enormous variation between hospitals in obstetric intervention rates. In four London hospitals, for example, the induction rate was 14 times higher in the highest-induction-rate- as compared with the lowest-induction-rate-hospital. The caesarean section rate went from zero to nearly one per 100 deliveries. Nobody seemed to know why the intervention rate varied so much, or was rising so rapidly, but it clearly had something to do with the increased medical surveillance of pregnancy, and with the battle that was being fought between the different professional groups interested in acquiring control over obstetric care. For example, and as Eardley Holland observed in 1935, many new hospitals were being built giving local GPs for the first time the opportunity to do obstetric operations.

The career of a medical innovation

At the end of the First World War, clinicians and health administrators had fastened on to the rising star of antenatal care as the light that would banish the darkness from a vast realm of death and disease. This was what John McKinlay has described as Stage 2 in the career of a medical innovation, namely its 'adoption by powerful interest groups ... professional associations, institutional structures and other resources' (McKinlay, 1981, p. 381). Stage 2 is followed by Stage 3, in which the innovation receives widespread public acceptance, indeed comes to be 'demanded' by the public, and Stage 4, in which the innovation achieves the status of becoming a standard procedure. However, since the procedure has not been subject to formal evaluation, there comes a time when doubts are raised as to its effectiveness. Eventually, often after more than a decade, 'an erosion of support begins to set in. The enthusiastic claims made for the innovation during its earlier stages are modified somewhat; it is not as universally applicable as once thought; it is useful only for certain groups of the population, or particular types of or stages in an illness' (McKinlay, 1981, p. 399).

The reasons why medical innovations enjoy such chequered careers are complex, but the pattern is a remarkably standard one across many specialisms, and many types of innovation. Thus it was with antenatal care — both as an overall screening programme, and as regards its component procedures (see chapters 7 and 8). The unbounded enthusiasm of the 1920s gave way to a more cautious approach in the 1930s. Few yet espoused the methodology of randomized controlled trials, so no one was very likely to propose evaluation of antenatal care on the basis of its random allocation to half the childbearing population.[1] Instead, doctors began to engage in a process of supposing that antenatal care just might have hazards as well as benefits. They inspected the field of all avoidable death and injury to see exactly which deaths and injuries were liable to be avoided by the judicious examination of the pregnant woman before the great unknown of labour.

The *Lancet* in a leader on 'The Risks of Childbirth' (13 August 1932) referred to Gibberd's analysis (see pp. 84–5) which had shown half of all sepsis deaths to follow normal labour. The very substantial contribution this group of deaths made to total maternal mortality could not reasonably be expected to be eliminated by antenatal care. The wearing of rubber gloves by those who deliver babies would be more likely to do that (though the *Lancet* thought the time was not ripe to insist on this outlandish measure). The point was well made by the author of a letter to the *Lancet* (29 December 1934) from an F. Neon Reynolds who contended that a precise proportion — 80 per cent — of maternal deaths were due to conditions (sepsis, haemorrhage, shock) not detectable antenatally. Citing the much lower mortality record of midwives, Reynolds declared that this was because they were not allowed to do anything. A *Lancet* editorial the same year took the view that an undiminished maternal mortality rate was not perhaps such a disgrace, given the fall in living standards of the late 1920s and early 1930s. Poverty was the most potent influence counteracting the benefit of antenatal care. 'It would be possible to argue that in view of the hard times we have come through, a maternal mortality rate which has not risen seriously is an achievement, some of the credit for which is due to antenatal work . . . *Supervision at an antenatal clinic will not by itself save life*' (*Lancet*, 24 November 1934, p. 379; italics added).

'A woman with human needs'

At another of the many conferences held that year on the same topic, this time under the auspices of the Association of Maternity and Child Welfare Centres, Dr Letitia Fairfield from the London County Council's Public Assistance Department, said the same thing in a different way. She drew attention to the misleading nature of the mechanical

---

1. Such an evaluation has since been proposed a number of times, but it has not yet been carried out.

model of women as reproducers that, with antenatalism, had crept insidiously into medical thinking:

> We need to get our antenatal work into focus, remembering that the process of childbirth is a continuous one . . . Antenatal care is an essential part of obstetrics, not a specialized stunt by itself, and the expectant mother is not an ambulant pelvis, but a woman with human needs, whose soul and body are closely interlocked . . . let us not forget the mother' (*Lancet*, 7 July 1934, p. 1198).

No, indeed not. The investigation carried out by the Women's Health Enquiry Committee and reported in Margery Spring Rice's *Working Class Wives* (1939), strongly suggested that the majority of British women experienced a pronounced drop in their standard of living when they became mothers. Of the 1,250 women who gave information in the investigation, an outstanding 31 per cent said 'no' or 'never' to the question 'Do you usually feel fit and well?' Nearly half the women were in poor or very bad health, and on average they had more pregnancies than women in apparently good or indifferent health, and were more likely to have a very low income. *Working Class Wives* produced statistics showing a linear relationship between income and the proportion of women in very bad health: 46 per cent of the lowest income group reported very bad health, as compared to 17 per cent in the highest income group.

Although it might have been thought that the nutritional supplementation policies of municipal authorities would, by the 1930s, have had some impact on the health of the poorest mothers, there were many practical problems with administering these policies. The women had to prove sufficient poverty, which was expensive in time and energy, if not shoe leather, and created a sense of stigma — not just in relation to the free milk, but also in relation to the antenatal clinics where eligibility for milk had to be proved. Moreover, different boroughs operated different income cut-off points, some simply did not have enough milk depots, and no one could be quite sure *who* in the family was actually drinking the milk or swallowing the supplemental vitamins or other food.

The picture in *Working Class Wives* is one of an unrelieved struggle to maintain a minimum standard of living, a struggle in which the remedial effects of medical care were an enormous irrelevance — even supposing medical care were an attainable end. Only 13 of the 1,250 women were insured under the National Insurance scheme through having a paid job. The rest had to pay for medical care, either directly or through a private insurance scheme, except during pregnancy when they were entitled to some free care. Only 8 per cent said they had used an antenatal clinic. Many women were sceptical about medical remedies — being told to rest or go into hospital for a costly operation when you had eight children to look after were impressively useless suggestions.

Moreover, 'A doctor cannot get employment for the husband, and unemployment is put down over and over again as the real cause of the wife's illness' (Spring Rice, 1939, p. 90). Unemployment in 1933 stood at 22 per cent. The move from productive to service industries charac-teristic of mid-industrial development created a new poor of jobless skilled people to stand beside the old poor, consisting of casual or unskilled labourers. Average earnings for men in 1938 were from 60 shillings to 70 shillings per week, for women 32–3 shillings (Cole and Postgate, 1961, p. 644). Seebohm Rowntree, in a revamped version of his book *The Human Needs of Labour* (1937) calculated the minimum budget for a three-child family as 53 shillings, and of a single woman living alone as 30 shillings 9 pence, a level that meant between one in ten and one in three of the working population fell below the so-called 'poverty line'. In 1936, Sir John Orr estimated that about half the British population was too poor to buy an adequate diet, and that up to a third suffered from serious dietary deficiencies.

In the second half of the decade abortion was also to become a prominent public health issue. The Women's Co-operative Guild pas-sed a resolution to legalize abortion in 1934, in 1936 the Abortion Law Reform Association was founded, and in 1935 a committee on abortion set up by the BMA recommended legalizing abortion in cases of rape or danger to the physical and mental health of the mother. Abortion was a significant cause of maternal death — 13 per cent of the maternal deaths occurring in 1934 were abortion deaths, mostly in married women and mostly following septic infection: indeed, more than a quarter of total maternal deaths from sepsis were sequelae of abortion.

In its 1937 *Report on an Investigation into Maternal Mortality* (which analysed by local inquiry all maternal deaths occurring in 1934) the Ministry of Health suspected the abortion rate of being a potent influ-ence on the mortality rate in any district. It observed that the rate of detected criminal abortion had nearly doubled between 1911–20 and 1930–33. There was little doubt that induced abortion was on the increase, and that many hundreds of British women died annually from their own attempts thus to prevent birth.

The 1937 Report was the last of a long line of broad national surveys, thereafter to be replaced by the more limited and discrete Confidential Enquiries into Maternal Deaths. Its difference from the earlier maternal mortality reports lay in the empirical nature of the investigation — six medical officers visiting those areas with an unusually high death rate, and enquiring both into the circumstances of each death and into the 'social, sanitary and economic factors of the district' by interviewing relevant individuals, including representatives of women's organizations and the local HM Inspector of Factories. Lacking Janet Campbell's expertise, the authors of the Report carried out an arid analysis of puerperal mortality in relation to occupation; showing a closer association with textile than with personal service work, they were mystified as to why the mortality rates in Liverpool, Bootle and Barrow on the one hand, and Blackpool and Southport on the other, should be so different. There was 'concurrent deviation' of unemployment and puerperal mortality rates, however. Overcrowding was not related. But climate was, to such an extent that when the Ministry showed a meteorologist a map of puerperal mortality in England and Wales he thought at first it was a map of the rainfall. (In fact, modern data do show some relationship between weather conditions and eclampsia as a possible cause of maternal deaths ('Weather and Eclampsia', leading article, *British Medical Journal* 12 April 1975, pp. 53–4).)

In its Report, the Ministry also saw fit to name some of the more diffuse characteristics of the age that must be relevant to women's reproductive function, though in some cases the connection could only be regarded as obscure:

> The sensationalism of the popular press, the emotional stimulus of the films, the never-ceasing impact of the radio, the speed of machines in factories and of the traffic in the streets, to which the physical reactions of men and women must be adjusted in this mechanical age, inevitably give rise to increased nervous tension. The fashion of 'slimming' and the habit of cigarette-smoking on the part of women are also features of the present age . . .
>
> The increased sensibility to pain and discomfort has led to the movement to secure for women of all classes the relief from pain in childbirth which was formerly accepted as part of the course of nature.
>
> Since the Great War there has been a loosening of the conventions which formerly governed the relations of the sexes . . . (Ministry of Health, 1937, p. 117).

A fair trial?

One of the three factors listed by F. J. Browne as responsible for the apparent failure of antenatal care to provide the magic answer was that it had not been given a 'fair trial'. There were three possible sources of error: (1) an insufficient proportion of the pregnant population attending for antenatal care; (2) not enough antenatal visits; (3) an inadequate standard of care.

The figures given for mothers attending municipal antenatal clinics in 1935 (288,000 mothers visiting 1596 clinics) represented nearly half the total number of births (CMO, 1937). During the 1930s, this figure had almost doubled, though there was great variation between different areas: some 73 per cent of mothers in London went to municipal antenatal clinics for example, but in the English counties only 17 per cent did so (PEP, 1937; see also Appendix I). No figures were available (except in the case of maternal deaths) for the proportion of women receiving private antenatal care. However, many local authorities, especially in rural areas, had, by this date, made arrangements to pay private practitioners for the antenatal care of women who could not afford it: in 1935, 8,866 mothers received antenatal care from private GPs under this arrangement (CMO, 1937).

Little can be deduced from these bare statistics of antenatal attendance. The average number of antenatal visits per woman was not known; G. F. McCleary (1935) reckoned it to be between three and six, but the *Lancet* (18 August 1934, p. 364) thought it more likely to be one or two. There is some evidence that many medical professionals of the time did not consider more than one or two visits necessary. The three antenatal examinations laid down in the 1937 Maternity Services (Scotland) Act, for example, were considered the *optimum* by many doctors (Baird, 1960).

What was done at these visits? The recommended equipment for an antenatal examining room in 1935 included a pelvimeter, stethescopes, a steel rule, a tape measure, a baumanometer for measuring blood pressure, a weighing machine, two sets of Sims's specula, a uterine sound, forceps of various kinds, 'rubber female catheters', an instrument known mysteriously as 'Playfair's probes', an enamelled instrument tray, a glass jar with a lid, three enamelled lotion basins, pessaries, five or six dressing cubicles, two or three lavatories, a clinical laboratory, an X-ray plant, and a well-ventilated waiting-room (Browne, 1935). Needless to say, most antenatal clinics of the period would have lacked many of these facilities.

Little data is available on the standard of antenatal clinical practice in the 1930s. Case-note material at the London Hospital shows that a sample of 100 women delivered by hospital staff in 1934–39 booked on average at 24.2 weeks and received 6.5 episodes of antenatal care (Table 4.1). The case-note format in use at the time had headings for the following information to be assembled: fundus, lie and presentation, fetal heart, relation of head to brim, blood pressure and urine. Seven lines were allowed for data entry, suggesting that not more than seven such examinations per pregnancy were anticipated. There was a line for pelvic measurements, which was rarely filled in. No blood tests, except for Wasserman tests in four of the 100 cases, were done. Records show that over the period 1934–50 there was a gradual increase in the number of visits and a decrease in the length of gestation at the first visit.

Table 4.2 gives slightly different data for the Glasgow Royal Maternity Hospital over the period from 1933–59. In 1933 women attended on average 2.6 times. They had their urine tested on average 4.6 times, their pelvises examined 1.3 times and their blood pressures taken 1.6 times. They had no blood tests and were not weighed. By 1949 there

Table 4.1 Antenatal Care at the London Hospital 1934–50[2]

| | *Year of delivery* | | |
	1934–9	*1942–5*	*1948–50*
Average number of hospital visits	6.5	7.8	9.1
Average time in pregnancy of booking (weeks)	24.2	21.8	18.9
Number of case notes in series	100	100	74

Table 4.2 Antenatal Care at Glasgow Royal Maternity Hospital 1933–59[3]

| | | *Year of delivery* | | |
Type of examination	*1933*	*1939* *1949* *Average no. of examinations*		*1959*
General examinations	2.6	2.7	3.8	5.7
Urine tests	4.5	4.8	7.4	7.0
Pelvic examinations	1.3	1.0	1.0	0.9
Blood pressures	1.6	4.8	7.7	7.0
Haemoglobin estimations	–	–	0.9	3.2
Blood group/rhesus factor tests	–	–	1.0	1.0
Times weighed	–	–	–	7.0
Number of case-notes in series	100	80	81	81

2. The data in this table were obtained from microfilm records held in the hospital. The first 100 cases delivering pre-1940 were taken, and the first 100 delivering between 1940 and 1942. The same total, of 100, could not be obtained for 1948–50, because there were only 74 complete records. Reproduced with the permission of the London Hospital (Mile End).

3. The same principle was used to obtain these data as for those in Table 4.1, i.e. the aim was to analyse the first 100 cases delivering in each of the years shown in the table. However, the three latter years yielded less than 100 cases. These records are also on microfilm, held at the Glasgow Royal Maternity Hospital. Reproduced with permission of Glasgow Royal Maternity Hospital.

had been a small rise in the average number of examinations, a large rise in urine tests (from 4.5 to 7.4) and in blood pressure estimations (from 1.6 to 7.7); and routine blood tests had begun to be done. The Glasgow notes required the position of the fetus to be recorded, together with the position and rate of the fetal heart, the height of the fundus, the relation of the presenting part to the pelvic inlet, and the pelvic measurements. A special space on the form (infrequently used) was allocated to 'X-ray and Pathological Reports'. The urine was to be tested for specific gravity, reaction, albumen, pus and sugar or blood. The colour and condition of the vaginal discharge was still considered extremely interesting ('red, brown, yellow, white, slight, profuse, offensive').

Ways of Seeing

But antenatal case notes in the 1930s did not reflect the fact that a revolution was under way which would ultimately enable obstetricians to claim an unprecedented degree of control over the hitherto mysterious workings of the womb. When R. W. Johnstone set himself the task of addressing 'Ballantyne's ghost' in 1947, he imagined Ballantyne listening 'with rapt attention as I am privileged to unfold the amazing story of the new physiology of the female reproductive organs'. Indeed, he claimed that more such knowledge had been attained in the span of a single generation than ever before. Johnstone was referring to a spate of endocrinological research which, in the years leading up to the second world war, had established the foundation of modern knowledge on the topic of female hormonal function in pregnancy. There were other developments too, notably in the understanding of the constitution of the blood and in chemotherapy, which profoundly altered the parameters of antenatal care. But it was the new understanding of reproductive hormones that most of all set the scene for the technological revolution.

The introduction of hormonal pregnancy tests

Following Hitschmann and Adler's work on the menstrual cycle in 1908, other researchers had pursued the mysterious link between cyclical changes in the ovaries and the pattern of menstrual bleeding and conception. In 1923 Allen and Doisy demonstrated that uterine bleeding followed a fall in the blood oestrogen level — this was the 'discovery' of the oestrogenic hormone. By 1931 the two hormonal entities oestrone and oestriol had been separated, though not yet named. The naming problem produced an international meeting sponsored by the Health Organization of the League of Nations which took place in Hampstead, London, in 1932 and was devoted to the matter of standardizing names for hormones. At this meeting there was much discussion of the need to collect reasonable amounts of the raw crystalline hormonal material, and offers in the region of 500 mg were made. Then a Frenchman, a Dr A. Girard, pulled out of his waistcoat, to everyone's amazement, and the benefit of future research, a bottle of 20 g of the stuff. From the point of view of understanding more about the properties, function and relationships of the new hormones, extracting enough of them was the problem. The Frenchman had discovered how to get them out of mare's urine; in 1936 Doisy and his colleagues reported the achievement of extracting a few milligrams of an oestrogenic substance from the liquor folliculi of four tons of sows' ovaries. Eventually, and not altogether happily as it turned out, something called diethystilboestrol (DES) was synthesized by Charles Dodds in 1938. DES was, of course, to play a sad role in antenatal care. Since its effectiveness and potential dangers were not evaluated, it was some years before it was eventually shown to be responsible for genital deformity and disease in the children of women treated with it in pregnancy (see pp. 194 and also Grant and Chalmers, forthcoming, for a discussion).

Progesterone, the other main relevant female hormone, was officially named in 1935, at a party near the Imperial Hotel in Russell Square on the eve of the second international conference on standardization of sex hormones. A number of researchers around the world had been investigating the substance produced in early pregnancy by the corpus luteum, and by 1935 had a number of different names for it — progesterone was the one adopted. Some nasty experiments on female rabbits in 1928: 'partial decerebration within 45 minutes of mating' (Parkes, 1966, p. xxvii), demonstrated the activity of pituitary hormones, the gonadotrophins. In 1930 Collip and his colleagues reported that the human placenta contained large amounts of a gonadotrophinic substance — human chorionic gonadotrophin.

The import of all this work to antenatal care was of course principally and simply that it paved the way for the first biological laboratory pregnancy test. A duo called Aschheim and Zondek made the observation in 1928 that pregnant women's urine was highly oestrogenic, and thereby gave their names to the first pregnancy test. The method, as described by F. J. Browne in his *Antenatal and Postnatal Care* in 1935, went as follows: five female mice three to four weeks old weighing 6–8 gm each were injected, usually in the buttock, twice a day for three days with morning urine. After 100 hours the mice were killed and the ovaries inspected. If they were enlarged and congested there was a 98 per cent chance that the woman from whom the specimen of morning urine came was pregnant. This process raised rodents (and female ones at that) to 'the rank of obstetrical consultants' in the inimitable words of R. W. Johnstone: clinicians were taught by Aschheim and Zondek 'to refer with assurance our doubts as to the existence of an early pregnancy to the arbitrament of young female mice' (Johnstone, 1947, p. 11).

The Aschheim–Zondek test was evaluated by Dr F. A. E. Crew, Director of the Animal Breeding Research Department at the University of Edinburgh, who set up in 1930 what he called a 'pregnancy diagnosis station' (PDS). Doctors all over the country sent their patients' urine specimens to the PDS which by 1946 had carried out 130,000 such tests. Crew reported (1930) that in about 1 per cent of cases the urine sample actually killed the experimental animal. Otherwise the tests done which could be followed up to establish whether or not the woman was pregnant gave a false result in only 3.04 per cent of cases.

In 1931 Friedman and Lapham substituted rabbits in testing for pregnancy, thereby making the procedure cheaper (rabbits were easier to get hold of than mice). Their version demanded what one writer called 'virginal rabbits of unimpeachable antecedents' (Henriksen, 1941, p. 573). The rabbits got morning urine in the ear for two days and were then killed. South African toads were also used in the Hogben test, but this apparently was a method restricted to England, since the toads in question were a scarce resource.[4] The advantage of the toad was that 'it is a more economical animal in that it gives its oracular answer by shedding its eggs and does not need to be killed and have its ovaries inspected' (Johnstone, 1950, p. 15).

By the time of the 1931 edition of Haultain and Fahmy's textbook on antenatal care, the Aschheim–Zondek (A–Z) test was mentioned as a new and important technique. By the mid-1930s it was resorted to by doctors when there was a particular reason for needing to know quickly whether or not a patient was pregnant. Dr Hope-Simpson, a rural GP, recalled:

We did use it if it was important to know. I can remember people coming and wanting to know if they were pregnant. And I would say 'I think you

---

4. In the Family Planning Association clinic in Sloane Street, London, the toads were kept in the basement and were regarded as a much-prized asset (Martin Richards, personal communication).

are' or 'I think you aren't.' Is it important that you should know before next month or whatever? And if there was some particular reason why they should know then we'd arrange an Aschheim–Zondek. It cost them a couple of quid (E. H. S. I).

The routine use of X-rays in antenatal work

However imperfect and expensive, the A–Z test launched the modern era in which obstetricians would eventually be able to claim a knowledge superior to that possessed by the owners of wombs themselves, as to the presence of a guest, invited or uninvited, within. One of the important, unforeseen, functions of the introduction of the A–Z test was that it helped to curtail, or at least offered an alternative to, a dangerous prevailing enthusiasm for diagnosing early pregnancy with X-rays. Röntgen's discovery (see pp. 27–8), delivered to the world before the turn of the century, had inspired clinicians in many different areas of medical work to re-examine the human body in the light of the new rays. Within a year of Röntgen's original work 48 books and over 1,000 articles on X-rays had been published (Reid, 1978). Some claims were obvious quackery, for example the announcement by a New York physician that the best way to become a doctor was to have X-rays of human anatomy projected into one's brain. The French characteristically tried out X-rays in the wine industry, and declared them to be an infallible method for separating true from false products (details of the test were, needless to say, never published).

By 1910, X-rays were being used to survey diseases of the alimentary tract, urinary system, lungs, and, of course, the bones and joints. The idea that they might be useful in obstetrics was slow to catch on, but, when finally directed to the womb, they were employed first of all to detail the stages in the growth of the fetal skeleton — in chimpanzees, and in 'man'. Some of the early experiments involved human fetuses from four weeks of gestation. The enormous detail with which the new technique of radioscopy, as it was sometimes called, was used to produce a developmental cartography of the fetal skeleton is clearly shown in figure 4.1; to every bone a birthday.

After seven weeks of pregnancy, X-rays were considered capable of revealing a good deal. They were thought, for example, to be an accurate method of assessing gestational age, although allowance had to be made for what, as early as 1908 had been recognized to be an important sex difference — bones showed up earlier on X-ray films of female fetuses. Assessments of pregnancy duration by X-ray were believed to be most reliable in early pregnancy, since centres of ossification appeared more frequently in the early months and their time of appearance was more constant. X-ray dating was said to be accurate

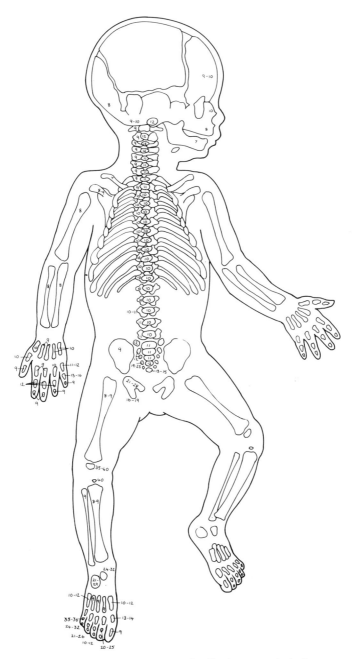

Figure 4.1   diagram of development of ossification centres in the fetus
source: Hess, J. The diagnosis of the age of the fetus by use of roentgenograms, *American Journal of Diseases of Children* 1917, p. 399. With permission of the American Medical Association.

within one week in the first half of pregnancy and within two weeks in the second half (Hess, 1917). By 1912 (Obata) the fetal crown-rump length (some half a century later to assume popularity in ultrasound investigation of pregnancy) was being measured. Abnormalities of skeletal development were an early focus of interest; spina bifida, a relatively common defect, was fairly easily identified. Fetal presentation and position in late pregnancy could be estimated, and the intrauterine death of a fetus was evidenced by a sign attributed to Spaulding in 1922 — the overlapping of the bones of the deceased fetal skull. The bony structures of the female pelvis in which the womb and its contents are located, was radiographed by Budin and Varnier in 1897, and had become 'an absorbing field of investigation', though yielding 'varying results', by the 1920s (Dorland and Hubeny, 1926, p. 215).

In the diagnosis of pregnancy itself, a field in which obstetricians had a major professional investment, but still little progress to report, X-rays were considered to be 'a very valuable aid' (Dorland and Hubeny, 1926, p. 259). They were thought especially useful in enabling clinicians to differentiate between those abdominal tumours due to pregnancy and those of a possibly more malignant kind.[5] Their *social* contribution was also significant, for with the help of X-rays, 'it may become possible at times to dissipate scandalous reports originated and circulated by venomous gossip-mongers when these reports affect single women or widows' (p. 259). The first legal ruling as to the admissibility of X-ray evidence was made in the USA less than a year after Röntgen's first announcement of X-rays (Reiser, 1978).

According to investigators in the USA, the uterine enlargement of pregnancy was discernible on X-rays by six weeks. A reliable diagnosis between six and ten weeks was claimed, although the clear picture required for diagnosis meant that the patient had to lie on her back with her pelvis elevated and with between 1.5 and 2 litres of carbonic gas injected into her peritoneal cavity — 'death, even, has resulted from this procedure' (Dorland and Hubeny, 1926, p. 261). It was also a good idea for the patient to have her bowels emptied first by means of castor oil, and for the fetus to be immobilized during the procedure by a band tied round the maternal abdomen. Somebody else advocated a totally different position, with the mother lying face downwards, her chest raised on pillows, and sandbags (for some unaccountable reason) placed on the backs of her thighs. A gentleman in Buenos Aires had found he could

---

5. See chapter 8, pp. 157–8 for a parallel motive in the development of obstetric ultrasound.

diagnose pregnancy during the first month by injecting iodated petrolatum into the uterus before taking the picture. But this method of diagnosis risked the termination of pregnancy — a profound disadvantage.

Detecting the presence of a fetus in the womb, and attempting to follow its progress, were activities that required the irradiation of considerable numbers of fetuses in early pregnancy. What the early radiographers saw when viewing fetuses is shown in Plate 4.I.

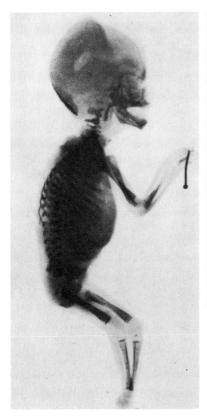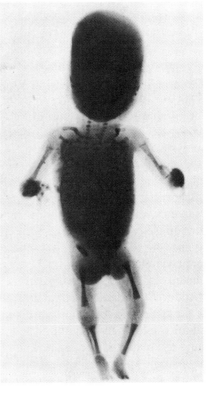

Plate 4.I X-rayed fetuses
source: Dorland and Hubeny, 1926, pp. 41–2

Fetal radiography was regarded by many as a fascinating field, with 'ascents and descents, turnings, twistings and writhings, rotations and revolutions' to be charted in the evolution of the embryo: 'Kidneys are rising and testicles descending' (Dorland and Hubeny, 1926, p. 71). It was also a field in which, by unhappily becoming martyrs to their own endeavours, the early explorers warned the world of the double-edged power of X-rays. Even as soon as the end of 1896, some workers were badly affected. An assistant of Thomas Edison's, Clarence Dally, died of cancer secondary to severe X-ray dermatitis; and by 1905 reports were coming in of other male X-ray workers rendered incapable of producing sperm. The evil effects of X-rays and radium on animal and plant life were also established early. Roots and seeds stopped growing, silkworms became restless, X-rayed cigarette beetle larvae refused to eat, the intestinal worms of horses became grossly mis-shapen, the X-rayed hind legs of puppies caused deformity in adult dog life, guinea pigs became infertile, and pregnant guinea pigs lost their babies. At the same time, the investment of those who worked with the new method of seeing inside the human body was so great that harmful effects were often strenuously denied. In Marie Curie's laboratory everyone knew radium could irreparably damage the body, yet they clung to the attitude that radium burns on the hands were medals won on the battlefield of science: the more scars, the greater the distinction (Reid, 1978).

By the early 1920s the sceptical were cautioning others (chiefly on the basis of the animal evidence) as to the real danger inherent in the use of X-rays in pregnancy. Brief exposure to the rays was advised (exposure time for the first X-rays was in the region of *one hour*), and the possibility was raised, indeed, of long-term damage to a child apparently normal at birth (Dorland and Hubeny, 1926, p. 25). But warnings of damage were counterbalanced by the attractiveness to the obstetrician of the information gained. Such warnings also were not communicated to those who in the 1920s and 1930s were responsible for referring for X-ray pregnant women as a routine part of antenatal work. Thus Dr John Sturrock recalls his own practice in Scotland during this period:

We used to X-ray everybody when I was first practising, and when we discovered it was an easy thing to measure the pelvis more accurately . . . Initially I don't think we had doubts as to safety. But it became obvious. I remember the fellow who started the department here, what a mess his hands were in . . . a friend of mine who took up radiology, he died of leukaemia. We didn't realize how *much* you should be protected (J. S. I.).

By 1924 the apparently invaluable access obtained by X-rays to the womb's sanctuary had already evoked the suggestion that every obstetric clinic should be equipped with an expert radiographer (Speidel and Turner, 1924). In 1935 L. N. Reece was not alone in proposing the 'routine use of X-rays in antenatal work'. 'It is suggested', said Reece, writing in the *Proceedings of the Royal Society of Medicine*, 'that antenatal work without the routine use of X-rays is no more justifiable than would be the treatment of fractures' (Reece, 1935, p. 489). Reece himself was a promoter of the art of fetal cephalometry (head measurements) and, having tried it out on 100 cases, declared that the fetal head grows exactly one tenth of an inch a week during the last eight weeks of pregnancy. The advantage of such information was, most significantly, in view of future developments (see chapter 8) said to be that it would facilitate 'an approach to scientific control of the time for labour'. If one knew how old the fetus was, one could deliver it by artificial methods without risking death or illness due to prematurity. That was one reason why all pregnant women should be X-rayed. The other was to determine the size of the pelvis. By this date X-rays were also being used for other obstetric purposes not foreseen by the early investigators. Placenta praevia (low-lying placenta) was diagnosable with X-rays — the favourite method, known as amniography, being the injection of a contrast medium such as strontium iodide through the maternal abdominal wall and into the amniotic sac (Burke, 1935).

In F. J. Browne's *Antenatal and Postnatal Care* the rise and fall of the fashion for antenatal X-rays is reflected in the inclusion of a separate chapter on the subject from the second (1937) to the ninth (1960) edition. (The tenth edition in 1970 is, not coincidentally, the first in which ultrasound gets a mention as an alternative way of seeing inside the uterus, see chapter 8, for some comparable statements about ultrasound.) In the first such chapter, R. W. A. Salmond, Director of the Radiological Department at London's University College Hospital, commented on the slow progress of X-rays in obstetrics compared with other branches of medicine, and attributed it to the confidence older obstetricians had in the information gained from clinical examination: 'The younger generation, on the other hand, seems to be more mechanically or laboratory minded, and makes more frequent use of these methods' (Salmond, 1937, p. 496). Figure 4.2, from R. W. A. Salmond's chapter, captures the directness of the gaze the mechanically-minded young men were thereby able to focus on the womb. As to safety: 'It has been frequently asked whether there is any danger to the life of the child by the passage of X rays through it; it can be said at once that there is none if the examination is carried out by a competent radiologist or radiographer' (p. 497). In the 1939 edition

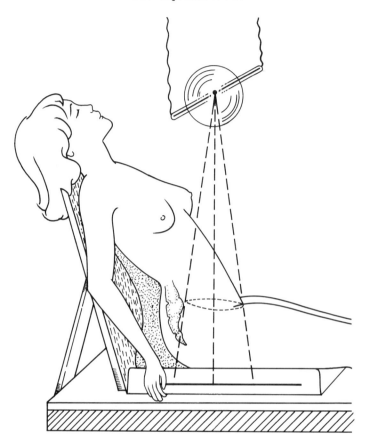

Figure 4.2 X-ray pelvimetry
source: after Salmond, R.W.A. The Uses and Value of Radiology in Obstetrics in Browne, F.J. and J.C. McC. (eds.) *Antenatal and Post-natal Care*, 1937, p. 508. With permission of publisher Churchill Livingstone.

Salmond was a little more circumspect on the question of safety, and the note of caution was confirmed and elaborated in the chapters of later editions (1955, 1960) written by Chassar Moir. The list of possible hazards detailed by Moir in 1960 ended with the findings published in 1956 by Alice Stewart and her co-workers in Oxford and implicating antenatal X-rays in the genesis of childhood cancer. Among 1,299 children who died from cancer before the age of ten, 13.7 per cent had been X-rayed *in utero*. Of a control group of living children only 7.2 per cent had undergone X-ray surveillance of their antenatal careers.

Stewart's findings — though subsequently criticized on methodological grounds (Campbell, 1977) — appear to have brought about a kind of
volte-face, which is rare in antenatal work. In 1957 the Annual Clinical
Report of Queen Charlotte's Maternity Hospital in London refers to a
'striking change' in radiological work at the hospital following the Stewart study:

> The effect of this publication has been sharply to limit the number of
> patients referred for X ray examination in the antenatal period, and thus
> the amount of radiological work dropped sharply in 1957. The techniques
> of examination were modified to lessen the amount of foetal irradiation.

Furthermore,

> The personnel of the Department has been very active in extracting from
> our records from 1943 to 1956 the information sought by the Statistical
> Research Unit of the Medical Research Council in a large enquiry (to
> which QCH will be a major contributor) into the validity of ascribing
> antenatal X ray examination as a factor in producing leukaemia (and other
> malignant disease) in children (p. 7).

Prior to the Oxford revelations, the annual number of antenatal
examinations as a proportion of patients delivered by hospital staff had
risen from 28.5 per cent in 1946 to 66.7 per cent in 1954, the particularly high figure in the latter year coinciding with the introduction of
new higher voltage X-ray equipment.

The advantages of dyeing leather red?

Three other technical developments affected antenatal care in the
1930s. These were the light thrown by Fullerton and Davidson and their
co-workers in 1933 on the relation between the haemoglobin level and
the increased volume of the blood in pregnancy, the new understanding
of, and facilities for, blood transfusions, and the chemotherapeutic
treatment of puerperal sepsis and other infections. Fullerton and Davidson's work led directly to the modern appraisal of what constitutes
anaemia in pregnancy, while the advance in blood transfusions effectively redefined the risks of obstetric intervention (such as caesarean
section) and offered a new response to the crises of antenatal and
postnatal haemorrhages. However, it did not really arrive on the clinical
scene until after the discovery of the rhesus blood groups by Land-

steiner and Wiener in 1940, and the refinement of transfusion technique developed during the Second World War (Farr, 1979).

The third advance, in chemotherapy, is one which is claimed to have
achieved what antenatal care had itself not been able to, and that is the
beginning of a sustained decline in the rate at which women died in
childbirth. By the 1930s the numerous aetiological theories concerning
puerperal sepsis had been condensed into one: infection. The possible
infective agents had also been reduced to one main one: the streptococcus, and to one primary group of streptococci, namely Group A. But
despite an increase in antiseptic measures, not much, if any, fall in the
incidence or case-fatality of sepsis could be seen. Prontosil was discovered in 1932 and introduced in 1935 cautiously on an experimental
and local basis. Its discoverer, the German doctor Gerhard Domagk, got
the Nobel prize for Medicine in 1939 (though Hitler imprisoned him for
it — he objected to Nobel prizes, since the last German to get one had
been the pacificist and anti-Nazi, Carl von Ossietzky, in 1936).

By one of those common serendipities of scientific discovery, the drug
prontosil was originally synthesized for quite a different purpose — in
fact for dyeing leather red, hence the name 'prontosil rubrum'. Domagk
tried it out on mice infected with haemolytic streptococci in 1932 with
striking results: mice given the dye by stomach tube all survived and
those without the dye did not. In 1935 he published his observations,
strengthened by his own use of the drug to cure his daughter of a
streptococcal infection derived from pricking herself with a needle. His
results were rapidly followed up all over the world. Prontosil proved
eventually to be effective against both streptococci and staphylococci,
and thus in the treatment of not only puerperal sepsis but pneumococcal
pneumonia, meningitis and gonorrhea.

English interest in prontosil dated from March 1935 when Sir Henry
Dale asked the German pharmaceutical firm I. G. Farbenindustrie to
send him some prontosil, so that he could place it at the disposal of the
Therapeutic Trials Committee. In January 1936 the first trials began at
Queen Charlotte's Hospital in London, and, later that year, Leonard
Colebrook and Méave Kenny reported in the *Lancet* (16 June 1936a)
their initial findings on a series of 38 patients with pueperal sepsis. Of
the 38, Colebrook and Kenny judged that 45 per cent could not have
been said to have been affected one way or the other by the drug. In
another 42 per cent of cases they felt the drug had probably aided
recovery. The death-rate was 8 per cent. But since the death-rate from
puerperal sepsis in the years 1931–34 averaged 22 per cent, it was
reasonable to assume that prontosil was working. The next series of 26

cases treated at Queen Charlotte's with prontosil, and reported on by Colebrook and Kenny in December 1936 (Colebrook and Kenny, 1936b), all survived. Colebrook and Kenny were still cautious in their judgement that the victory was due to prontosil. They considered whether the cases treated had been unusually mild — they had not been. Yet there *was* evidence suggesting a decline in the virulence of the infection that was occurring independently of the new drug treatment — the case-fatality rate was falling among non-prontosil cases at Queen Charlotte's and elsewhere, for example among puerperal fever cases admitted to the North Western Fever Hospital in London, where it fell from 22 per cent in 1933, to 11 per cent in 1934, to 7.8 per cent in 1935, to 5.3 per cent in the first half of 1936 (no prontosil was used in these cases). In Scotland the case-fatality rate for puerperal sepsis rose until 1928, after which it began an uninterrupted decline: the rate of *notification* of the disease, however, increased until 1934 (Douglas, 1955).

Training for battle

Speaking at the Royal Sanitary Institute in 1935, Eardley Holland called antenatal care 'a remarkable record of high endeavour'. Everything, he went on:

> has in fact been done but the one essential thing. Imagine the British Admiralty sending a battleship into action with an improvised crew. But that is just what has been done in the battle which has been joined against the maternal mortality-rate. The necessary personnel has not been trained, and until this has been done there is not the slightest chance of victory (Holland, 1935, p. 973).

The military metaphor first appeared in medicine in the 1880s, and it reflects both the social preoccupation with war and the masculinity of those who practised medicine (Sontag, 1977). But what did Holland mean? He meant three things: first, that the requisite trained staff for an effective and efficient maternity service were not being produced, secondly, that there was not enough emphasis on the basic principles of good midwifery, and, thirdly, that there was hopeless administrative confusion and division of responsibility as to whose responsibility the medical care of pregnant women really was — Britain needed a *national* maternity service.

Midwives and handywomen

One problem discussed from the beginning of antenatal care concerned the inadequate training and technical resources of midwives. Midwifery training made no reference to antenatal (or postnatal) care until 1916. In 1919 the Board of Education secured approval from the Treasury to contribute towards the cost of training midwives. In those years the number of untrained but bona fide practising midwives was quite high. In fact it remained legal until 1937 in England and Wales for an unqualified woman in bona fide practice to be admitted to the roll of the Central Midwives Board (CMB), and 1947 was the first year in which there were no midwives in practice admitted under this clause. The Central Midwives Board reported in 1916 that 25 per cent of the women on the Midwives' Roll in that year were untrained, and an impressive 44 per cent of *practising* midwives were untrained. The Board's Report discussed a practice that was causing some concern, which was that of the 'covering' by medical practitioners of uncertified women acting as midwives. The woman would deliver the patient and then send for the doctor, who notified the birth and signed the maternity benefit form: the woman gave the doctor a small fee in return for his guarantee that if any trouble ensued the patient was his. The other arrangement was for the doctor to book the patient but arrange with an uncertified woman that she should only call him if problems developed. He would claim, if challenged, that the woman was acting as his nurse, and that he was unavoidably prevented from conducting the delivery. (This was a good sign of the overwhelming reluctance of many medical practitioners to become involved in maternity work, the 'Cinderella' of medicine.)

By 1923, when Janet Campbell reported for the Ministry of Health on *The Training of Midwives*, the majority of training schools recognized the need for instructing pupils in antenatal work, but in six of 71 schools visited by a colleague of Janet Campbell's in the Ministry of Health, Dr Jane Turnbull, pupil midwives were instructed solely to quiz pregnant women as to their previous history and present health, not to examine them. In 1923 the different agencies providing midwifery instruction included:

(1) Maternity wards of hospitals;
(2) Ministry of Health-subsidized maternity homes;
(3) Poor Law institutions (which were not subject to the supervision of the CMB);
(4) District Nursing Associations;
(5) practising midwives approved by the CMB as teachers.

The training period was six months for unqualified women and four months for trained nurses (before 1916 it was three months). Campbell recommended extending these periods by six months and two months respectively (this happened in 1924), and suggested that the curriculum should be revised to make it more comprehensive and standardized. By 1933, a mere 3 per cent of midwives on the Roll of the CMB and 4 per cent of those practising midwifery were without formal training; in 1937, the period of training was raised from 6 to 12 months for SRNs and from 12 to 24 months for all other entrants. Campbell recommended, too, the registration with the local supervising authority of all women practising as monthly nurses or handywomen, so that these groups, who still played a key role in the total pattern of care, might be subject, along with midwives, to the supervision of the inspector of midwives.

The province of the midwife in the mid-1930s was ill-defined. By and large the emphasis on professional training was a welcome development, but its impact on the midwife's status all too often acted to reduce her autonomy. Lady Forber, alias Janet Lane-Claypon, MD, the author of a comprehensive volume on the *Child Health Movement* (1920), wrote in 1936 of the midwife's uncomfortable position, 'surrounded as she is by numerous agencies and persons who are all anxious to attend the mother or take her into an institution' (Forber, 1936, p. 107).

Yet not everybody was anxious to erode the midwife's autonomy, and some took active steps to bolster it. Dr Ivor Cookson, practising in Gloucestershire, had, like many of his fellow rural practitioners, a great respect for midwives:

I never took on the delivery if I could avoid it; the babies were delivered by the midwife even in the pre-NHS days when the only normal deliveries I attended were those of fee-paying patients. This was important. If a doctor has a reputation for taking over deliveries which the midwife could manage herself, he is not called to the delivery, or is called too late. In my village there was only one midwife who dealt with all the patients herself unless she was away and a relief took over. She must have delivered 80 to 90 percent herself and although I was there if needed, often I had little to do, except to encourage and admire. Before the NHS she could send patients to a doctor only for two antenatal examinations, and could call him to the delivery only if it were abnormal. Afterwards he could give full antenatal care, and also attend all deliveries if he had a good liaison with a co-operative midwife who would call him in time (I. C. I.).

Although Queen Victoria had eulogized in 1853 about pain relief during childbirth, only women who could pay for a doctor's attendance were able to secure the comforts of chloroform. Midwives had no analgesia to offer mothers until R. J. Minnitt of Liverpool Maternity Hospital designed in 1932 a portable apparatus for delivering gas and air. From 1936 on (1946 in Scotland), midwives were able to use gas and air analgesia, provided a doctor had certified the patient as fit to receive it, and the midwife could show she had been trained to use it. However, the necessary instruction was not actually incorporated into standard midwifery training until 1946. In that year only one in five practising midwives were qualified to administer gas and air, and they had to have another qualified person or pupil midwife present. The implications of this limitation were recalled by Cookson:

> My senior partner first had a trilene inhaler in 1947, and we had a more advanced model in 1948. At first I gave the trilene myself, then I taught the midwife to give it. When we had acquired a good deal of experience and were sure of the safety of it when used by the midwife herself, I took the responsibility of letting her use it before I arrived. This was years before the CMB approved its use by midwives. Then, my midwife had to attend a course and acquire a certificate of competence before she could have an inhaler to use on her own responsibility. The same applies to pethidine. I took the responsibility of supplying an ampoule for her to use when she so decided, years before the CMB allowed her to use it on her own responsibility (I. C. I.).

The 1936 Midwives' Act (the 1937 Maternity Services Act in Scotland) established what many people felt was an absolute necessity for more effective maternity care — a salaried midwifery service under the administration of local authorities. Under the terms of the Act, local authorities could either employ midwives directly, or by paying voluntary associations to do so. By this date, the policy-makers seemed to have agreed that midwives should, as far as possible, be recruited from the pool of women with a nursing training. It was thought that this would improve care. It may have done, but what it also represented was the beginning of the end of British midwifery as a profession concerned with the *normal* physiology of childbearing. The insidiousness of this move was hidden beneath statistics that evoked a picture of the midwife's continuing ascendancy: in 1946, 90 per cent of deliveries in England and Wales were conducted in the presence of a midwife, who in 75 per cent of cases took full responsibility (Political and Economic Planning, 1946). Figure A.11 (p. 304) gives the overall trend in numbers of midwives practising in England and Wales from 1908 to 1981.

Teaching the doctors

Medical training was equally slow to incorporate the new theory and practice of antenatalism. Instruction in antenatal conditions, diagnosis and treatment, was not included in the medical curriculum until 1923, and even then the amount of instruction was minimal. Dr Hope-Simpson refers to the humble state of ignorance in which doctors at the time typically emerged from medical training: 'I can remember the District Nurse telling me, the first time I put on forceps, you know, Doctor, we usually use the blade the other way round. I learnt from my District Nurses all sorts of things. They gave us 20 births in the hospital, but that wasn't much to learn on' (E. H. S. I). From 1928 attendance in an antenatal department was made obligatory in some medical schools. Some years later, in Scotland, Dugald Baird recalled:

> A man called Fairbairn, from one of the London hospitals, came up to examine in the finals just about 1936, just before I left Aberdeen and he said, but where are the antenatal cases? Have you no antenatal beds? I said they're never used for examination purposes. You may not believe this, but this is absolute fact . . . it was round about the late 1930s that the students were shown women with antenatal complications. Aberdeen may have been particularly backward but I've no reason to believe that (D. B. I).

One route out of this conundrum was to raise the status of the art (science?) of medical midwifery, and to this end, the British College of Obstetricians and Gynaecologists was founded in 1929. The idea was that a college equivalent in standing to the Royal College of Physicians (1548) and the Royal College of Surgeons (1540) would do for obstetrics and gynaecology what had been done for medicine and surgery.

In the latter part of the nineteenth century most successful obstetricians were Fellows of the RCP, but around the turn of the century a move in favour of the FRCS began to manifest itself. The problem was to create an institution that would establish both medicine and surgery as necessary credentials for those who wished to supervise the reproductive capacities of women. According to its originator, William Fletcher Shaw (1954), another reason for the founding of the College was precisely to combat the claims of the public campaigners who associated maternal mortality with poor medical care.

The plan for such an institution was cemented during a shooting party on the fells of North Lancashire in the early 1920s. There were nine signatories to the articles of association all of whom were men. The formal certificate of registration was received on 13 September 1929. The College established a diploma for GPs in 1931 (now the Dip. Obst. RCOG), and a membership examination for consultants in 1939. The jocular claim was made (Kerr, et al., 1954, p. 282) that the founding of the College was the factor that finally led to the much-desired fall in maternal mortality.[6]

The founding of a British College of Obstetricians and Gynaecologists (it received its Royal Charter in 1938), was thus a most significant move in the medicalization of childbirth. It was an overt attempt to provide would-be obstetricians with that degree of professional status and instruction which would, in the end, ensure an effective challenge to all other professional groups involved in the clinical care of childbearing women.

Competing for business

In the 1920s and 1930s, the maternity care field was thus shared by untrained women, trained women (midwives), municipal clinic medical officers, GPs and specialist obstetricians. There were also maternity nurses and health visitors in there somewhere fighting for their own bit of legitimate terrain.

It was difficult to evaluate the proficiency of the different groups. In Dorset in the mid-1940s, Dr Hope-Simpson went to deliver a baby in a little village called Hook:

> I didn't know she was pregnant. She was living in a house which I later heard was known locally as the harem. The man was not her husband, and his wife was acting as a sort of Sarah Gamp to deliver the baby. There was no midwife there at all, and the baby was born, the mother was having acute diarrhoea at the time, and I had to wash everything up and clean up the Mum. Didn't have a moment's trouble. Not a rise of temperature, no trouble with the baby, nothing at all.
>
> The ones [handywomen] we knew were quite good. Mind you, they had all sorts of strange ideas, but they weren't dangerous ideas, most of them (E. H. S. I).

---

6. The same vision of an easy institutional answer to complex problems was responsible for the claim made in the late 1970s that the founding of the National Perinatal Epidemiology Unit in Oxford accounted for a drop in Britain's perinatal mortality.

Apart from the women they delivered, and some of the local medical practitioners, no one liked handywomen. They were regarded as vestiges of an outdated system of community care which was, of course, exactly what they were. The trend of the time was towards professionalism. Experience and familiarity could not be regarded as appropriate qualifications for the new providers of pregnancy and delivery care, despite the fact that sufficient experience was exactly what many of the new providers lacked, and that by the 1930s many critics of the maternity services had begun to bemoan the new alienation of the childbearing woman from her professional attendants.

GPs were not, at the time, accused so much of alienation, as of lack of interest in the adequate supervision of pregnancy. Nowhere was this conclusion more startlingly realized than in the maternal death inquiries. Doctors' cases predominated in fatal maternities, and this was by no means solely because they got the lion's share of difficult cases. Moreover, it seemed from various surveys that the mortality and morbidity rates attained by a domiciliary midwifery service in which there was a relatively small element of specialist referral, were often very good. The J. S. Fairbairn mentioned by Dugald Baird (p. 111) examined in 1927 the records of the Queen Victoria's Jubilee Institute — a national organization providing delivery care and working through county nursing associations. He found that over a number of years mortality in the midwives' cases was under half the general rate for England and Wales. He, like others, found an increasing tendency among midwives to call for medical aid. This was not associated with an improvement in the mortality rate of mothers, but did surely demonstrate the birth of a less self-reliant midwifery profession.

At a time when the BCOG and the BMA were staking a claim against the protection of midwives as independent managers of normal childbearing, midwives therefore had their defenders in the medical press. In the country areas, moreover, GPs often had a healthy respect for the midwife's expertise. The crux of the matter was good local collaboration. There had been many conflicts between midwives and doctors in the early days of antenatal care. The municipal clinic antenatal schemes depended on midwives for the referral of cases, since the new system of care was imposed on the old one, which was midwife-controlled. 'The first object', said the Ministry of Health's 1929 Report on Midwives, 'must be to remove any suspicion from the mind of the midwife to the effect that the medical officer of health and his staff exist for the purpose of finding fault with her and harassing the midwife in her work' (Ministry of Health, 1929b, p. 49). Midwives were not happy about referring patients to clinics since (aside from not wanting to admit professional defeat), they were reluctant to lose their fee; even as late as 1936 some local authorities had not yet initiated an appropriate system of financial compensation for this.

As for the GPs, they could hardly avoid realizing that they were caught in an uneasy — and inescapable — trap between the specialist hospitals and the midwives (not to mention the municipal maternity clinics). Only they and the midwives could offer what was regarded at the time as an absolute necessity of good care — continuity: the same person attending the mother in pregnancy, labour and delivery, and afterwards. Some people argued that public health authorities and specialists entirely overlooked the psychological benefit of continuous GP family-oriented maternity care. As Dr Dale Logan remarked:

> Unless antenatal work is carried out by the family doctor it will probably be done in a routine, stereotyped way, and the patient treated as a case, not as an individual, in the usual institutional manner . . . To separate the antenatal supervision of a patient from the conduct of the confinement is simply ridiculous. Yet this is being done regularly all over the country and is one of the most serious disadvantages of the present method of running antenatal schemes (Logan, 1934, p. 1141).

Throughout the 1930s, the BMA campaigned tirelessly against municipal clinic care and in favour of GP care, arguing that the growth of the former had actually increased maternal mortality. The attack on local authority care centred on three shortcomings of that system: (1) the whole-time medical officers who staffed the clinics often had little or no practical experience of obstetrics — and 'once they enter the service of a local authority they may never see a woman in labour' (PEP, 1946, p. 9); (2) as we have seen, they were not allowed to provide treatment for any of the complications they diagnosed, for fear of treading on the toes of the private practitioners; (3) the system was quite antithetical to the principle of continuity of care. The pregnant woman was not delivered by the person who had surveyed her pregnancy. Crucial too, was the fact that there was no system of transferring the information gained about her condition antenatally in the local authority clinic to the person responsible for delivering her.

As with other such moments in medical history, the force of the attack in the 1930s on municipally-provided antenatal care did not necessarily bear much relation to evidence about the quality of the work done. The 1937 *Report on an Investigation into Maternal Mortality*, for example, commented that comparing the 14 per cent of cases attended antenatally by local authority medical officers with the 56 per cent attended by GPs: 'The proportion of cases in which the antenatal care exercised by the municipal clinics was good appeared to be much higher than that for which GPs were responsible, and reference by medical officers of the clinics of patients in whom signs of illness or abnormality were detected for consultant advice or for admission to hospital was more frequent' (Ministry of Health, 1937, p. 189). In one sense it did not appear to matter very much what local authority medical officers did. Their time had passed, and the emphasis in antenatal care was moving away from community care and into the hospital. The introduction of the NHS in 1948, together with the growing concentration of deliveries in hospital, was to sound the final death knell for local authority antenatal care.

5

Fighting for Health: the Second World War and antenatal care 1939–45

It would . . . be true to say that by the end of the Second World War the Government had . . . assumed and developed a measure of direct concern for the health and wellbeing of the population which, by contrast with the role of Government in the 1930s, was little short of remarkable.

Titmuss, 1959, p. 506

In the early months of the Second World War the Ministry of Health became concerned about the incidence of head louse infestation among children. According to one survey, around a half of pre-school children living in industrial areas had lousy heads. At the age of fourteen, 50 per cent of girls, but only 20 per cent of boys, were infested (Ministry of Health, circular 2306). Although throughout the war a surprisingly high incidence among girls and women was reported,[1] overall the head louse seemed increasingly to be losing the battle.

The louse's fate drew attention to three changes in the health arena that had implications for antenatal care. First, the social dislocations of war for the civilian population gave a new visibility to health as an aspect of lifestyle rather than simply a medical care product. Second, greater visibility ensured better data — the wartime prevalence of lice on the heads of children was probably no new phenomenon, it was just that they had not been counted so carefully before. Third, and most important, the Government, faced directly in time of war with such evidence as to the state of the public health, could no longer afford to pass the buck: a new conception of national responsibility for the welfare of the people had to be formulated.

The Second World War was the first modern war — the definition of a modern war being that everyone was involved in it; indeed, up until

---

1. The sex difference wasn't explained. Perhaps it was due to the louse's preference for frequently washed hair?

D-day in 1944, more civilians than soldiers died. Before the outbreak of war, in 1939, Government officials were already grappling with the problems they foresaw would result from civilian injury and death, but it was Churchill who pointed out, in 1934, that the dislocation of the civilian population (due to bombing) was likely to be the worst problem. Thus it was necessary for the state to take positive action to mitigate the worst effects of war. Warfare led to welfare.

The evacuation of pregnant women was carried out with a red and blue card system. Pregnant women in the evacuation areas could register at any maternity and child welfare centre, where they would be issued with either a red or blue card. Those with blue cards were the ones whose babies were imminent, and they travelled by road in the company of midwives; the others, the red card-holders, went by train. It sounded deceptively simple, but in fact the existing policy of 'divided rule' obtaining in the maternity services at that date made it far from simple. Over 400 welfare authorities in England and Wales provided such services as clinics and health visiting. There were 188 supervisory authorities for domiciliary midwifery. Beds for institutional confinement were held at two types of hospital — municipal and voluntary. The health visitor, the domiciliary midwife and the hospital, supposed to work hand in hand, were often responsible to different authorities. Both the clinic medical officers and general practitioners were cut off from one another and from the other services. The phrase 'a national maternity service' had begun to be heard in the early 1920s; it was above all a demand for unification in maternity-service provision, and for putting the financing of the service on a sound basis. In 1930 Arthur Greenwood, then Minister of Health, calculated the cost of a national maternity service as £2,750,000 per annum, approximately the same sum as the yearly expenditure on public baths and wash-houses, and a sum which even the Labour Government of the time decided it could not afford.

Since the major response to civilian bombing (apart from direct injury) was predicted to be a panicky, disorderly exodus from the cities, the major remedy was planned evacuation. This was the policy that was most directly to affect the medical care and general welfare of mothers and children.

Evacuation was not to be compulsory and the country was divided into three: evacuation, reception and neutral areas. The 'priority classes' who needed to be evacuated were defined as

(1) schoolchildren;
(2) younger children;

(3) expectant mothers;

(4) blind people and cripples.

The working figures used in the lead-up to the war were four million —
in other words, it was predicted that four million people would choose
(or have chosen for them by parents or schools) evacuation as the
answer.

It was into this network of piecemeal provision that the wartime
evacuation of pregnant women had somehow to be slotted. Where would
they go? The plan was to accommodate them in private homes for a few
weeks before the birth, then to arrange for the delivery and a postnatal
stay of about two weeks in a maternity home. But in fact private
householders were not especially anxious to have pregnant women
billeted on them; there was no guarantee that they would make it to the
maternity home in time, and they would hardly count as additions of
productive labour (in the accepted sense) to the household. Descriptions
of the first meetings between evacuees and hosts in the reception areas
as resembling 'an early Roman slave market and Selfridges' bargain
basement' (in the words of one evacuation officer quoted in Titmuss,
1950, p. 111), did not omit to mention the fact that the hosts chose the
strong-looking lads and the clean nicely-dressed children first, and the
pregnant women last. To overcome this problem householders were
paid more for taking in a pregnant woman.

Then there was the problem of providing enough maternity beds in
the reception areas. Not until eight days before the evacuation scheme
began were the reception authorities authorized to get on with the job of
adapting and equipping houses as emergency maternity homes. 'All over
the country, bathrooms, sluices, gas stoves and radiators were hastily
installed in dozens of houses and mansions' (Ferguson and Fitzgerald,
1954, p. 32). The improvised accommodation included a two-bed unit
in an occupied private house, four beds in a midwife's house, and some
in a farmhouse, a boys' club, and a disused block of a public assistance
institution. In Glasgow, the Department of Health for Scotland com-
mandeered Lennox Castle (125 beds in 1943) as an emergency maternity home. When the Medical Officer of Health asked the mothers how
they liked it, they said it was a grand idea because they could get a
holiday at the same time (MacGregor, 1967).

By the end of 1939, some 6,000 confinements all over the country had
taken place in these emergency homes whose lasting significance was
that they introduced many women for the first time to the experience of
an institutional delivery. In Glasgow, for instance, the proportion of

births taking place in an institution rose by 20 per cent between 1939 and the early months of the war. In this way, it is probable that the shape of the wartime maternity services was at least a contributory factor in the sharp post-war upturn in the institutional delivery rate.

Wartime plans naturally upset the smooth running of existing maternity hospitals. The General Lying-in Hospital in London, for example, was instructed by the Ministry to close its door to in-patients because it was located in a vulnerable area. The hospital took over and staffed three buildings in St Albans, one of them said to be a former Bishop's Palace, and commonly referred to by hospital staff as 'just around the corner'. This was probably Diocesan House in Verulam Road, which enjoyed a later career as a nunnery. Hospital staff also took over the running of two other units, at Radlett and at Great Gaddesden, for the reception of expectant evacuees under the Government scheme. They kept on with local domiciliary work, though, which meant that 'In many instances babies were born during raids in basements or cellars, and antenatal visits were made to patients who had sought protection in public shelters' (Rhodes, 1977, p. 311). The hospital sought for Ministry permission to reopen the London antenatal clinic for those mothers who 'persistently' applied for help and who were willing to go to St Albans for the actual delivery. The request came during the period of the 'phoney war', when the expected attack on civilians did not materialize, and the evacuated mothers-to-be trekked back to their London homes. The clinic was duly reopened, and a scheme worked out whereby the mothers attending it were taken by London County Council ambulance to St Albans about two weeks before their due date 'to a house practically adjoining the hospital, which we furnished for the purpose, and where the mothers enjoy a restful home life under the kindly eye of the Assistant Matron prior to being sent to the hospital building for the actual confinement' (p. 306). The Hospital's Annual Report for 1940 called this arrangement beneficial to 'the peace of mind of the patient and of the husband, who is perhaps a member of the Forces, or away from home engaged in work of national importance and unable to give his moral support' (p. 310).

The General Lying-in Hospital's services were extremely popular, and by 1943 it was recorded that so great was the demand for them that many mothers were booking eight months in advance. In June 1946 the St Albans department was closed, and bomb damage repairs on the York Road building in London meant an opportunity to adapt the ordinary peace-time accommodation so as to raise the total number of beds, carry out improvements in lighting and heating, and supply a new resource referred to in the minutes of the Committee of Management as 'Babies' Bathrooms'.

The number of emergency maternity beds in England and Wales provided during the war reached a peak of 3,150 in 1941, when 27,868 babies were born in them. However, the occupancy rate was never more than two-thirds; mothers failed to use them as much as they might have done. Records of these emergency maternity homes show that the stillbirth and maternal and infant mortality rates were all respectably, even surprisingly, low. The Ministry also arranged hostel accommodation antenatally and postnatally. There were 17 antenatal hostels providing 308 beds in 1939, 58 with 1,360 beds in 1941, and, during the busiest year, 1944, 176 with 3,819 beds. By then hostel accommodation had virtually replaced private billets. But, throughout the period of emergency, the Ministry faced a problem to which it never found an answer — the reluctance of expectant mothers to avail themselves of the new arrangements. Supply exceeded demand by a politically uncomfortable margin every year of the war. In fact, the gap between the numbers of people in the priority classes entitled to evacuation and the number who chose to go was some three and a half million. In contrast to the four million evacuees predicted, less than half a million actually materialized.

The problem was evident from the first day of the evacuation scheme. Instead of the expected 140,000 pregnant women, only 12,300 turned up. Many mothers-to-be were simply less afraid of bombs than of unfamiliar surroundings. Moreover, many changed their minds and left the reception areas for home before the delivery. Others removed themselves as soon as possible after the birth. The result was chaos and confusion: 'Secondary schoolboys of 17 were presented at billets in place of mothers with young children, while mothers in the last weeks and even hours of pregnancy, arrived instead of unaccompanied schoolchildren' (Titmuss, 1950, p. 107). Midwifery training schools moved to the reception areas found themselves without teaching material, or in the cities mothers who refused to leave found themselves without midwives. Many maternity and child welfare centres became civil defence posts. By mid-1942, mothers who attended antenatal clinics and were expected to have normal confinements were refused hospital beds. They either had to have their babies at home or be evacuated. Some accepted what was close to a compulsory evacuation policy, while others were most indignant at this curtailment of their freedom of choice, and as a mark of protest refused all antenatal care and made no arrangements for the confinement. Another protest strategy, used by some 20 per cent of eligible women, was to register for evacuation and then not appear. Most of these women ended up being admitted as emergency cases to their nearest hospitals when labour had started, a form of gatecrashing that added to the dislocation in the services, and was not appreciated by those who had the job of ensuring their smooth functioning.

Educating people about motherhood

Despite the hiccoughs, there is no doubt that the exercise of organizing temporary homes and care for large numbers of mothers and children displaced from their normal environments was educational, in both an administrative and a wider social sense. Administratively, the evacuation scheme was a nightmare executed with superlative efficiency on the basis of such thoroughly imbibed trivia as railway timetables and the holding capacities of the bladders of children of different ages. Socially, the meeting of town and country, of working class and middle class, starkly exposed the nation for the first time to an awareness of the condition of all its people: 'Conservative and Labour supporters, Roman Catholics and Presbyterians, lonely spinsters and loud-mouthed, boisterous mothers, the rich and the poor, city-bred Jews and agricultural labourers, the lazy and the hard-working, the sensitive and the tough, were thrown into daily intimate contact' (Titmuss, 1950, p. 112). In particular, the condition of evacuated mothers and children came as a shock to many, and not only because of the prevalence of lice on the evacuated heads. The policy of evacuation led to a perceptible, almost measurable widening of government responsibility for the alleviation of distress of all kinds among all classes. It was in this sense that the war was, in Richard Titmuss's phrase (p. 509), 'most fruitful for social policy and action'. One cause of its fruitfulness was that, instead of relying on 'the family' to provide for individual health and subsistence needs, the government had to step in and do so instead. At the peak of the war some two and a half million husbands were living away from their wives and children. In a whole variety of ways, families were no longer self-sufficient. With many wives and mothers out at work, the traditional burden of community care for the young, the old, and the ill could not be assumed to lie on women's shoulders alone. Applications from men away in the army for 'compassionate leave' — an interesting concept — were one sign of strain: these ran at a persistently high level throughout the war (and less than 60 per cent were granted) (Ferguson and Fitzgerald, 1954, p. 9).

If the goals of welfare were thus advanced during the war, it was a broad conception of welfare that was at stake. Not surprisingly, then, this same soil nourished a broad conception of antenatal care also. In the official histories of the war there is scarcely any mention of the import-ance (or extent) of clinical antenatal care. According to some commenta-tors on this period of Britain's history, women during the war did on the whole take their antenatal care responsibilities seriously, and begin to attend earlier in pregnancy (see Winter, 1981; Duncan, et al., 1952); but the evidence is sparse. They needed to attend in order to have their priority food certificates signed, but what impact, if any, this had on their clinical care we do not know. There was not likely to have been an increase in the amount of antenatal care carried out by doctors, since one of the direct effects of the war was a doctor shortage: between 1939 and 1943, the number of doctors in the public health services fell by over 20 per cent. GPs were reduced by a third, and 10 per cent of those still working were over seventy (Titmuss, 1950, p. 530).

Feeding 'the raw material of the race'

What did happen was, in a sense, a return to pre-twentieth century notions of antenatal care. Although medical authorities after the turn of the century had continued to emphasize the importance attached in the nineteenth century to a holistic approach to pregnancy care (a good diet, sufficient rest and exercise, etc.), the tide had gradually been moving away from this view and towards a more mechanical notion of antenatal care. During the war the Government reversed this trend, and implemented policies of commitment to a broader definition of what constitutes good antenatal care.

Diet was the first matter requiring attention. The national milk scheme was introduced in July 1940, with the aim of providing for every child under five, and for all expectant and nursing mothers in Britain, a pint of milk daily at 2d a pint instead of the normal 4½d; very low-income families got the milk free. The cost of the scheme was borne by the Exchequer and it was administered by the Ministry of Food, a body established in May 1940 to ensure the equitable distribution of food in wartime. The transfer of responsibility for food policy to the Ministry of Food came as something of a relief to the Ministry of Health, which had been worried about the failure of an earlier scheme to supply cheap/free milk via the maternity and child welfare authorities. The interest of both Ministries in the matter was continuous with the stress given from the early days of the infant welfare movement on the key role of dietary supplementation, especially milk, in promoting health.

At the time the National Milk Scheme was introduced, per capita consumption of milk in Britain was little higher than it had been before the First World War, but the middle classes consumed about three times more than the working classes. The scheme was instantly successful. Unlike the wartime maternity bed situation, demand was far in excess of what was anticipated. By 1945, take-up of the milk was running at 178 million gallons, as against an estimated 60–70 million. About 70 per cent of those entitled to participate were doing so: the figure for 1943 was even higher, 90 per cent. Intriguing evidence of the decline in poverty over the period of the war was provided by the fact that the proportion of families in the low income category who received the milk free, fell from 30 per cent in 1940 to 2 per cent in 1945, despite the fact that the 'means' test applied made no allowance for increases in the cost of living. The milk scheme, together with the school milk and meals provision, did, very definitely, bring about a more equitable national distribution of available resources. Milk consumption rose relatively little (5–20 per cent) over the period 1935–1944 in the more wealthy South of England towns, but by a much larger amount (200–400 per cent) in Northern industrial towns.

From August 1940 the liquid milk was supplemented by the addition of a 'national dried milk' for babies, a substance that was still popular among mothers some 30 years later. The subsidy on national dried milk made it from a half to a third the price of commercial baby food, which angered the manufacturers a good deal. From 1944 the milk was fortified with vitamin D on the advice of the British Paediatric Association, and again contrary to the interests of the commercial manufacturers, who saw this as a subtle move to transform the milk into a 'composite food'. Vitamin supplements were themselves provided under a second national scheme. The vitamin welfare scheme was introduced in December 1941, because of worries about the possible shortage of vitamins in the diets of young children due to the scarcity of certain foods, especially oranges, butter and eggs. The scheme started with free blackcurrant syrup or purée (for which purpose the Ministry took over the entire 1941 national blackcurrant crop), and cod liver oil for the under twos. A few months later orange juice was substituted for the blackcurrant syrup and a low price charged. The orange juice, in concentrated form, was obtained from the USA on lease lend, and also survived for many years, becoming popular among the wealthier classes as an additive to gin in their pre-dinner drinks.[2]

---

2. Pamela Craig, personal communication. It seems that in some areas at least the blackcurrant syrup continued to be available.

In 1942 the vitamin welfare scheme was extended, so that all expectant and nursing mothers and under fives who were getting free or cheap milk would also get free or cheap orange juice and cod liver oil. Since pregnant women sometimes found the oil unpalatable, vitamin A and D tablets were introduced as an alternative. The Ministry of Food defined the principle underlying these schemes with admirable clarity; it was the determination to supply to pregnant women and young children 'whatever they needed, not only for an adequate, but for a full diet ... The raw material of the race is too valuable to be put at risk' (House of Commons Debate, 1943, cited in Ferguson and Fitzgerald, 1954, p. 162).

The national milk and vitamin welfare schemes took their place within the framework of broad schemes for the wartime distribution of all scarce resources according to need. Indeed, so wide was the Ministry of Health's concern that it kept an anxious eye on many of the supply shortages that more properly fell under the aegis of the Board of Trade — for example prams, rubber teats and knickers, chamber pots and sanitary towels. Teats, especially, became a problem in the summer of 1944, due partly to an insufficient appreciation of the effect women's mobilization would have on the breastfeeding rate. The supply of condoms also suffered in the rubber shortage, but this, although undoubtedly a matter of great concern to the civilian population, embarrassed the Government to such an extent that the Minister was forced to declare 'No direct concern in the matter' (Ferguson and Fitzgerald, 1954, p. 12).

Rationing of food could less obliquely highlight the special needs of the fertile population; for example, the normal weekly allocation for an adult was one egg, but expectant mothers and under fives received an allocation of four. Take-up of rationed food was 100 per cent but take-up of the cheap or free vitamins was not as good as had been the case with the milk scheme. The Ministry of Health gave the overall figures at the end of the war as 46 per cent for fruit juice, 21 per cent for cod liver oil and 34 per cent for vitamin tablets (CMO, 1946). The Ministry of Food gave somewhat higher figures — 57 per cent, 30 per cent and 45 per cent respectively (quoted in Titmuss, 1950, p. 514). But even citing the lower figure, the Ministry felt able to declare that

The national provision of milk and vitamin supplements to the priority groups has probably done more than any other single factor to promote the health of expectant mothers and young children during the war, and this scheme, together with rationing and the greatly improved nutritional qualities of the national loaf has contributed to the gradual decline in the maternal, neonatal and infant mortality and stillbirth rates, so noteworthy in the last five years (quoted in Titmuss, 1950, p. 93).

The healthy effect of war

In 1944 no less a person than the Minister of Health had declared that he was proud to hold office at a time when the infant mortality rate was the lowest on record; the neonatal mortality rate was the lowest on record; the maternal mortality rate was the lowest on record; the still-birth rate was the lowest on record; and the birth-rate was the highest for 15 years. (See figures A.1–A.5, pp. 296–298.) According to these indices, the Second World War was the best thing that had happened to pregnant women for a long time, indeed, since the First World War, which had itself gestated the idea of antenatal care.

What had accounted for this dramatic improvement in survival chances for mothers and babies? 'This cannot be just an accident' muttered the Chief Medical Officer at the Ministry of Health, 'All that's been done to safeguard mothers and children must have had some effect' (Ferguson and Fitzgerald, 1954, p. 171). Nevertheless proof is hard to come by. The first conclusion it is safe to draw is that, contrary to expectation and despite the enormous dislocation in medical care services for pregnant women, the war did not make things substantially worse. Over the period from 1939–42 deaths to older babies (post-neonatal and infant mortality rates) rose slightly, probably reflecting an impact of the social hazards of war — it is known that these rates are especially responsive to social conditions. In this respect it is possible that the war caused a temporary deterioration in what was a long-term downward trend in infant mortality, which was successfully re-established in the second half of the war, from 1943–45. By 1939 improvements in mortality and associated improvements in the national diet were certainly already being commented on by policy-makers (Winter, 1979). But during the first half of the war, neonatal mortality did not alter, nor did the death-rate for illegitimate infants, nor did maternal mortality, and nor did the stillbirth rate. The stillbirth rate, however, had fallen dramatically by the end of the war — by about 30 per cent in England and Wales, the largest fall ever recorded. The greatest improvement took place in the mining regions of South Wales and in industrial

Lancashire and Cheshire. The wartime improvement in the stillbirth rate was a world-wide phenomenon, and can be seen in most countries for which reliable data exist. After the end of the war the improvement slowed down everywhere, hesitated or even reversed itself. A consistently downward trend in neonatal mortality was also noted during the war in some other countries (Duncan, et al., 1952).

What was the cause of the contrast between 1939–42 and 1943–45, and why did the stillbirth rate improve so markedly and consistently? It was during the latter period of the war that the economic and social policies of the Coalition Government were most likely to have had an effect — not only the milk and vitamin schemes, but also the control of inflation. From late 1942, and as a result of the Government's action to keep prices down, the index of weekly wage rates overtook the cost of living index. A progressive tax structure simultaneously helped to redistribute income away from the middle classes and towards the waged working class. There was, of course, full employment at home, and employment among women was unusually high: about 800,000 women who would not ordinarily have gone out to work had joined the labour force by 1943 (Central Office of Information, 1944). The war challenged gender stereotypes and conventions — nearly two million workers in munitions factories changed sex in the USA; 'Rosie the Riveter', the woman with an acetylene torch, became a national heroine, and for the first time in British history, service women became eligible to receive military decorations. It is most unlikely that women's psychological health did not benefit in many subtle and not-so-subtle ways from this temporary liberation.

When the nature of the fall in the stillbirth rate is examined, it is clear that the main fall took place in the 'ill-defined and unknown' causes of death, suggesting that the basic advance was in the physiological efficiency with which pregnant women were gestating fetuses (as well as an enhanced statistical interest in defining the different causes of death). Ian Sutherland, an Oxford epidemiologist, published in 1949 an analysis of the epidemiology of stillbirths in which he attempted to answer the question as to whether antenatal care itself could have been responsible for the wartime improvement. He obtained from Medical Officers of Health in the county boroughs of England and Wales returns on the total number of antenatal clinic attendances and home visits to pregnant women for each year from 1934 to 1945. He then constructed complex indices of the quantity of antenatal care, and looked at these indices in relation to mean stillbirth rates. To his surprise, he found no correlation. 'The indices of antenatal care have imperfections', he conceded, 'but it is extremely doubtful whether they are so imperfect as to account for the entire lack of correlation' (Sutherland, 1949, p. 74).

There are thus three basic explanations of the apparently beneficial effect of the war on national health: (1) the underlying long-term trend towards more national health care and social service provision (of which clinical antenatal care was but a small part); (2) the specific income- and diet-equalizing policies of the wartime Government; (3) longer-term changes — in the ages and obstetric experiences of mothers, affecting the overall risks of death, as well as changes in nutrition, and in other factors in mothers' own childhoods, showing their benefit a generation later. The three explanations are not, of course, necessarily in competition with one another: all are likely to be right. Beneficient forces of many kinds joined hands during the Second World War to protect the health of mothers and children: full employment, food subsidies, price controls, welfare foods, no disastrous epidemic (a piece of extraordinary good luck). The strange fact that, despite the repeated bombing of water mains and sewers, no single case of typhoid attributable to the water supply was recorded during the war, was evidence of *generational* improvements in the nation's health and resistance to disease.

The population in 1940 was simply in better health than the population in 1920 or 1910. Thus, in contrast to the dismal unfitness of army recruits at the time of the Boer War (discussed in chapter 2), only 2.3 per cent of army applicants in 1939 were pronounced unfit. In England and Wales in 1901–10, expectation of life at birth stood at 48.5 years for a boy and 52.4 years for a girl; by 1939, the figures were 60.2 and 64.4 years. Mothers who were bearing children in the late 1940s were almost certainly fitter than those who were doing so in the 1920s or early 1900s. The legacy of infantile rickets and pelvic deformity was on the decline, and there were signs that mothers were becoming more resistant to some of the traditional scourges of childbearing (the drop in the case-fatality rate of puerperal sepsis being one example).

In its 1944 *Report on a National Maternity Service*, the Royal College of Obstetricians and Gynaecologists favoured the interpretation that social and economic factors, especially increased purchasing power and the food subsidies, had played an important role in the lowered stillbirth and neonatal mortality rate, and to some extent in the decline in maternal mortality. They published in this connection a rather interesting table which appeared originally in the 1930 Registrar-General's decennial supplement on occupational mortality. The table shows a higher mortality in Social Class I (by husband's occupation) than Social Class V for all causes of puerperal death except haemorrhage during the years

1930–2. The Committee found itself quite unable to explain the meaning of the table, beyond noting that Social Class I and II mothers tended to have their babies at an older and hence less favourable age than Social Class V mothers; but this reversal of the usual rule that being middle class was better for one's health was widely regarded as truly alarming. It was also seen as evidence relevant to the wartime debate about the strength of environmental versus medical care effects on health.

A country fit for babies

In a book suitably entitled *Battle for Health* and published in 1944, a Dr Stephen Taylor wrote about a different kind of war, the war for health that was synonymous with civilization:

> The battle for health is not fought only in hospitals and laboratories, and at the bedside of sick people. It is fought in Parliament and on the Borough Council, in the factory and in the mine, in fields where food is grown, and shops where it is sold, in the school and in the home . . . We are all of us in this war (Taylor, 1944, p. 9).

Taylor's book was a plea for health to be seen as a social as well as a medical product: in both respects it reflected the mood of the times. Everybody wanted the wartime improvement in health to be maintained after the end of hostilities. Saving mothers was not mentioned by Taylor, but saving babies was: he included tables showing the well-known pattern of international and intranational social class differences in infant mortality, and he went on to ask:

> What are we to do to save our babies? What must Spain and Portugal, Malta and India do to save theirs? First, we must get rid of overcrowding; and we must do it without producing poverty by raising rents in the process. This is a battle we must all fight — the battle for better homes. These homes must have proper washing facilities, food-storage space, and drainage. Next, we must feed our expectant mothers and their babies.
> In Britain this is not something new but a continuation of what we are doing now. In the world, it means to each nation what food it needs; not what it can afford. German babies have not sinned; we shall have to feed them too (Taylor, 1944, p. 111).

Babies were in the news again:

> From one end of Britain to another; from the gay, smooth opulence of

London's West End flats to the massed, grimy towns of Lancashire; from the inarticulate bravery of the Rhondda Valley to the glowing homeliness of huddled English villages, men and women are having smaller and smaller families. Millions of parents are revolting against parenthood and these millions of individual decisions are collectively expressed in a falling birth-rate pointing ultimately to extinction (Titmuss and Titmuss, 1942, p. 11).

The Minister of Health may have congratulated himself in 1944 that the birth-rate was higher than it had been for 15 years, but there was no doubt that the long-term trend was downward. This was a public fact by 1936, when the prospect of a dwindling population led to the Population Investigation Committee, consisting of an assortment of specialists from various fields, and headed by the future director of the London School of Economics, Professor A. M. Carr-Saunders. This Committee, jointly with the RCOG, was to commission the first national survey of maternity in Britain in 1946. By March 1944 the perceived problem of the falling birth-rate had become so urgent that a Royal Commission on Population was appointed to find out what was really going on, and why, and what could be done about it. In phrases reminiscent of that earlier concern with population quantity and quality (see p. 34) the Royal Commission, in a statement in September 1945, referred to the far-reaching effects of a continued fall in the birth-rate on 'British social and economic life, on migration to the Dominions, and on Britain's position among the nations'. Behind all such considerations, opined the Commission, 'lies the ultimate threat of a gradual fading out of the British people' (Royal Commission on the Population, 1945, p. 5).

Why was there such a shortage of babies — a puzzle of direct relevance to antenatal care? That champion of the cause of infant welfare, G. F. McCleary, returned to the fray with a book called *Race Suicide* published in the same year (1945). In this he disputed the 'density theory' propounded at the time, apparently by reference to the behaviour of fruit flies reared on banana pulp in bottles of known cubic capacity. The fruit flies eventually stopped multiplying, and human beings, said McCleary, would ultimately do the same. Birth control was not the cause of the decline — no more than was the weapon with which Othello stabbed himself the cause of his suicide. *The Times* sided with the view that a family allowance system was desirable to raise the number of babies, but observed there was more than a single reason for family limitation. 'The care of children adds greatly to the duties and ties of the home and restricts opportunities for social life and leisure; and the home without children, or with no more than one child, has come to be the end of marriage for numbers of married people' (*The Times*, 25 June 1942). Margery Spring Rice (author of *Working Class Wives*) in 'An Essay on Population', published in the *Fortnightly Review* (August 1942), doubted that a family allowance of 5s a week per child would actually constitute sufficient inducement for people to have children. At the Health Congress of the Royal Sanitary Institute in 1938, it was said, not inappropriately, that the tendency to have fewer children would not be halted until the tendency for maternity to become a major operation was itself halted (*The Times*, 6 July 1938).

It was, of course, a topic on which everyone felt qualified to comment. The Workers' Educational Association (WEA) produced a pamphlet, 'The Future of the Family', in which they gave their own reasons for the decline — criminal abortion, fear of pregnancy and childbirth (the remedy for which they suggested, with an enlightened air, was not more analgesia but training in 'natural childbirth'), increasing 'neurasthenia' leading to avoidance of sex, knowing too much about the dangers of reproduction, the emancipation of women, the relative attraction of motor cars as opposed to babies (the annual cost of running a car being said to equal the annual upkeep of one or two children) (WEA, n.d.).

Determined to penetrate the fog of these conflicting theories, Mass Observation carried out a survey of *Britain and her Birth Rate* in 1945. They interviewed 1,000 married women, aged between twenty and forty-five, in London and in Gloucestershire. In the East End of London 12 per cent of the women interviewed said they would want more children if they did not have to go through so much in the process of birth. Fear of the pain of labour and of the chances of dying were mentioned as they had not been earlier in the century (for instance, in *Maternity: Letters from Working Women* in 1915) — thus giving weight to the WEA theory. Younger women protested about the lack of facilities for the poor — the lack of beds and of analgesia:

> The hospitals for poor people should be made as comfortable as the rich nursing homes are. Rich people don't suffer, why should we? And they should make more beds available *now*.

> What is being done to make childbirth easier? Is anything being done? Or are all our brilliant doctors and specialists still content to tell us that childbrith is a 'natural function'? (Mass Observation, 1945, p. 113).

Around a quarter of the women interviewed for the Mass Observation study gave insufficient money as a deterrent, about one in six the responsi-bility and work of children. Lack of domestic help was very important — Britain was rapidly entering the phase when the only servant a man of any class could expect to keep was his wife (Galbraith, 1974). A third of the Mass Observation women said having more help in the house would make a difference to their desired family size.

The public debate in the late 1930s and 1940s about the population problem was not a debate about antenatal care, but it did engender a very full discussion of all aspects of parenthood, and this had the effect of placing the supposed benefits of medical care in pregnancy and childbirth squarely in the context of the overall meaning of maternity to women, to families and to the nation. It put into perspective the myopic vision of the 1920s and early 1930s, when clinical antenatal care was hailed as the miracle answer to an elastic range of problems. It paved the way for the NHS, which was born in the post-war eulogy of mother and child: 'The birth rate may have fallen in Britain, but we are still proud of our babies' (Leybourne-White and White, 1945, p. 33). The purpose of the NHS was to create a better and still healthier world for Britain's babies — and a world in which women would be happy to bear them.

6
Doctors' Dilemmas: antenatal care
1945–60

Perhaps the young lady was right when, to the question, 'with whom would you like to be wrecked on a desert island?' she replied 'an obstetrician'. She may have been voicing the opinion of the public, who are making a great demand on hospital confinement and specialist care, because they know it is safer.

Russell, 1956, p. 682

In 1937, 40 per cent of British babies were born in institutions: by 1959 this figure had risen to 64 per cent. Place of birth and the organization of antenatal care are intimately linked. When most babies are born at home, the logic of intranatal and antenatal care vests control with the community services — with the GPs, the midwives and the Medical Officers of the local health authorities. With the centralization of care in hospital, antenatal care itself eventually becomes an increasingly hospital-based service.

A survey of motherhood: maternity in Great Britain in 1946

In the spring of 1946, 13,687 newly-delivered British mothers were interviewed by health visitors about their experiences of maternity. The focus of this first exercise in national perinatal surveillance was in many ways unique; it represented an attempt to find out what impact the maternity services had upon the women who used them, particularly whether the services helped women 'to regard childbearing as a normal process' and what it cost parents to have a baby.

Maternity in Great Britain began with antenatal care. As its authors observed, the criticisms made of antenatal care were, by 1946, old hat, but 'it is remarkable that there is an almost total lack of reliable statistics to enable the achievements of the service to be measured' (Joint Committee, 1948, p. 23). The only national statistics available were published by the Ministry of Health, and gave figures for the number of

pregnant women attending antenatal clinics or coming under GP antenatal schemes. No national data were available on the clinical content of
antenatal care.

Table 6.1 shows type of antenatal supervision for the *Maternity in
Great Britain* mothers. Only 0.9 per cent of women did not receive any
antenatal care, and of those who did receive care, about three-quarters
obtained it from local authority sources. Interpretation of the figures
sent in by the health authorities[1] was complicated by the fact that many
submitted figures for the number of women attending for antenatal care
which were higher than the number of notified births. This discrepancy
led to the realization that even the crude data supplied by the Ministry
were unreliable, since the yearly figure included women whose first
attendance had been in the previous year but were still on the books.[2]

Table 6.1 Antenatal Supervision: Maternity in Great Britain Survey 1946

% of mothers receiving antenatal care from:								
Local Authorities			Private Sources					
								No.
	GP	Mid-			Mid-			of
Clinics	Schemes	Wives	Specialists	Practitioners	Wives	Nobody	Total	cases
%	%	%	%	%	%	%	%	
54.4	5.0	13.5	1.4	22.5	2.3	0.9	100.0	13,650
	72.9			26.2				

source: Joint Committee of the Royal College of Obstetricians and Gynaecologists, *Maternity in
Great Britain*, 1948, p. 26. With Permission of the publisher Oxford University Press.

The health visitors who did the interviewing for *Maternity in Great
Britain* asked mothers when in pregnancy they first went for antenatal
care and how many times they did so. The average time for the first
attendance varied from 19 to 24 weeks before delivery, and the average
number of attendances per pregnancy was eight. Private doctors and
hospital antenatal clinics 'achieved' the highest proportions of first
trimester attendances — 51.3 per cent and 41.2 per cent respectively.
Social factors were important: early attendance for antenatal care was

1. Local health authorities sent in to the Ministry of Health annual figures for antenatal
   attendances. Since there was some confusion about the basis on which these figures were
   calculated, for *Maternity in Great Britain* the MOHs for ten country boroughs were asked how
   they interpreted the Ministry's question (which was one about the 'total number of women who
   [attended] clinics during the year').

2. This qualification needs to be borne in mind wherever these figures are cited in this book.

more a first pregnancy, higher social class, than a fourth pregnancy, lower social class habit. The authors of *Maternity in Great Britain* noted that these differences would be difficult to iron out, since they reflected characteristics of a universal nature: a survey done in Michigan, USA, a decade before had come up with very similar findings.

As to the *content* of antenatal care, the 1946 surveyors of British motherhood did not feel that mothers could be regarded as reliable sources of data on this matter. 'Field studies' were consequently done in five maternity and child welfare authorities to fill the information gap. These indicated that

> Judging by the entries on record cards in the five authorities visited, blood-pressures are taken and urines tested at the majority, but not at all attendances at antenatal clinics. Additional examinations were carried out by some authorities; thus, in Kent, nearly all primigravidae were rhesus-grouped and, at the thirty-second week, had X-ray measurements taken of their pelves (Joint Committee, 1948, pp. 44–5).

The local health authorities varied in the number of times an expectant mother was examined by a doctor. However, it was pointed out by the authors of *Maternity in Great Britain*, that it could not be assumed that frequent examination by a doctor was a good thing; indeed, there was a 'danger that, if there is a doctor's consultation at each visit, the abnormal side of pregnancy will be emphasized. In addition, midwives will be deprived of an interesting and useful side of their work. Most important of all, however, this practice tends to hurried and inadequate consultations' (p. 45). One such unlucky subject was a 16-week pregnant primigravida, attending for the first time. The doctor who saw her had already seen 29 women in 80 minutes:

> A health visitor interviewed the expectant mother outside the consultation room and recorded details of her history and present symptoms. The woman then removed her stockings and knickers behind a screen and, otherwise fully clothed, entered the consultation room attended by her midwife and the health visitor. Here she lay on a couch, her dress was pulled up, and her abdomen hurriedly palpated. The doctor listened to the foetal heart and asked two or three questions about a minor symptom of which she was complaining. No further examination was made and the doctor took no detailed history. It was three minutes from the time she entered the consulting-room till the time she left (Joint Committee, p. 45).

As we shall see, there is a startling continuity in descriptions of such doctor–patient encounters in antenatal care over the whole period from 1946 to 1982.

On the matter of effectiveness, *Maternity in Great Britain* lapsed into a methodological simple-mindedness that has since achieved notoriety among epidemiologists. The analysis selected the proportion of mothers breastfeeding at eight weeks as an index of antenatal care's effectiveness (on the dubious grounds that infant feeding method varies little with social class and that the promotion of breastfeeding should be an important function of antenatal care). Since a linear relationship was found between frequency of antenatal supervision and the proportion breastfeeding (the most supervised women being the most lactating ones) it was concluded that frequent antenatal care is a cause of high breastfeeding rates. This provoked the alarming conclusion that the quality of antenatal supervision was a more important influence on breastfeeding than any other factor 'biological, social or economic' (*Maternity in Great Britain*, p. 162). (See Appendix 2 on this subject.)

Antenatal care and the National Health Service

The idea of an integrated health service which would be free to the user at the time of use was not new when the NHS Act was passed in 1946 (1947 in Scotland). It had been publicly debated in one form or another for more than 25 years (Ross, 1952; Honigsbaum, 1979; Abel-Smith, 1964). So far as the maternity services were concerned, comprehensive health care removed from the constraints of the insurance principle had long been envisaged by some groups as the only workable solution to the problem of improving reproductive survival and health.

The form the Health Service took when the Act came into operation on 5 July 1948, represented the outcome of a long process of negotiation and struggle between central and local government and the various branches of the medical profession (see Gill, 1980; Honigsbaum, 1979; Stevens, 1966). It also marked, and gave administrative expression to, a longer historical process of growing divisions within medicine. These divisions were to prove a particular embarrassment to the smooth running of the Health Service's maternity care sector; indeed, the balance of power between GP, specialist hospital obstetrician and local health authority providers (the 'tripartite' structure) manifested in the NHS Act was to set the stage for an enduring conflict between the different providers of maternity care (see Gill, 1971).

Under the NHS Act, responsibility for maternity care was divided between hospital authorities, local executive councils (representing the GPs) and local health authorities. The hospital authorities were responsible for hospital maternity beds and out-patient antenatal and postnatal treatment. The hospitals provided antenatal and postnatal care for their own booked patients, an out-patient consultation service for others, and specialist domiciliary consultations and emergency obstetric services ('flying squads'). The executive councils made contracts with GPs providing maternity medical services, which covered antenatal and postnatal care and delivery in some cases. GPs on the obstetric list could provide care for any patient who applied to them, while those not on the obstetric list could give maternity medical services only to their own patients. (On the other hand, they could choose not to do so.) The matter of an obstetric list differentiating between two classes of GPs was fiercely resisted by the BMA in the pre-NHS Act negotiations, and for many years afterwards, on the grounds that every GP was legally qualified to practise midwifery.[3]

The local health authorities provided domiciliary midwifery services — antenatal and postnatal and delivery care, ambulance, health visitor and home-help services. Local authority antenatal clinics gave care both to domiciliary midwife-booked cases, as well as interim antenatal care for hospital-booked cases and some GP-booked cases. This meant theoretically that a pregnant woman could receive antenatal care from three sources — the municipal clinic, the hospital and the GP, each of which might be doing something different, and none of which was obliged to communicate with the others. Lack of communication between the local authority clinic, the GP and the hospital services, always a problem, became even more of one under the NHS, since there were many more women involved in more than one type of care. Not until 1958 did some local health authorities introduce maternity co-operation cards, and in that year in only 18 per cent of local health authorities was co-ordination of maternity services considered by the Ministry to be satisfactory (CMO, 1959). The disjointed picture of antenatal provision characterising the 1950s and 1960s is illustrated in figure A.9 p. 303 and figure A.13, p. 305.

As the Committee of Enquiry into the Cost of the NHS in 1956 (the Guillebaud Committee) and the Report of the Maternity Services Committee in 1959 (the Cranbrook Report) both noted, the working of the tripartite structure produced a most confused situation. There were

---

3. GPs in Scotland did not have to have a special obstetric qualification in order to undertake maternity work.

regional differences in the degree and type of confusion. In some places GPs actually staffed the local authority antenatal clinics on a sessional basis. In other places the local authority antenatal clinics had ceased to provide any medical care, concentrating solely on education. Or GPs might use the local authority clinic midwives at their own clinics — and so on. And who paid for the services of a GP called in an emergency in a home delivery of a patient for whom she/he had not undertaken to provide care? The local authority or the executive council?[4]

A dying breed: the local authority antenatal clinic

Within a few years of its birth, it was recognized that the NHS had effectively killed the local authority antenatal clinic as the main structure providing for the clinical surveillance of pregnancy in Britain.

Before the NHS, the municipal clinics had constituted the only source of free antenatal care for most childbearing women. They provided a type of care that integrated social, educational and clinical aspects over the whole period of pregnancy and early motherhood. They existed in the community, and, for the most part, were easily accessible to their clients. Their clinical and educational curricula may have been guided by a somewhat patronizing view of mothers — as needing to be 'educated' into motherhood — but at least their location in the community meant that the service they offered was based on some appreciation of mothers' actual circumstances and needs. The NHS altered this situation overnight by providing two competing venues for free antenatal care — the GP's surgery and the hospital clinic.

The result was evident in Ministry of Health figures: total antenatal attendances at local authority clinics fell by 21 per cent between 1949 and 1955 (Cranbrook Report, 1959), and by 1955 there were almost a million more hospital than local authority antenatal clinic attendances yearly. Payments for GP maternity work showed a big increase over the same period, 1948–55, though figures were not available for the total annual number of antenatal visits made to GPs (CMO, 1964). Of those local authority clinical antenatal sessions that did still take place, a third were attended by midwives alone, and the average number of attendances per patient was less than five, suggesting that at best the local authority sector was merely supplementing GP and hospital ante-

---

4. The local authority.

natal care (Godber, 1963). By the time of the second big national survey of maternity in Britain in 1958, only 15 per cent of births had been preceded by any local authority antenatal care (Butler and Bonham, 1963) — a decline of 58 per cent since 1946. On figure A.9, p. 303, the line 'women attending community clinics' shows a decline from the late 1940s which accelerates in the early 1960s.

Most important of all the factors responsible for the demise of local authority care was that pregnant women could now exercise some choice as to the type of care they wanted. Choice made the disadvantages (sometimes offsetting the advantages) of local authority antenatal care more obvious — the inability of the local authority medical officer to treat any disease or complication diagnosed, the discontinuity between the personnel carrying out pregnancy care and attending delivery. By choosing to go to her GP for antenatal care, a woman stood a better chance of assuring for herself continuity of care.

In the face of this changed reality, the local authority medical officers at first sought a new alliance with GPs. Instead of trying to keep GPs out of public health work, now they tried to get them in. They asked for more GP beds, more home deliveries, and for an administrative structure that would divide responsibility for the maternity services between the three sectors equally, rather than giving a disproportionate share to the hospital specialists. They knew that it would only be with the co-operation of GPs that maternity care in the public health sector would survive at all.

Increasing the power of the GP in this particular battle, and also widening the medical care horizons of many childbearing women, was the provision of the NHS Act that both a midwife and a doctor might now be booked for a normal delivery. (In Scotland this innovation had been introduced some years before, in the Maternity Services (Scotland) Act of 1937.) Before 1948 in England and Wales, midwives had been able to call a doctor to a confinement under the 'medical aid' rule of the CMB. As we saw in chapter 4, 'medical aid' cases were increasing in the 1930s, a development that probably signified a certain loss of confidence on the part of midwives in their ability to secure a normal delivery. But in 1948 most women having babies at home began to book a doctor for the delivery. This development immediately (though temporarily, as it turned out) gave more prominence and power to the role of the GP in maternity care.

Opponents of public health antenatal care had already before 1948 suggested that it should be limited to a purely educational exercise. After 1948, this suggestion acquired the force of a new dogma. 'What is the future for the local authority medical officer?' asked two commentators on the situation in 1954: 'It would be churlish not to pay tribute to the work of the clinic doctors' they conceded, 'who came into existence to provide adequate antenatal care at a time when this was not otherwise available, and it is no reflection on them to suggest that the work should be done by the patient's own GP where this is feasible. Moreover, the local health authority should continue to provide very important educational facilities — by holding mothercraft classes and antenatal exercise and relaxation sessions in the centre' (Redman and Walker, 1954, p. 43). The only letter responding to this plan, from doctors W. C. W. Nixon and Shîla G. Ransom (*British Medical Journal* 31 July 1954, p. 300) charitably observed that 'It seems a pity that "relaxation sessions" should be thrown to the local health authorities as a sort of consolation for its dwindling responsibility.' Figure A.10, p. 304, gives some information about the state of local authority provision for 'mothercraft' in the 1960s. The line is more or less level, though total births were falling, so there did indeed turn out to be some expansion in this field.

If an official lid still needed to be placed on the notion of local authority antenatal care, the Cranbrook Committee achieved this in its 1959 Report. 'We should like to pay a very warm tribute to the local authority medical officers for the maternity work done by them over a long period' recorded the Committee (pp. 41–2), again damning with faint praise. Though the Committee anticipated (rightly) that hospitals would ultimately share the maternity education function, in 1959 it could see no place apart from the local authority clinic where women booked for home delivery would be exposed to motherhood instruction.

The rise (and fall) of the GP

In the 1930s, it had looked as though the GP's stake in antenatal care might be lost altogether — particularly as unemployment drove increasing numbers of women to seek the free care of the public health system. Even chloroform, the GP's main countervailing attraction, was not sufficient at that time to assure her or him a safe niche in antenatal care. Instead, the niche was largely that of an 'emergency service in support of midwives' — fine for midwives, but not for GPs whose professional credibility demanded a more central role in maternity work.

The NHS reversed this trend, and gave both women and GPs a new and strong incentive to develop GP antenatal care. In fact, the NHS was nothing short of 'revolutionary' to GPs in giving the patient a direct route to GP care independently of both the specialist obstetrician and the midwife. Uniquely, too, the GPs were to receive a separate fee for midwifery services: the more cynical could thus point to the financial incentive GPs had to become good midwives. As a matter of fact, it was a provision of conditions of maternity work for GPs under the NHS that the fee was paid *irrespective* of whether the GP actually, in the event, attended the delivery. 'Time and multiparae wait for no man', observed a *Lancet* leader in 1949 (1 October, p. 611). The GP got his/her seven guineas for two antenatal and one postnatal examinations, and for going to the delivery *when necessary*. When E. V. Kuenssberg and S. A. Sklaroff sent questionnaires to Scottish GPs in 1956, they found that, of the 162 doing maternity work, 108 said they liked it. Presumably the remaining 54 were in it for the money, or out of a sense of duty (Kuenssberg and Sklaroff, 1958).

During the 1950s a number of surveys of the GPs' work showed how GPs had capitalized on the new opportunities. One of the first was an analysis by a Kent GP, Dr E. Tuckman, of midwifery work in a four-doctor partnership. In this practice the doctors had decided that one of them would specialize in obstetrics. After an initial examination by her own GP (including the testing of blood for haemoglobin estimation, blood grouping, Wasserman and Kahn tests and referral for a routine chest X-ray) every pregnant woman was seen by the practice's GP–obstetrician. Between September 1950 and August 1952, 94.7 per cent of the births occurring to patients on the lists of the four doctors were preceded by exclusively GP antenatal care. The first antenatal attendance took place before eight weeks in 21 per cent of these women; by 20 weeks, 81 per cent had been seen. The number of visits ranged from five to fifteen for 80 per cent of the women:

> At the first examination the GP obstetrician confirmed the diagnosis of pregnancy and carried out a general obstetric examination. Advice on the management of nausea and vomiting of early pregnancy was given in numerous cases, strengthened by the prescribing of anti-histamines in 32 patients (8.5 per cent). Drug treatment was continued beyond the 16th week in only 4 of these. Elastic stockings for varicose veins were prescribed for 13 patients, and 35 were given breast shields for the treatment of mal-developed nipples. Haemoglobin levels below 10gm per cent were found in 85 patients (22.5 per cent) and ferrous sulphate was prescribed. Forty-five women were Rhesus negative, and of 25 of the husbands of these patients tested, 21 were Rhesus positive (Tuckman, 1953, p. 467).

Tuckman's practice was not confined to clinical care. It was the custom for the doctors also to try to give the mothers confidence in themselves and their attendants. In other words, the mothers were talked to and 'simple explanations were offered'. There were, additionally, three courses of formal talks including diagrams, pictures and X-rays with titles such as 'What Goes On Inside You'.

This analysis of GP midwifery work showed one important feature of the GP's new role under the NHS: deciding which patients were not suitable for GP antenatal care, and which patients should merit a hospital delivery. As Dr Cookson put it, recalling his own evidence to the Cranbrook Committee on the desirability of GPs retaining normal deliveries, '70 per cent of patients can be delivered by a policeman in the back of a taxi, and get away with it. The only thing is to decide which 70 per cent' (I. C. I). The satisfactoriness of the GP's role in maternity care was increasingly judged on how effectively this exercise of risk-selection was carried out. GPs who wished to defend their role in maternity care began to publish analyses of the cases they had supervised, examining the overall safety of GP care (see, for example, Cookson, 1954; Howard, 1962; MacGregor and Martin, 1961). The issue was by this time not whether GP–obstetricians should exist, but what exactly it was safe to let them do. There were also those who defended the midway position of institutional care by the GP. Thus, Drs Jameson and Handfield-Jones (1954) wrote glowingly of the advantages of GP maternity work in a Cottage Hospital setting: doctors in four practices used it, they held their antenatal clinics in the hospital 'out-patient room', 'the day being chosen to fit in with the local bus services'.

The degree of commitment to maternity work among some GPs in this period was undoubtedly very high. Those with the highest levels of commitment invariably wanted a higher proportion of their patients to be delivered at home. Defence of GP obstetrics in the period following the beginning of the NHS thus tended to be linked to a defence of home delivery. But there were problems, one of which was GPs' lack of knowledge and skill. There were even some who suggested that the relative lack of trend in the stillbirth rate in the late 1940s and early 1950s was the fault of inefficient GPs. C. S. Russell, Professor of Obstetrics and Gynaecology at Sheffield University, referred to this in the following terms:

Some years ago a senior resident in a maternity hospital was asked on the telephone to take in a midwifery case. He was rather short of beds and thought he ought to ask the general practitioner some questions. He learned that the patient was in mountainous labour, but some of the other replies were so equivocal that finally, in desperation, he asked just what was presenting; was it a vertex? 'Oh, no', came the reply, 'nothing abnormal like that' (Russell, 1956, p. 682).

In a memorable reflection Russell concluded:

> I would like to push out of domiciliary midwifery those who are afraid of it, for they have no courage, and those who are not afraid of it, for they have no imagination; those who say there is nothing to it, and are prepared to go and do a case now and then, just to keep their hand in, for they have no understanding; and those who have no interest — for they have no soul (p. 684).

Having a soul meant tolerating conditions of work which, from the early 1960s on, many GPs were not prepared to tolerate. 'I remember one time', said Dr Cookson, staunch defender of GP obstetrics, 'when my wife was cutting sandwiches to go out for the day on a Sunday and the telephone rang and it was somebody in labour. So without saying a word she just stopped cutting sandwiches and started cooking the Sunday dinner. You don't get wives like that nowadays' (I. C. I).

Whatever happened to the midwife?

In many countries, including Britain, the antenatal care movement disturbed a long-established tradition of maternity care in which childbearing (whether normal or not) was the province of midwives. Following the 1902 Midwives' Act, and with the development of ante-natal care during the First World War, the proper sphere of midwives became that segment of childbearing which could be considered as 'normal'. In the early years of this century, a division thus developed *within* childbearing between the normal and the abnormal. Midwives became practitioners in the art of the normal, obstetricians in that of the abnormal. The matter did not rest there, however, because although the normal/abnormal distinction was to be consistently held to over many years, the boundaries round the two notions were to shift constantly. Whereas a breech delivery would have been normal, and thus handled by a midwife in 1918, it would be considered abnormal and the province of the obstetrician today (requiring a caesarean section in some places). While 70 per cent of childbirths were thought normal enough to be delivered at home in the 1930s, 70 per cent were identified as abnormal enough to be delivered in hospital in the 1950s (figure A.6, p. 299).

Changes in the age and parity of the childbearing population, or underlying changes in the condition of the nation's health, do not explain such large variations.

Before the NHS, midwives retained much of their traditional control over childbearing: they were the cheapest deliverers, opportunities for independent practice existed, and partly because they still had a considerable hold over maternity care, their activities and influence were respected by many doctors. When the NHS began, the situation for the midwife was not altogether clear. In one way the rot had set in, because the new NHS regulations codified the practice whereby a midwife attending a delivery at which a supervising doctor was also present stopped being a midwife: she became a 'maternity nurse'. Another consequence of the NHS for midwives was that the first point of contact for most pregnant women in future was not likely to be the midwife but the GP. The NHS gave women direct access to a doctor 'not only when the midwife arranged it'. This seemingly trivial administrative arrangement radically and permanently altered the midwives' control over maternity care. Dr Cookson recalls the impact of the NHS Act on midwives in his area:

> When the NHS gave patients the opportunity to go to a general practitioner for maternity services some midwives were dismayed. A senior midwife told me that they were 'bitterly disappointed but as it is in the regulations we shall have to conform'. But the midwives who encouraged their patients to go to a GP were in the minority. How did the patients react? If the general practitioner was interested in obstetrics they were glad to go to him, more so if the midwife approved. We have to remember that pre-NHS conditions ensured that some GPs were not experienced in obstetrics and might well refer their patients to midwives or clinics. (I. C. I.).

A Working Party was set up in 1947 to enquire into the reasons for a problem identified in the midwifery profession prior to the NHS, namely the shortage of midwives. The Report of this Working Party, which was published in 1949, was the first on the subject for two decades — since Janet Campbell's Report of the Departmental Committee on the Training and Employment of Midwives in 1929.

The Report, asking, 'What is the proper duty of a midwife?', provided the following answer:

> She should be the practitioner of normal midwifery: the expert in normal childbearing in all its varied aspects. The doctor is her partner in the

detection and treatment of abnormalities, the health visitor in public health and health education and in the rearing of the child whose immediate post-natal existence she has seen firmly established. We would emphasize here that, in our view the midwife is no mere 'delivery woman' whose prime function is the skilful delivery of a live child. This is indeed the climax of her task, but it started months before, early in pregnancy (Ministry of Health, 1949, p. 25).

The key issue identified was 'whether a service based on the midwife with the doctor behind her can be regarded as inferior to one based on the doctor working with a maternity nurse', and the answer given in the 1949 Report was 'no'.

Since the Report was based on evidence collected before the foundation of the NHS, it throws little light on the difficulties of the new 'partnership' between midwives and GPs. Nevertheless, it revealed that younger midwives, qualifying in 1945–46, tended to be dissatisfied with the attitude of the medical profession. Their complaint was that GPs were often simply ignorant about midwifery, and that midwives should be able to refer their patients directly to specialists.

By the time of the evidence given to the Cranbrook Committee in the late 1950s, the Central Midwives Board was well entitled to complain that midwives were fast becoming 'welfare agents'. The Board advocated a system where the midwife would be the first person in a district to be told of a pregnancy and would be responsible for arranging and supervising all the care received by the childbearing woman. It sounded rather a pie-in-the-sky recommendation by then, but the CMB was, naturally, quite correct in supposing that only if midwives could be reinstated to a position of control could the ultimate death of an independent midwifery service be avoided.

Hospital obstetrics: the pattern of the future

Behind these developments in the maternity work of GPs and midwives lay the pattern of the future: the rising star of hospital obstetrics. By the late 1950s, as we have seen, antenatal attendances at hospital clinics were far in excess of those at local health authority clinics, and twice as many births took place in hospital as at home.

In the early struggle by male midwives for ascendancy over the traditional female birth attendant in the eighteenth century, access to hospital practice had been important in providing would-be-obstetricians with clinical experience, a (relatively) passive clientele, and an organizational basis for the construction of professional medical-midwifery hierarchies. Hospitals, by aligning normal parturition with the confinement of the sick, created a medical label for pregnancy, a feat which had to be accomplished if pregnancy was to be regarded in the future as a legitimate subject for medical discourse and treatment. While conditions in the mid-twentieth century were very different from those under which the early male midwives worked, the underlying problem was in essence the same. Who controlled — should control — the surveillance of pregnancy and childbirth? The female midwives were still there, and were still claiming the right to manage normal pregnancy and labour. Beside them now were the GPs, with a new financial incentive to take on maternity work; and in the shadows lurked the public health doctors siding with whichever group seemed most likely to present the vestiges of a case for the definition of pregnancy as a public health matter. In the face of these conflicts, removal of pregnancy to hospital was an answer with at least the merits of simplicity.

However, simplicity has rarely been the reason for any significant development in the history of medicine — or any other history. The years leading up to the establishment of the NHS saw the specialists, including the obstetricians, in a relatively strong bargaining position. Their skills were, at the time, regarded as scarce; the BMA had insisted to the Government that none of its members would enter the Health Service unless all hospitals were removed from the control of municipal government and voluntary organizations, thus establishing for the specialists a very substantial degree of control over the hospital sector. On this basis the specialists were able to negotiate a favourable position for themselves with respect to conditions of service, pay, control over appointments and promotion, and the merit awards system, and the right to continue in a private practice which, perhaps most incredibly of all, was to include access to NHS beds.

These were years in which childbearing women in Britain still possessed two important rights which they were fighting to hold on to and have since lost: the right to refer themselves directly to a hospital antenatal clinic (without first seeing the community midwife or GP), and the right to book a hospital bed without a medical recommendation. They were also years which saw the beginning of the articulation of consumer 'choice' in maternity care, and the outright recognition of consumer dissatisfaction with hospital care.

Evaluating antenatal care: the invention of perinatal epidemiology

A development of mixed blessing to the rising star of hospital-based, specialist obstetrics was that represented by the 1946 and 1958 surveys of British natality: the new epidemiological interest in 'perinatal' medicine. Epidemiology stepped in during the post-war era with the tools to evaluate on a 'scientific' basis the contribution, if any, made to the safety of mother and child by such procedures as antenatal care.

The inherent impossibility of reaching any definite conclusion about the effectiveness of antenatal care on the basis of hospital or GP populations had been demonstrated over and over again in the 1920s, 1930s and 1940s. The difficulty with such data-bases was that selection biases could not be ruled out: one could never be sure whether the clientele of a particular hospital or general practice was representative of the general population of women having babies. Also needed was a more discriminating index of mortality. By the 1950s maternal mortality was no longer any good as an outcome variable because of its relative scarcity — 0.76 per 1,000 total births in England and Wales in 1951, a fall of over 80 per cent since 1931. Infant mortality — deaths within the first year of life — had never been regarded as a good indicator of medical care in pregnancy and at birth because of the long period after birth during which social influences could take their toll, masking any possible effect of medical care. The term 'perinatal period' was used by the German paediatrician, Pfaundler, in 1936. In the 1930s, inquirers into obstetric mortality had noted the tendency for stillbirths and intrapartum and early neonatal deaths, to be united by the same set of causes — for example, failures in the function of the placenta to support healthy growth, and congenital malformations. From the mid-1940s the term 'perinatal mortality' was increasingly used as a new composite index (Pfaundler, 1936; Baird, et al., 1953; WHO, 1957). By 1953 it was creeping into the language of reports: the Annual Clinical Report for Queen Charlotte's Maternity Hospital used it for the first time (1953, p. 83), and the Chief Medical Officer at the Ministry of Health in his Annual Report (CMO, 1955, p. 123) acknowledged that 'The term "perinatal mortality" is being increasingly used in referring to the total loss of infant life before, during and shortly after birth', although 'there is as yet no generally accepted definition of the term'. Perinatal mortality did, of course, come eventually to be defined by international agreement as the number of stillbirths (fetal deaths of 28 weeks or more gestation) and the number of deaths within the first week of life per 1,000 total (live plus still) births (WHO, 1974). In Figure A.3, p. 297, the 'perinatal mortality' rate is shown as a generally declining index from 1930 to 1980.

The concept of 'perinatal mortality' ineluctably linked the antenatal with the intranatal and the postnatal, a move in the realm of ideology which was to further the same association in the realm of the physical organization of care. But what could epidemiologists in the 1950s say about the role of medical care in perinatal mortality? Was it possible to identify which place of birth and which type of antenatal care were conducive to the lowering of perinatal mortality rates? Although interpretation of the statistics is sufficiently complex for the matter still to be debated (see, for example, Tew, 1977), it did appear from the 1958 survey of 24,855 British births that the safest place to have a baby was a hospital consultant unit, and after that there wasn't much to choose between a GP unit, a private nursing home, one's own bed, or the back of a taxi (Butler and Bonham, 1963). Then, as now, there are two very different groups of women having babies at home and running different risks of mortality. Perinatal mortality among home births to married women in their late twenties and early thirties is low, but among illegitimate births to mothers in their teens it is high (Campbell, et al., 1982). As to antenatal care — oddly called by the authors of the volume reporting these findings 'prenatal' care after the American fashion — the perinatal mortality of babies whose mothers had no antenatal care was five times the national figure. The unsolved problems with all such tabulations is that mothers who deliver prematurely and are liable to lose their babies will have chalked up fewer antenatal visits, although some of those with a high number of attendances will also run a higher-than-average risk of losing their babies, due to underlying medical problems responsible for the high attendance rate. The Report also discussed the type ('grade') of prenatal care and mortality. The mortality of 'hospital only' prenatal care was about the national average, despite including, presumably, a fair proportion of high-risk cases. 'Hospital in part' had a higher mortality. As to the variation in mortality in the grades 'GP only' 'LHA only' (intermediate mortality), 'GP and midwife' (highest mortality), and 'midwife only' (lowest mortality), the comment was that this 'is difficult to explain' (Butler and Bonham 1963, p. 66). On the face of it, and according to table 6.2, it did not seem as though the explanation lay in the greater technical efficiency of the low mortality grades of prenatal care.

For some reason not explained, table 6.2 does not give a figure for 'midwife only' care: nevertheless, substantial differences in the frequency with which three routine antenatal tests were carried out are apparent. The proportion of women not having their haemoglobin or

Table 6.2 Routine Prenatal Tests, 1958 Survey.

Grade of prenatal care	No haemoglobin test	Blood pressure not always tested	Rh. type: no test and no record
Hospital only	4.7	1.6	0.7
Hospital in part	18.4	17.2	1.7
LHA clinic throughout or in part	35.2	18.6	4.8
GP only	60.0	17.8	12.0
GP and Midwife	67.9	25.4	13.0
All cases	33.3	15.9	5.5

source: Butler and Bonham, *Perinatal Mortality* 1963, p. 76. With permission of the publishers Churchill Livingstone.

their rhesus group tested or their blood pressure taken was highest in the 'GP and midwife' and lowest in the 'hospital only' group.

The information on the technical efficiency of antenatal care in 1958 produced by the survey was certainly interesting. One in three pregnant women in Britain in 1958 did not have their haemoglobin tested in pregnancy, one in six did not always have their blood pressure taken, and one in 17 did not have their blood examined for its rhesus type. Despite the fact that the 1952 Report of the Chief Medical Officer at the Ministry of Health observed that blood tests were now accepted as routine in pregnancy (CMO, 1953), technological innovation — the acquisition of new forms of knowledge and new skills — is one thing: the diffusion of this innovation in practice is yet another.

Changing standards

The practice of antenatal care was changing during the years from 1945–60. Two indices of this change were described in Chapter 4: antenatal care at the London Hospital from 1934–50 and at the Glasgow Royal Maternity Hospital from 1933–59. The picture was one of an increasing number of hospital visits per pregnancy, an earlier time of first attendance, and the introduction of blood tests on a (more or less) routine basis. We may supplement this data with three further data-sets relating to rural English General Practice over the period 1946–57 (Table 6.3), General Practice in Wales from 1946–70 (Table 6.4) and antenatal care at Queen Charlotte's Maternity Hospital from 1948 to 1978 (Table 6.5). Again, we see a pattern of earlier, more frequent visits, and the increased administration of specialized tests. In 1953–4 pregnant women were weighed for the first time — a new custom which had also been introduced into hospital practice in Glasgow by 1959 (p. 95). Height, recorded for only about 1 in 10 patients in 1946–50, was recorded for almost all by 1969–70 (table 6.4).

Table 6.3 Antenatal Care in Rural English General Practice 1946–57[5]

	1946–8	1949–50	1951–2	1953–4	1955–7
First visit					
(weeks pregnant)	21.8	18.3	17.2	15.8	13.9
Number of visits	6.5	9.8	9.9	8.6	9.1
Blood pressure					
measurements	4.6	8.5	7.7	7.9	8.1
Urine tests	3.1	6.5	5.9	6.1	7.6
Blood tests	0.17	2.42	2.81	2.9	2.8
Weighing	0	0	0	4.8	7.1
Number of case-notes					
in series	35	45	77	100	109

Table 6.4 Antenatal Care in a Rural Welsh General Practice 1946–70[6]

	1946–50 %	1951–60 %	1961–70 %
Attending at three months			
or before	51.3	58.8	71.9
Blood examination in early			
pregnancy*	39.1	71.9	100.0
in late pregnancy**	5.7	9.5	58.9
Regular blood pressure			
and urine examination	98.7	95.9	96.8
Weekly abdominal			
examinations in last			
four weeks	98.7	93.9	90.3
Height recorded	12.8	59.8	98.4
Regular weight record	3.2	37.2	96.2
Number of case-notes			
in series	156	296	185

*Blood group, rhesus factor, haemoglobin, Kahn.
**Rhesus factor, haemoglobin.

5. Data taken from the case-books of Dr Ivor Cookson, who generously made them available for this purpose.

6. Dr L. A. C. Wood kindly provided the data shown in this table.

F

The Captured Womb

Table 6.5 Antenatal Care at Queen Charlotte's Maternity Hospital, 1948–78[7]

	1948–50	*1957–58*	*1967–68*	*1977–78*
First visit	17.6	16.1	17.2	16.2
(weeks pregnant)				
No. of visits	8.1	10.2	10.8	10.4
No. of inpatient	0.1	0.3	0.3	0.4
admissions				
No. of antenatal	1.5	3.4	5.4	9.5
tests/procedures				
Inductions (%)	3	8	27	24
Number of case-notes in	100	100	100	100
series				

In the table relating to Queen Charlotte's Hospital practice, Table 6.5, antenatal tests and procedures are lumped together in the penultimate line which shows a doubling over the decade from the late 1940s to the late 1950s.

This much can de deduced from the available evidence. But what of the evidence that is harder to obtain — the experiences of the women in Britain who in the years from 1945 to 1960 gave birth and underwent (or avoided) antenatal care? One of the first babies cared for antenatally under the NHS was Phillip Campion, born in March 1949. In a unusual and valuable document, *National Baby*, Phillip's mother recorded her experiences with antenatal care:

> Today there is nobody I know, and I languish rather boredly on a series of benches and chairs, worming my slow way up to the head of the queue. Owing to a slight misunderstanding with a 49 bus, I arrive later than usual; and at this place ten minutes' difference in arriving may set you back an hour in departing. My un-algebraic mind has never fathomed the Why of this; it just *is* so.
>
> I sit, and knit, for the first half-hour . . . At the end of the corridor the silhouette of a very, very pregnant Mum in nothing but her vest is seen gravely mounting the weighing machine . . . The nurse who does the blood pressure is . . . restraining a toddler from climbing into his mother's lap . . . and telling other Mums where to go, all as usual . . .
>
> Now it is my turn to go in to Doctor. He is in a hurry, and spends precisely two and a half minutes in discovering that I am in perfect health and do not need his ministrations. I know it is two and a half minutes, for

---

7. Data obtained from Medical Records Department, Queen Charlotte's Maternity Hospital. For each of the years shown in the table the first 50 complete sets of notes were taken out and analysed. Data reproduced with the permission of the Joint Medical Committee.

he says at the end, dismissing me, that I have wasted just that much of his time.

Waiting in yet another queue to get my paper back from Sister, I take a dim view of this remark. One can legitimately look at the matter in another way, and say that he has wasted two and a half hours of my time (Campion, 1950, pp. 40–3).

After the baby was born, Sarah Campion calculated the financial costs of NHS antenatal and delivery care: £5 4s 4d, as against a minimum outlay of £180 for private care.

Not until the 1960s did systematic surveys begin to be done of the 'consumer' point of view. Meanwhile, we can only attempt to capture from surviving case-notes the quality of her experience. Mrs Baker (a fictional name) became pregnant in the first half of March 1948. On 12 August she went to her GP who recorded

> Lack of energy and occasional weak turns. Nausea but not vomiting. Appetite good, L.M.P. [last menstrual period] 22 April. No vaginal discharge. Frequency of micturition. (Grandmother died of diabetes). On exam. lower abdo. obese. No fundus felt. Collostrum [sic] expressed from breasts. To wait and see. (Hope-Simpson, case-notes)

A vitamin syrup, liquid paraffin for constipation and iron tablets were prescribed. On 17 August Mrs Baker's urine was tested for albumin and sugar. On 25 August the doctor wrote 'Has had a few weak turns since. Always in the kitchen when she is getting meals. Has a small stuffy, ill-ventilated flat. On examination abdomen does not appear bigger. Collustrum expressed from breasts. To review in a month.' She was given another prescription for vitamins. She went back on 16 September, saying she felt fetal movements, but the GP could not find a fetal heart. He reckoned the expected delivery date as 25 January, and referred her to the local nursing home for delivery (the notes give no reason why). She had another urine test on 2 October: all clear. On 4 October the doctor signed a certificate of pregnancy for the housing authorities. Mrs Baker's next visit was on 16 November when the fundus seemed to be about six months and the fetal heart still could not be heard, although movements were 'marked'. By 9 December she had swollen ankles and complained of giddy attacks. But her urine was clear: she was advised to rest. At the end of the month, 30 December, her ankles remained puffy and her blood pressure was 170/100; she was prescribed phenobarbitone and told to stay in bed for a week. On 6 January a urinary infection was diagnosed, but the baby pipped the GP's clinical acumen to the post by being born the day before the test result arrived, weighing in at four pounds seven ounces.

Part II
The Reign of Technology: antenatal care 1960–80

7

Getting to Know the Fetus

I forget just which psychiatrist or psychologist it was who, in categorizing the various medical specialties in terms of the psychologic traits of their practitioners, decided that obstetricians were compensating for an ungratifed childhood curiosity to know where babies come from. If that is true, then many . . . today could be said to have handsomely overcompensated.

Liley, 1976, p. 70

By 1940, hormonal pregnancy tests could establish the highly probable existence of a fetus. Its heart could be heard with a stethescope. Its skeleton could be visualized with X-rays, though not without a risk of long-term damage. But otherwise knowledge of the fetus could only be acquired through knowledge of the mother — by asking her questions, by clinically examining her abdomen and by laboratory examination of her metabolic products. By 1960, not much advance on this situation was to be seen in the routine practice of antenatal care in Britain and other industrialized nations. Yet many developments which were to revolutionize antenatal care were by that time underway.

The revolution in antenatal care has taken place as part of an overall spurt of growth in professional techniques for managing reproduction, and, in that sense, the developments of the past two decades in antenatal, intranatal and postnatal care should be taken together. Yet the new interventions relating to antenatal care are by far the most revolutionary in character. They are revolutionary because, for the first time, they enable obstetricians to dispense with mothers as intermediaries, as necessary informants on fetal status and life-style. It is now possible to make direct contact with the fetus, and to acquire a quite detailed knowledge of her or his physiology and personality before the moment of the official transition to personhood — the time of birth.

This chapter looks at some of these new ways of finding out about fetuses, beginning with ultrasound. Ultrasound is interesting not only as a new clinical strategy in itself, but because its rise from unknown procedure to routine use illustrates the essential character of techno-logical innovation in antenatal care — to some extent in medicine itself. The development of obstetric ultrasound in Britain is thus spelt out in some detail below for two reasons: (1) because the character of its development provides an object lesson in the development of all such technologies; and (2) because possessing a window on the womb has always been a powerful motive for the professional providers of maternity care.

The fetus as submarine or seeing with sound

In 1958 an article was published in the *Lancet* with the dryly unpromis-ing title, 'Investigation of Abdominal Masses by Pulsed Ultrasound'. Its authors were Ian Donald, then Regius Professor of Midwifery at the University of Glasgow, J. MacVicar, Gynaecological Registrar at the Glasgow Western Infirmary, and T. G. Brown, a representative of Kel-vin Hughes Ltd, a local engineering firm. The three men described in their article the use of ultrasonic sound waves to study living human tissue. The principle of abdominal ultrasound was that short pulses of high frequency energy from a piezo-electric crystal were transmitted 50 times a second into the body through the skin of the abdominal wall. When this energy beam encountered a surface or interface, the reflected part returned to the crystal; this, in turn, was converted into an electrical signal which was transferred to a cathode ray tube. As it developed, ultrasound was to go through a long series of mechanical refinements. Eventually, the technique was to diversify into A-mode (one-dimensional) and B-mode (two-dimensional) scanning. The B-mode would ultimately be used to produce something described as 'real-time scans' — true to name, as used in obstetrics, these were scans which showed on the screen life in the uterus as it was really going on. A third technique, Doppler ultrasound, is a continuous, rather than pulsed, ultrasonic beam useful for demonstrating rhythmic intrauterine happen-ings such as the beating of the fetal heart.

Ultrasound, or 'sonar', as Ian Donald preferred to call it — an acronym for 'sound navigation and ranging' — developed originally as a technique for detecting submarines during the First World War in 1916–7. (See Langevin, 1928; Chilowsky and Langevin, 1916.) The implica-tions of the technique for fetuses as pseudo-submarines were not immediately picked up, although any imaginative person might have been expected to observe that 'There is not so much difference after all between a fetus in utero and a submarine at sea' (Donald, 1969, p. 618). We must remind ourselves that in the post First World War era X-rays were still thought to provide that window on the womb Ballantyne had anticipated earlier in the century as a vital technical adjunct to the obstetrician's work. The incentive for the great research investment in obstetric ultrasound came in the mid-1950s, when Alice Stewart's work on the long-term hazards of X-rays provided an incentive for the development of an alternative method of viewing intrauterine life.

After the war the technique of ultrasonic echo sounding was turned to such innocent purposes as sounding the ocean floor for depth measurements of use in shipping and navigation, and for locating deep sea herring shoals. The pioneer work on soft tissue ultrasonography was done in the U.S. in the late 1940s and early 50s by Douglass Howry at the University of Colorado Medical Center, John Wild at the University of Minnesota and George Ludwig of the Naval Medical Research Institute, University of Pennsylvania. Much of this early work had limited application to living human beings, since the experimental material came from the postmortem room or consisted of dead dogs' intestines. In Ian Donald's own words,

> The translation into obstetrics came rather as a spin-off . . . I started with a very well-known clinical problem, especially in Glasgow — of the enormously distended female abdomen. Glasgow was stiff with them in those days — when I first came here in 1954. I don't know whether women ate more, or they ate more sweets or their husbands didn't love them and they ate to comfort themselves — it was a common sight to see women with their jaws working all the time at the bus-stops. They were so fat, unbelievably fat, you just couldn't tell what on earth was going on inside . . . (one) woman was so fat she was bedridden. She lay like a turtle on her back with flippers, and the nurses had to use all their strength to roll her over . . . the physicians looking after her could not believe that such abdominal distension didn't have a tumour behind it. I sunk my hands up to the metacarpals in loads and loads of fat but even I couldn't be convinced . . . (I. D. I.)

That was the clinical problem. Donald's own determination to solve it had several origins:

> I've always been an engineer at heart, I suppose. My wife says it's because I only had daughters — no sons — and therefore nobody to play trains with. There's something in that. None of my daughters would play trains with me — they did it occasionally just to humour me, but you could see they wanted to get back to their dolls . . . (I. D. I.)

Another key factor was Donald's location in Glasgow, a city with heavy engineering commitments, already practising the art of ultrasound in the metallurgical industry. When Donald arrived in Glasgow, he was familiar with the existing techniques of metal flaw detection and determined to investigate their applications to human tissues. He read a textbook of ultrasonic physics and then operated on the wife of an engineer, a research director of a firm manufacturing atomic boilers. The woman gratefully survived a hysterectomy and introduced Donald to her husband:

I told him what I was interested in and I said I would like to see whether his metal flaw detecting equipment could show anything different between one kind of tumour and another. It seemed a reasonable thing to try — if you can do it on metal you can do it on human tissue. So he said okay . . .

Those were the days, as I said, of huge lumps and bumps and cysts and so on. We took down in the boots of two cars all these lumps which we'd kept — we pushed them into the boots of our cars and drove down to this factory on a hot July day. Me and my registrar . . . And I went behind locked and closed doors and he got out his metal flaw detecting equipment. They hadn't even got any photographic equipment for photographing anything on the cathode ray tube. They had to call in the factory artist to sketch what he saw on the tube . . . It was as bad as that. But there was no doubt about it — that you got different echoes from different tumours. And this firm, they were a very nice crowd, even provided a gorgeous fat lump of steak as a control material. At the end of it we said, well, who's going to take it home. And nobody would. They just didn't like the idea of it having been mixed with all these tumours from all these unfortunate women — they thought it was rather like cannibalism . . .

July 21st 1955, a hot Friday afternoon. I shall never forget it, because that was when I realized we'd struck oil . . . this was it. There was no getting away from it. So I lost no time in applying it to my patients. They'd come along with a big lump inside and I used their metal flaw detector which I borrowed from their factory. We even used the same kind of disgusting gear oil on their tummies to act as an acoustic coupling medium. We used transformer oil . . .

After a few blind starts with a variety of machines, much-needed clinical success arrived in the form of a woman patient Donald was invited to see. The patient had an enormously bloated abdomen; she had had a barium meal X-ray and stomach cancer had been diagnosed. The outlook was considered hopeless. On examining the patient, Donald agreed with the physicians' diagnosis. But ultrasound revealed instead a gigantic benign cyst, which was duly removed (the patient recovered and emigrated to New Zealand).

Diagnosing the tumour of pregnancy

As Donald and many other obstetricians and gynaecologists have
observed, the commonest abdominal tumour in women is pregnancy. It
is therefore perhaps somewhat surprising that ultrasound was applied
relatively late in its development to obstetric problems. Application of
ultrasound to obstetrics in the beginning in Glasgow was hampered by
the geographical separation between the gynaecology department in the
Western Infirmary and the obstetrical department at the Royal Maternity Hospital in Rottenrow. The first set of apparatus was held at the
Infirmary, so a duplicate set was needed for the obstetric department,
and obtained in 1957. Plate 7.1 shows a pregnant woman lying under the
Glasgow ultrasound machine in that year; plates 7.2 and 7.3 show the
emerging relationships between the pregnant bodies of women and
ultrasonic equipment and its operators. The male figure in Plate 7.2 is
Ian Donald. The 'patient' in plate 7.3 is a full-sized adult doll, thus
positioned for an exhibition at Olympia in London. The representation
of pregnant women as objects of mechanical surveillance rather than
recipients of antenatal 'care' is an obvious message of these pictures.

Soon after ultrasound apparatus was acquired at Rottenrow, and
while doing his antenatal ward round on Friday mornings, Donald was

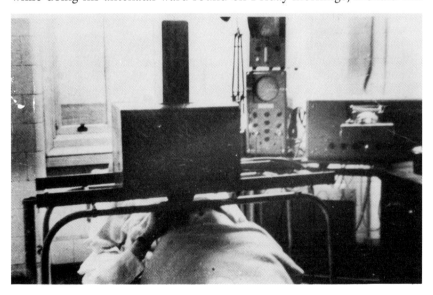

Plate 7.1 Ultrasound in Glasgow in 1957
source: Donald, I. *Sonar — its Present Status in Medicine* 1980, p. 18. Reproduced by permission of
the author.

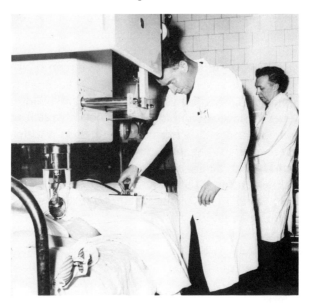

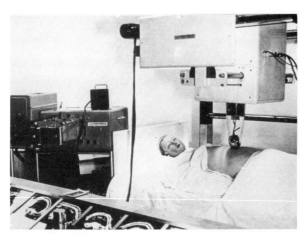

Plate 7.2 and 7.3 The first automatic ultrasound scanner for obstetric use completed in 1960
source: Donald, 1980, p. 19. With permission of the author.

puzzled when his staff nurse, Marjorie Marr (later to become Matron of the new Queen Mother's Hospital in Glasgow), always seemed to know which way up the fetuses were. It turned out that she had developed the habit of using the portable ultrasound apparatus in advance of the ward round in order to determine the presentation of the fetus. Once Donald had thus realized how easy it was to get a picture of the fetal skull, he had the idea of measuring the fetal biparietal diameter (BPD: skull width). The idea was to plot and monitor intrauterine growth, and to work out fetal skull size in relation to the all-important bony capacity of the mother's pelvis.

By 1963 Donald and his team had turned their minds more specifically to the question of early pregnancy diagnosis. Examination of 135 cases of pregnancy under 20 weeks was reported in a paper published that year, with the earliest diagnosis made now at eight and a half weeks (MacVicar and Donald, 1963). Yet seeing inside the small just-pregnant uterus with ultrasound was technically difficult, and the breakthrough here came quite accidentally, as the result of a further 'chance' observation, as Donald described:

> sometimes these patients were rather frightened, because by now we had an automatic machine about the size of a grand piano . . . There was this little patient who was very nervous, so nervous in fact her bladder filled up to bursting point and she said, please can I go to the loo? Normally the nurses say make sure your bladder is empty before you see the doctor. And this woman came in fit to burst, there was her full bladder, recognized that easily, we knew *that* one, but behind it was the uterus . . . you could see it in all its outlines, contours, length, dimensions, the lot — the sound waves just went straight through the bladder and gave you a kind of viewing technique — a window into the pelvis . . . What happens, you see, the sound waves travel very well in water and therefore very well in urine. Beautiful view you get (I. D. I.).

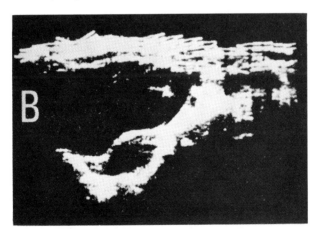

Figure 7.1 Full bladder (B) test to visualize the empty uterus behind
source: Donald, I. Diagnostic uses of sonar in obstetrics and gynaecology in *Journal of Ob. and Gyn. Br. Comm. 72* 1965, p. 908. With permission of the author.

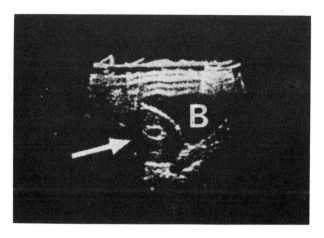

Figure 7.2 Very early intrauterine pregnancy behind a semi-full bladder (B)
source: Donald, I. Ultrasonics in Obstetrics in *British Medical Bulletin* 24, 1, 1968, p. 72. With permission of the author.

Inspired by the view (reproduced in figure 7.2), Donald's enthusiasm for ultrasound leapt unbounded further towards the beginning of it all, the moment of conception:

> And then a woman came along to see me, four miscarriages, no children, and she didn't even know if she was pregnant. Put her on the couch and there was the full bladder and this time I was looking just more or less to see if there were any fibroids in the uterus or something funny like that. I wasn't thinking about pregnancy.
> And there was a little ring inside. I didn't recognize what it was at first. A very early gestation sac — seven weeks. [Figure 7.2 gives an idea of what Donald saw.] The urine test hadn't even been done. She didn't know she was pregnant. She said her period was a bit late, but she wasn't sure. So I re-examined her — the thing was bigger. And then I went to New York and I addressed the New York obstetrical society, and I said, just look at this! . . . And they all looked totally unbelieving. I said that ring's a gestation sac — that's a pregnancy, and my God, it was. I delivered that baby with my own lilywhite hands at term — a perfectly healthy baby, her first (I. D. I.).

The team now began to glimpse a new panorama of detail about the early life of the fetus. Soon afterwards came the episode of the blighted ovum in the womb of one of Donald's own registrars:

> She turned up from Canada one day. I said, nice to see you, what do you want?

So she says, well, I'm pregnant, will you have a look at me? She'd got two children already (two sons) and [was] very keen to have a daughter . . . So I put her on the screen and of course she knew my ultrasonic work backwards — she runs an ultrasonic unit in Canada — and she looked at this screen and I didn't say a word . . .

She got off that couch blind with fury, she got dressed . . . She booked a plane straight for Canada, she booked a seat next to the aisle, right near the back of the plane and the loo. Sure enough, about half way across the Atlantic, she starts to bleed. So she goes into the loo and she passes something. Now this is the bit I like her so much for, bless her. Instead of turning on all that blue stuff that goes down the loo, she picked it out and put it in a bottle, if you please. She then got to her destination, not only did she have it examined in the path lab, she had it photographed under water and sent me a photograph. Then she had it examined by the cytogeneticist and it would have been a mongol. And it's in my book: 'By kind permission of the mother, herself a gynaecologist' [see figure 7.3] (I. D. I.).

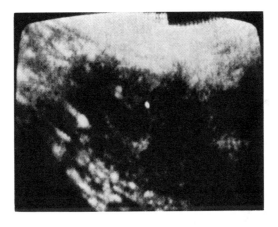

Figure 7.3 Blighted ovum. (By kind permission — the mother, herself a gynaecologist) *source*: Donald, I. *Practical Obstetric Problems* 1979, p. 1024. With permission of the publisher Lloyd-Luke (Medical Books).

In 1964 the group published a paper on 'fetal cephalometry by ultrasound' (Willocks, et al., 1964). The paper began by affirming the great investment obstetricians have in ascertaining the size and observing the growth of the fetus *in utero*, and referring to earlier (not very successful) attempts to plot normal growth curves for the fetal head. The problem as it was defined in 1964 was that obstetricians might suspect intrauterine fetal growth retardation from the presence of maternal toxaemia, or other factors or from clinical examination, but they could not *know*. From the measurements Donald and his co-workers did with ultrasonic cephalometry, it was decided that abnormal growth patterns could indeed be diagnosed from ultrasonic measurements of the fetal head.

Table 7.1 shows the 'success rate' of ultrasonograms performed over the previous five years in Glasgow. 'We continue to learn the hard way' Donald observed.

Table 7.1 Ultrasonograms in Glasgow 1960–65

Diagnosis	Correct	Incorrect	Inconclusive	Total
Pregnancy	220	37	31	288
Hydatidiform mole	26	1	—	27
Fibroid	62	12	15	89
Ovarian tumour	77	36	9	122
Liver and spleen	6	2	4	12
Ascites	22	9	2	33
Miscellaneous	20	13	15	48
Normal	35	3	4	42

source: Donald, 1965, p. 907. With permission of the author.

One nut the team had not yet cracked was the localization of the placenta by ultrasound. By 1967 they were more hopeful on this score, and in 1968 they reported on 675 cases exposed to ultrasonic placentography for a variety of indications including antepartum haemorrhage, amniocentesis and 'high free presenting part'.

The routine use of ultrasound in antenatal care

By 1966, the ultrasound case-load in Glasgow had become nearly 'unmanageable', with as many as ten patients a day (28 per cent of all QMH patients) being examined in the 'comprehensive ultrasonic department' situated alongside the department of radiology (still itself examining 23 per cent of QMH patients). By 1970, the clear predominance of obstetric indications (95.7 per cent of the total) for ultrasound was evidenced in the department's statistics, and the list of obstetric indications for ultrasound ran to no less than 20 items.

Many technical innovations in medicine begin life with the professional cold shoulder. The initial professional objections to obstetric ultrasound were that (1) it might be dangerous, (2) it was expensive, and (3) clinical examination was sufficient or superior: 'One of my alleged friends' recalled Donald (1976, p. 21) 'from the rival city of Edinburgh rewarded our hospitality by declaring to a hilarious group of students that in Glasgow we were employing a machine costing more than £10,000 in order to diagnose an ovarian cyst which he could feel with a twopenny glove'.[1] Donald himself made the comparison between his own efforts to launch ultrasound on the one hand, and Semmelweiss's to reduce the contagiousness of puerperal fever and Simpson's to control the pain of childbirth, on the other (Donald, 1969).

The first reference to ultrasound in Browne's textbook on *Antenatal and Postnatal Care* occurs in the 1970 edition (p. 9): 'The apparatus is costly and not yet available in many clinics, but it undoubtedly has great value, especially in difficult cases.' Around this time proponents of perinatal medicine were already recommending the routine use of ultrasound in early pregnancy (Huntingford, et al., 1971). There was much talk of the new vistas ultrasound had opened up, and of the 'great promise' it held for being 'a safe non-invasive method of fetal evaluation from the earliest gestational stages' (Kaback 1976, p. 2). By 1974, and despite continuing opposition among some obstetricians, the first question on the examination paper for the MRCOG diploma was one about ultrasound (Donald, 1976). By 1978 the ascent of ultrasonography had reached such peaks it was said that modern obstetrics and gynaecology could not be practised without it: 'The quality and quantity of diagnostic information obtained by ultrasonography far exceeds anything previously available and has had a revolutionary impact on the management of patients' (Hassani, 1978, p. vii). Two years later the advent of routine scans throughout pregnancy was heralded 'irrespective of the place of antenatal care', and the optimum number of scans in a normal pregnancy was set as 'at least five' (Law, 1980, p. 127). 'There is no doubt', confirmed Stuart Campbell and D.J. Little, 'that the development of the real-time scanner has transformed prenatal care. Ultrasound is now no longer a diagnostic test applied to a few pregnancies regarded on clinical grounds as being at risk. *It ... should be regarded as an integral part of prenatal care*' (Campbell and Little, 1980, p. 27: italics added). Indeed, the time had come for experts such as Campbell and Little to advise obstetricians on which machines to buy — a kind of *Which?* guide to the market, and one justified by the multitude of commercial interests

---

1. The offending gentleman was Clifford Kennedy.

involved in producing scanners — quite the reverse of the lack of commercial interest of which Donald had complained more than ten years before. The market in scanners was now such that the real-time machines cost anything from £9,000 to £18,000, and those that required the taking of polaroid photographs would add an odd £8,000 or so per year to the running costs. Ultrasound machines, said Campbell and Little, could be expected to pay for themselves by reducing unnecessary admissions to hospital (in fact it seems likely that routine ultrasound screening has the opposite effect — see p. 171).

A second generation of ultrasonically-trained and technology-minded obstetricians was now on the loose. One of Donald's disciples, Stuart Campbell, had taken the new technology south of the border to Queen Charlotte's Maternity Hospital (QCMH) in 1968. Within one year of ultrasound's arrival at QCMH, it had become a routine method for estimating fetal maturity and growth and for localizing the placenta. No figures of the number of women getting ultrasound were given until 1973, when the Annual Report included for the first time a section on 'fetal monitoring in pregnancy'. In that year, 48 per cent of patients received ultrasound. Between 1973 and 1974, the proportion of patients at QCMH receiving ultrasound rose to 62 per cent. By 1978, the figure was 97 per cent.

Not all hospitals in Britain had followed the QCMH lead quite so wholeheartedly: table 7.2 gives statistics for various antenatal procedures used at the London Hospital from 1973–80. In 1978 when nearly 100 per cent of QCMH patients had ultrasound, the figure at the London Hospital was rather less than two-thirds.

As well as the rise (and slight fall) in the career of ultrasound, table 7.2 alerts us to the fates of some of the other new technical procedures — for instance HPL (human placental lactogen) screening and monitoring the fetal heart (see pp. 178–80); a persisting degree of referral for X-rays is also evident.

By the late 1970s, obstetric ultrasound had thus become a common method of fetal surveillance. Internationally, it was popular too: according to a recent WHO study of prenatal care in Europe, ultrasound is performed in 22 European countries for which information is available, and in three of these it is a routine part of prenatal care (Pusch and Schmidt, 1983). Where the health care system is insurance-based, and in private practice, the existence of the technique has substantially boosted the profits to be made from pregnancy surveillance as an area of medical work.

These newly-surveyed fetuses have yielded new types of information

Table 7.2 Various antenatal procedures at the London Hospital 1973–80

Procedure	Percentage of pregnant women receiving in							
	1973	1974	1975	1976	1977	1978	1979	1980
Ultrasound	26.5	40.1	42.2	42.8	53.0	61.5	51.3	50.6
X-ray (all sites)	7.5	11.9	10.6	8.7	8.1	5.4	5.5	5.6
Oestriol	0	0	0	0	0	15.9	14.8	22.5
HPL	5.8	16.6	18.5	18.0	22.9	9.3	3.3	3.7
Amniocentesis	0	0	0	0	0	1.2	1.6	1.6
Fetal heart monitor	0	0.2	0.9	0.4	4.6	7.3	10.5	8.6

Reproduced with permission of the London Hospital (Mile End).

about their private lives. Fetal breathing movements, first suspected in 1543 by Vesalius[2] and described in 1888 by Ahlfeld (1905), were detected by ultrasound in 1971 (Boddy and Robinson, 1971). In 1972 Boddy and Mantell reported a total of 24 per cent at 26–34 weeks and 38 per cent at 35–42 weeks of pregnancy, of maternal abdominal movements due to fetal respiration. Patterns of fetal activity in normal and growth-retarded fetuses also came to be exposed to scrutiny. One group of researchers, aware of the need to know how normal fetuses behave, took 229 ultrasonic recordings from 21 pregnant women without known pregnancy complications. They found fetal breathing movements present for a mean of 31 per cent of the time, fetal trunk movements for 18 per cent of the time, and total fetal activity (TFA) for a mean of 48 per cent of the period observed. All types of movement showed diurnal variation, and seven women's fetuses had attacks of hiccups lasting for five to 20 minutes. By comparison, 20 growth-retarded fetuses were responsible for a significantly different incidence of intrauterine activity: breathing movements 16 per cent of the time, trunk movements 12 per cent and TFA 28 per cent (Roberts, et al., 1980). One tactic for working out how fetuses move is to push them around *in utero* through the mother's abdominal wall, this test of fetal vitality being termed one of 'motor provocation'.

In Denmark it was found that the known sex difference in birth size may be demonstrated by eight to twelve weeks of pregnancy (Pedersen, 1980). Researchers in Oxford in 1981 (Visser, et al., 1981) discovered that fetuses empty their bladders at 110-minute intervals. In the Netherlands, Wladimiroff and co-workers (1980) established that it usually

2. According to the orthodox medical–historical account. The number of pregnant women before that date who suspected fetal breathing movements is not known.

takes fetuses between 10 and 30 minutes to fill their stomachs, and they do so more urgently after their mothers have themselves dined. Also in the Netherlands, another group of researchers detected fetal eye movements with ultrasound (Bots, et al., 1981), adding yet another phenomenon to the mounting list of fetal characteristics now 'known' to exist *in utero*. Attention shifted during this period away from the fetal biparietal diameter as the crucial index of intrauterine growth to a variety of others, for example the size of the fetal liver: apparently, retarded liver growth occurs 10 to 20 weeks before the fall-off in the growth of the head circumference among 'compromised' fetuses. By 1982 it was confidently said that ultrasound can reliably detect more than 80 congenital abnormalities (*British Medical Journal*, 25 September 1982, p. 878). Those who practice ultrasound had acquired, by this time, the benefit of specialist journals and newly-certified diplomas of one kind or another (Kossoff, 1980).

How safe is safe?

This question was the substance of some of the early professional opposition to ultrasound. Ian Donald himself was old enough to remember some of the dreadful effects of X-rays and his own appalling lack of caution in handling the technique.

In 1974, he observed that the literature on the potential hazards of ultrasound was now so vast that it could not easily be summarized,

> except to state that the evidence to date would appear to indicate that sonar, as in present apparatus, is without known harmful effect. Nevertheless, I very much fear that if energies are increased with more sophisticated apparatus in the future, a threshold level may be reached, if, in fact, any such exists. It is also likely that the threshold may be different for different types of tissue which have many different susceptibilities (Donald, 1974b, p. 210).

Elsewhere, he admitted that on this point

> head waggers must be expected. After all, it took the best part of half a century before the use of X-rays in pregnancy was associated with a significant increase in the incidence of leukaemia and malignant disease in later childhood of the irradiated fetus. The possibility of hazard would have been much more quickly recognized had all babies shown the disability, but, in fact, it was only the collection and review of mass statistics which were able to show that although the majority of babies

came to no harm a statistically significant number were affected as compared with a population of children not exposed (Donald, 1974a, p. 304).

Ultrasound had been tested on animals (kittens, frog spawn and rodents) and on *in vitro* human cells during the same period as its early clinical uses developed. The alarm generated by a 'Preliminary Communication' from two workers in Cape Town to the effect that continuous Doppler ultrasound was capable of inducing chromosome aberrations in human blood cultures (Macintosh and Davey, 1970) was not confirmed by further incriminating evidence of the same kind. An article by Donald and his team the following year (Boyd, et al., 1971) reported a similar study to Macintosh and Davey's done some years earlier and showing contradictory findings. It was suggested that Macintosh and Davey's findings might be attributable to poorly controlled experimental conditions, for instance toxic substances released by ultrasound from polythene materials used in the experiment or gross variations in ultrasound power within the cell-containing solution. Other contradictory studies appeared; the matter could not be settled.

The list of possibly hazardous effects of ultrasound is legion (see Stratmeyer, 1980; Bang, 1980, for a discussion). As with other medical monitoring or treatment techniques, the appropriate methodology for assessing both the benefits and hazards of ultrasound scanning in pregnancy is that of a randomized controlled trial, with a sufficient period of follow-up to determine the presence or absence of long-term morbidity during the childhoods and adulthoods of fetuses ultrasonically surveyed *in utero*. However, it can be very difficult to set up this sort of evaluation once a practice has become established in clinical work. Robin Mole, Director of the Medical Research Council's (MRC) Radiobiology Unit at Harwell from 1969 to 1977, was concerned in the attempt to get underway in the early 1970s what was probably, world-wide, the first projected multicentre trial of obstetric ultrasound. The planned study was to be a randomized controlled trial of ultrasound, using a number of centres. The pregnant women who would be randomly allocated to ultrasound or no-ultrasound groups were to be those about whom individual obstetricians felt uncertain as to whether or not ultrasound would be of value. The babies were to be followed up by the child health service, in school medical examinations. In the run-up to planning the trial, remembers Mole:

---

3. Technically speaking, the issue of possibly rare long-term effects may not most appropriately be addressed with an RCT, but rather with a case-control study.

. . . there were problems with obstetricians and there were problems with paediatricians . . . But people who were interested in populations were all for this survey of ultrasound, and they agreed with me when I said anything that's going to be introduced into medicine on a really large scale must have a prospective trial of some sort . . . you really ought to take pains to try to measure the possible harm and the possible value. Even at that time people knew the health services were going to be short of money, and if you're going to buy these machines, and buy people to work them, then you're going to commit yourself to a lot of money. And there are so many things that I've seen in my life when something was started, on perfectly understandable grounds, but turned out to be totally useless, yet you have to go on using it because you become "negligent" when you don't . . .there's a great deal in medicine like that.

But the obstetricians and paediatricians didn't look at it like that at all. They felt they'd got to do the best thing they could for the individual who presented herself to them. They could say, well we know that ultrasound is going to do good . . . and the other people, they're only talking about *hypothetical* harm.

Everything would have been alright in the days when ultrasound machines were so uncommon that only some women could be ultrasonated. However, it took three years of meetings to hammer this through. It really was very wearing. Some paediatricians walked out and wouldn't have anything more to do with it, they thought it was morally wrong and so on . . . but we finally got sufficient agreement . . . We got Council to agree to put by a quarter of a million pounds on condition that we did a satisfactory pilot study. (R. M. I.).

The calculations for the size of the study had originally been done using the model of X-rays and childhood cancer: how many pregnant women would need to be entered into the trial in order to have a reasonable chance of detecting an effect of the same order of magnitude? This turned out to be too expensive, so the sums were redone and the size of the study scaled down. Mole's own theories about possible adverse effects focused on damage to vision or hearing and on Down's syndrome in the children of female fetuses receiving ultrasound *in utero*. The pilot study of the obstetric aspects was duly completed with total success, and the protocol for the main study was then laid before the MRC, who turned it down. As Mole recalled:

By then the membership of the Cell Board [the particular subdivision of the MRC dealing with this area of medicine] had changed. Scientists who worked with test-tubes now said this wasn't a proper scientific investigation. They asked, what are they going to look for? We had to say we didn't know, but that we wanted to follow children up . . . And all we'd really got to do was to get a list where one woman was ultrasonated and the other wasn't and we thought they were the same in every other respect. Once we had that catalogue of names we could think of other things to follow up — we'd got our randomly set up population. But because we couldn't say precisely what we were looking for, they said that isn't science. And that isn't stupid. But of course you can't be that sort of a scientist if you're engaged in medicine. You can never wait for all the evidence, it's never complete. Whatever advances are made, you still don't know everything and you have to make a judgement. (R. M. I.)

Since the failure of the British MRC trial there have been some studies of the costs and benefits of ultrasound. Wladimiroff and Laar (1980) found that a single ultrasound examination could detect babies that were both small- and large-for-dates, but they did not demonstrate any difference in pregnancy 'management' or perinatal mortality and morbidity with ultrasound, and no long-term follow-up data were available on the childhood health of these ultrasounded fetuses. A recently completed trial in Norway shows no overall benefit substantive enough to justify ultrasonic screening of all pregnancies. A notable cost was that the women screened with ultrasound spent more than twice as long in hospital during pregnancy than the unscreened women (Bakketeig, et al, 1984).

Intrauterine fetal visualization

Ultrasound is one, but not the only, way of seeing the fetus, of representing her or him as a patient — indeed, determining whether it *is* a her or a him is one objective of the new surveillance methods.

During the late 1960s and early 1970s a variety of other methods were developed for revealing the status and intrauterine living conditions of fetuses. These have contributed their own momentum to the revolution in antenatal care.

The phrase 'intrauterine fetal visualization' is the title of a book published in 1976 (Kaback and Valenti); the papers in the book were given at a conference in California on the subject of an activity known as fetoscopy. (Allied to this are two other techniques known — for obvious reasons — as hysteroscopy and amnioscopy.) These new strategies for access to the womb started in the 1950s when Westin (1954) introduced into the cervical canals of pregnant women an instrument called an endoscope.

The aim of the original exercise was to see the fetus and study its oxygenation. By means of fetoscopy, obstetricians could actually look at bits of the fetus and its environment — and in real-life colour — rather than having to interpret a series of electrical signals on a black and white screen. The technique of fetoscopy, described as offering 'unlimited diagnostic potential' (Devore and Hobbins 1980, p. 76) was later improved by Valenti (1972) and Scrimgeour (1974). As a broad means of diagnosing congenital malformations, the method was, however, rapidly overtaken by ultrasound and by direct sampling of the amniotic fluid by inserting a needle through the maternal abdominal wall (this overtaking of one method by another merely, of course, serving to index the intensely competitive nature of the race to pioneer the best way of getting to know the fetus). However, the drawback of amniotic fluid as a guide to fetal condition is that over 90 per cent of the fetal cells it contains are dead. There are thus some genetic disorders which are not detectable by this method.

The technique of fetoscopy permitted direct access in early pregnancy to what Kaback (1976, p. 1) called 'human fetal material'. To start with, researchers examined fetuses before electively aborting them, using a 5–6 mm diameter paediatric cystoscope: 'Unfortunately, most pregnancies sampled were associated with interruption because of the size of the instrument used' (Devore and Hobbins, 1980, p. 62). The mother normally has a local anaesthetic at the site of insertion. 'Intrauterine viewing time' (p. 63) is 10–50 minutes, and there is little point in doing it before 15–20 weeks, because the uterus is too small. Ultrasound is used to determine placental site and fetal position and lie; and, if fetal movements obstruct the view, diazepam (valium) may be used to sedate her or him. If the fetoscopist is unable to see the desired bit of the fetus, then the fetus may be 'manipulated' into view.

Fetoscopy thus opened up the route to another brave new world, that of antenatal fetal surgery. Such surgery can have either diagnostic or treatment objectives. In the former category came fetoscopy to biopsy fetal blood cells, or chorionic villi (placental connections to the wall of the uterus), suspected of harbouring congenitally inherited blood disorders (Alter, 1981; Williamson, et al., 1981), or other genetically-determined malformations such as ectrodactyl (split hands and feet), and severe immunodeficiency disease (Hoyer, et al., 1979; Henrion, et al., 1980; Durandy, et al., 1982). The first successful surgical *treatment* procedure on the fetus *in utero* was reported in 1981 at the University of California when surgeons catheterized the bladder of a twin born two weeks later (*Guardian* 28 July 1981).

Although amniotic fluid is the container of many dead fetal cells, it remains useful in other ways. For example, looking at its colour with amnioscopy will inform the clinician as to whether the fetus is passing meconium (bowel movements) which could signal its distress. Such observations were documented by Saling in 1962, although he was not the first to notice the association. In 1972, Brock and Sutcliffe in Edinburgh carried amniotic fluid research a step further when they noted a high concentration of a particular fetal protein, subsequently named alphafetoprotein (AFP) in the amniotic fluids of fetuses with neural tube defects — either anencephaly (failure of the brain to develop) or spina bifida (literally 'divided spine'). Brock and Sutcliffe's original observations were made on samples of amniotic fluids collected for other research and frozen for three years — yet another example of a serendipitous pathway to the development of new techniques.

To secure samples of amniotic fluid, a procedure called amniocentesis began to be performed with increasing frequency. (It appears first in 1978 in Table 7.2 charting the development of antenatal care at the London Hospital.) In amniocentesis, a sample of fluid surrounding the fetus is withdrawn by a needle inserted through the mother's abdominal wall. The procedure carries the possible hazards of spontaneous abortion, neonatal respiratory problems and orthopaedic postural deformities (MRC Working Party, 1978; Standing Medical Advisory Committee, 1979). Because of these hazards, and because of the idea that AFP screening might be used in all pregnancies to prevent the birth of all (or nearly all)[4] fetuses with neural-tube defects, maternal blood samples eventually came to be the preferred medium for examining AFP levels. The presence of AFP in the sera of pregnant women was first demonstrated by Foy, et al., in 1970.

In 1971 yet another biochemical mystery of amniotic fluid was revealed to the world when Gluck and his co-workers were credited with the discovery that ammotic fluid contains information about the maturation of the fetal lung, about the readiness of the fetus to emerge into the breathing world. Fetuses matured in this manner are better able to survive independently of their mothers, since they are less likely to have breathing problems after birth. The clinical need for information about fetal maturity depends on obstetricians' ability safely and reliably to intervene and terminate pregnancy by inducing labour, and by this date the fashion for inducing labour was increasing. Obstetricians needed

---

4. Ethical objections by parents to elective termination of pregnancy will probably always be an important constraint here.

more than ever to know that they were not about to precipitate into the world persons unable to breathe.

The argument put forward by Gluck and his co-workers was that changes in amniotic fluid phospholipids reflect what is happening inside the fetal lung. A sudden rise in the concentration of one such compound, lecithin, after 35 weeks' gestation was thought to signal the maturity of the alveolar lining of the fetal lung. With 1–5cc. samples of amniotic fluid a process known as thin-layer chromatography (TLC) provided assessments of fetal lung maturation: these assessments were described as lecithin/sphingomyelin ratios. Sphingomyelin was also a phospholipid found inside the lung, but unlike lecithin its concentration in the amniotic fluid appeared to be relatively stable throughout pregnancy; the crucial ratio was one in which on the TLC test the lecithin spot was bigger than the sphingomyelin one. Although the L/S ratio test was eagerly espoused by some centres, like all such tests it turned out, not unexpectedly to have problems. Quite a lot of fetuses expected to develop respiratory distress syndrome (RDS) neonatally because of an inadequate L/S ratio did not do so — in fact between a third and two thirds in different places (Holton, 1976). There were also some who, according to the test should have been alright, but weren't. If the mother had diabetes, the pregnancy was complicated by rhesus haemolytic disease, or the AF sample contained fragments of blood or meconium, then the test was not reliable either.

The fetoplacental unit or the maternal supply line

The ultrasonic application of marine metaphors to the womb, and excursions into the fetal marine environment with fetoscopy and amniocentesis have provided us over the past 20 years with a whole new way of describing pregnancy. Other new antenatal metaphors have also been created. From the ocean to the stars, and a rather astronautical view of the fetus, seen as floating gravity-less and attached by its supply line to the spaceship of its mother: figure 7.4 (a diagram from a textbook on *The Placenta and Its Maternal Supply Line*) alludes to the unmistakable parallel between the fetus and the cosmonaut, whose own supply line to the mother spaceship is the very source and support of life itself. A similar characterization is apparent in other technical literature of the period. Thus Barnes (1975, p. i) referring to the respiratory function of the placenta, employs the analogy of 'an hermetically sealed room with a single occupant and a slowly closing porthole'; and Frank

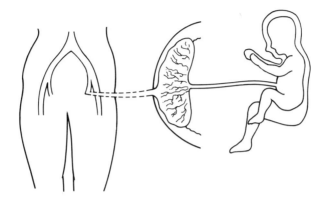

Figure 7.4 The fetal cosmonaut
source: Gruenwald, P. *The Placenta and its Maternal Supply Line* 1975, p. 4. With permission of the publisher MTP Press Ltd.

Hytten in a chapter called 'Metabolic Adaptations of Pregnancy' (1976, p. 35) describes the fetus thus:

> The fetus is an egoist, and by no means an endearing and helpless little dependent as his [sic] mother may fondly think.[5] As soon as he has plugged himself into the uterine wall he sets out to make certain that his needs are served, regardless of any inconvenience he may cause. He does this by almost completely altering the mother's physiology, usually by fiddling with her control mechanisms.

Spaceships may imagine they're important to astronauts, but in reality astronauts have the upper hand.

The function of the placenta in relation to the mother on one side and the fetus on the other has mystified people for centuries. With the recent development of a more complex and sophisticated understanding of pregnancy, it has become abundantly clear that, whatever else the placenta is, it is not merely an 'afterbirth'. It may be described as a tumour whose growth offers a clue to immunological mechanisms at work in the promotion and prevention of cancer (Dilman, 1977), or as an organ so inseparably linked to the fetus that the two may only have one name — the fetoplacental unit (Curry and Hewitt, 1974). Not only is the placenta's physiological role unclear, but its social status is most

---

5. It is not known whether mothers *en masse* think of fetuses thus; or how they think of them.

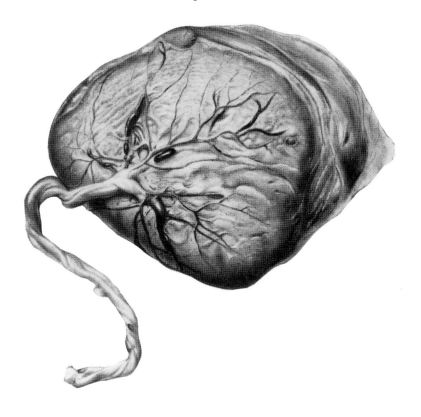

Figure 7.5 The marginal placenta
source: Klopper and Diczfalusy, *Foetus and Placenta* 1969, Frontispiece. With permission of the
authors and Blackwell Scientific Publications.

ill-defined (figure 7.5 also from a textbook, shows it, in turn, suspended
in space). In some cultures the placenta is the twin of the newborn,
regarded as almost human, yet Western obstetricians do not draw the
same conclusion from their designation of the placenta as integral with
the fetus. It seems that where professionalized medicine has become the
department of society managing reproduction, then the placenta, though
fascinating before birth, becomes afterwards merely a bit of tissue to be
extracted from the mother. It is not regarded as important for mothers to
see their placentas, and the plea of some natural childbirthers not only to
see but eat or bury theirs, raises the interesting question as to who *owns*
the placenta. It has to be part of that capturing of the womb by the
professional managers of childbirth that in law it is the duty of the

professional deliverer at least to dispose of this marginal, fairly unpleasant, but undoubtedly useful, organ.[6]

Why do fetuses need placentas? What can placentas tell us about fetuses? How is it possible to monitor the status and functioning of the placenta in the womb? These basic questions have stimulated yet another new research area within obstetrics, naturally enough known as placentology (with its own specialist journal since 1980). The questions are both theoretically interesting, and of practical importance. The practical importance to antenatal care of finding out about placental function derives from the placenta's burden as the all-provident mother-spaceship; organizing the physical and emotional state of the fetus, feeding, breathing and excreting for it. All goes well when the placenta does its (her?) task efficiently. But like real mothers and real spaceships, placentas sometimes misfunction: hence the concept of 'placental insufficiency'. It was (once again) Ballantyne who observed a 'wasting condition of the newborn that 30 years later Runge in Germany proposed might be due to impairment of the nutrient supply line to the fetus: the two gave their name to the Ballantyne–Runge syndrome, a condition now more commonly called intrauterine growth retardation (IUGR), small-for-dates (SFD), or small-for-gestational-age (SGA). Thus placental failure or 'insufficiency' came into view as a main cause of impoverished growth and nutrition in the just-born. The concept itself is a veritable rag-bag of causal aspersions and implications. To blame the placenta is to exonerate the mother, and this, as Gruenwald (1975) observes, in turn implies that nothing can be done; whereas it is important for obstetricians to believe that *something* can be done.

Vast numbers of investigations have been carried out since the 1940s on the chemical constituents, blood flow, metabolic processes and structure of the placenta. The desire to know how the placenta transmits, or does not transmit, various substances through to the fetus has inspired a plethora of experiments in which mothers have been injected with such materials as atrophine (Hellman, et al., 1963) or radioactive amino-acids (Garrow and Douglas, 1968), and the impact on the fetus studied. In one such experiment, 20 pregnant women had a wide-bore needle inserted into their femoral arteries, below the groin, and inflated pneumatic cuffs round their upper thighs to obstruct circulation to the

---

6. The placenta is a crucial source of various hormones used in clinical practice or manufactured commercially. A related and more recently-reported use is that of the amniotic membranes to heal ulcers and burns (Faulk, et al., 1980).

legs. Through the needle a contrast medium was injected very rapidly and under very high pressure so that a series of X-rays could be taken of the uterine and placental blood vessels (Solesh, et al., 1961). In another experiment (Browne and Veall, 1953) radioactive sodium chloride was injected directly into the space behind the placenta in normal and toxaemic women, and the rate at which radioactivity disappeared was measured. By 1963 this test, of which many clinicians apparently had high hopes, had fallen into disuse because the information on radioactivity-disappearance time did not seem to relate consistently to anything else (Klopper, 1969).

In terms of evolving a reliable test of placental function for routine use in pregnancy, interest has centred on the ever-fascinating subject of hormones. The importance of the placenta as a hormone factory was first recognized in 1905 by Halban in Germany. The technology for the laboratory study of placental hormones was available from the early 1930s (Smith and Smith, 1933), but did not become popular until it was simplified some 30 years later from a complicated bioassay to an easier and speedier chemical one. In 1969 Diczfalusy and Mancuso, surveying the topic of oestrogen metabolism in pregnancy, listed 27 different oestrogens which had been isolated and detected in human pregnancy urine — urine being the golden medium for studying these particular secrets of the womb. By 1970, the number of different procedures for carrying out hormonal assays of maternal urine was more than 50 (Kubli, 1971). The most popular of these have been a substance named human placental lactogen (HPL) which appears in maternal blood (Letchworth and Chard, 1972), and an oestrogen called oestriol, most popularly collected by asking mothers to centralize their urine in plastic containers over periods of 24 hours at a time (see Bergsjø, et al., 1973).

The pattern of antenatal monitoring displayed in Table 7.3 shows the point at which both oestrogen assays and ultrasound were introduced into the fetal surveillance of one geographically defined population — the residents of Cardiff. In Table 7.2 earlier showing data from the London Hospital, 'oestriol' tests are first coded in 1978.

A person at heart

Finally, in this, no doubt as yet unfinished, sequence of fetal surveillance techniques, we come to the heart.

By 1972 only 48 days of pregnancy were needed to demonstrate ultrasonically the presence of an embryonic beating heart. But this was

Table 7.3 Antenatal monitoring among parturients resident in Cardiff 1967–74

	1967	1968	1969	1970	1971	1972	1973	1974
Oestrogen assay	—	3.0	3.2	9.0	19.1	19.7	17.6	16.4
Mean no. of assays per case	—	2.6	2.8	2.5	2.9	2.8	3.2	3.6
Ultrasound	—	—	—	0.7	10.1	14.3	20.0	21.0
Mean no. of examinations per case	—	—	—	1.0	2.1	2.3	2.5	2.2

source: Davies et al., Predicting Fetal Death, *British Medical Journal* 12 Feb. 1977, p. 443. With permission of the BMJ and the authors.

by no means the beginning of obstetricians' interest in the fetal heart rate as an index of wellbeing. There are many reports before this time of experiments with antenatal cardiotocography, such experiments being designed to see whether changes in fetal heart rate frequency or rhythm can be taken as reliable warning signs of fetal distress *in utero* (see for example Hammacher, et al., 1968; and also the review in Greene, et al., 1965). The principle on which antenatal cardiotocography is based — the emission of electrical activity by the heart — was first observed by Cremer in 1906 — by accident (again). In the late 1950s and early 1960s experiments were conducted with therapeutically aborted fetuses[7] in which the presence of electrical activity in the heart was demonstrated by the implantation of electrodes (Stern, et al., 1961; Miller and Marini, 1958).

The use of fetal heart rate recording during pregnancy has had the principal benefit of enabling obstetricians 'to discover as a reality the rhythm hidden behind intermittent auscultation of heart sounds' (Melchoir, 1969, p. 107). Since the 1960s, continuous fetal heart rate monitoring in labour has emerged as a new technique, the object being that of picking up fetal distress in time for the fetus to be saved by rapid delivery (Beard and Campbell, 1977). Fetal heart monitoring in labour can be done using either internal or external methods. With the former, an electrode is fixed to the 'presenting part' of the fetus, normally the scalp. The external method involves locating an instrument on the outside of the mother's abdomen. Ultrasound may be used for this (with a transducer placed on the abdomen), and some women now receive what is called Doppler ultrasound to monitor their fetal hearts for many hours during labour.

7. Who owns the aborted fetus?

The Captured Womb

A pregnant woman in receipt of antenatal cardiotocography as the technique was employed in 1969 is shown in figure 7.6. She is smiling — though whether women actually enjoy the test is unknown. Some advocates of the method have proposed 'stressing' the fetus (with, for instance, oxytocin, as in a procedure known as the oxytocin challenge test), or at least waking it up so the heart rate rhythms may be correlated with fetal activity. ('The stimulus can be produced with sonic instruments, by external palpation or vaginal examination, so that the fetus reacts with reflex movements' (Hammacher, 1969, p. 85).) There are endless reasons why obstetricians should make fetuses move, and the era of the womb's sanctity as a private, peaceful place is, indeed, over. There are also many routes to provoking fetuses — one of which is simply sending doctors into the room: Myers (1979) found increases in the fetal heart rate with the entry of four or more doctors into the mother's room (the 'white coat' effect).

The general usefulness of non-stress antepartum fetal heart monitoring has recently been surveyed by Grant and Mohide (1982) who, after examining the evidence of many available studies, reached the conclusion that there is no basis for recommending it as a routine screening procedure. There are technical problems to do with standardizing both the procedure and the interpretation of the resulting heart rate traces. Grant cites the four RCT's so far carried out of this method of fetal

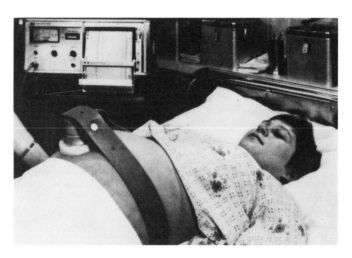

Figure 7.6 Antepartum cardiotocography
source: Whitfield, C.R. The Significance of methods for monitoring the fetal heart in Huntingford et al. *Perinatal Medicine, Proceedings of the First European Congress*, Berlin 1969, p. 81. With permission of the publisher Georg Thieme Verlag.

surveillance. The women studied in all four trials were considered high-risk: the technique did not significantly decrease perinatal mortality or morbidity. The most interesting result was that there were more deaths from causes other than lethal congenital abnormalities in the group of cases for which clinicians had access to the test results than in the group for which they did not.

'He is borne(e) before he is born'

In 1914 Ballantyne's book *Expectant Motherhood* regretted the profound invisibility of fetal life. Comparing the infant's first step Ballantyne deemed

> this initial phenomenon of erect locomotion . . . commonplace, almost insignificant, when compared with the first throb of the developing heart of the embryo and the first discernible flow of blood in his [sic] vessels.
> The building of a ship is more wonderful than the launching of it on its first cruise; the sculpturing of a statue is a greater thing than the unveiling of it; and so the making and growth of the infant in the womb are more momentous than its entrance into the life that follows birth . . . Birth is not the beginning of life . . . A mother carries, or bears her child for nine months before she gives birth to him; he is borne before he is born (Ballantyne, 1914, pp. 6–9).

This perspective on the human condition led Ballantyne to philosophize along the following lines, quoted here in full because they precisely anticipate the recent technological revolution in antenatal care:

> Could we throw upon the screen in kinematographic fashion the embryo as he [sic] passes from the simplicity of two or three rows of similar cells into the complexity of many interacting and interwoven systems of organs and tissues, all recognisably different; could we see the unborn infant as he quadruples his weight in one month of ante-natal life and doubles his length in another month of the same marvellous time; could we watch the first performances of functions such as the circulation of the blood, the formation of the bile, and the reflex actions of the brain and spinal cord, we should be compelled to cast away such ordinary expressions of surprise as 'wonderful', 'amazing', 'incredible', and 'unsurpassed', and seek to coin new terms to body forth the ideas which would be forming in our minds (Ballantyne, 1914, p. 5).

This is, indeed, what has come to pass. New technical representations of the fetus have spawned a new vocabulary of antenatal care. The 'verit-able iron curtain' (Donald, 1969, p. 326) of the mother has been swept aside and 'The expanding armamentarium of the laboratory — ranging from the electron microscope to radioimmune assays, from ultrasonics to binding site analysis — has been brought to bear on the study of the maternal–fetal relationship' (Barnes, 1975, p. i) — with the conse-quence that *'Today the infant at birth is no longer an unknown patient'* (Saling, 1969, p. 1; my italics).

Reviewing some of the newly-carved routes to fetal patienthood in this chapter, I have remarked how energetically and single-mindedly the goal of seeing and knowing the fetus (often irrespective of the mother's own inclination) has been pursued in recent decades. Another message of my survey is that the process of technological innovation in antenatal care has enjoyed a career spectacularly unhampered by the potential brake of clinical evaluation; new technologies have been dreamt up (albeit often serendipitously), introduced experimentally, and then rapidly non-experimentally into clinical practice. At times it has seemed that the nature and limits of technological innovation have been inspired 'simply' by a global impulse to expose as much of the fetus's intrauterine life to the physician's gaze as is both technically and humanly possible. For example, as Tulchinsky said, in 1974:

> Hormones are presently used for the assessment of fetal well-being only because of our present inability to get access into the fetal compartment and to determine other biochemical and physiologic indices of fetal wellbeing . . . Difficulties in interpreting results of such studies are numerous. Despite all these problems, the clinician *has* to depend on these tests because they are one of few *objective* criteria which the clinician presently has at hand (Tulchinsky, 1974, p. 98; italics added).

When 'subjective' criteria were the only ones around, obstetricians experienced an unwelcome dependence: 'Recent advances have greatly enhanced the obstetrician's ability to monitor fetal maturity. Until [this point] . . . the physician was *forced* to utilize last menstrual period dates, [and] onset of fetal activity' (Quilligan and Freeman, 1969, p. 150). The underlying motive of obstetricians to acquaint themselves with fetuses was described thus by Browne:

> It is becoming essential for those most closely concerned with reproduc-tion (obstetricians) to pass from empirical intervention in the course of pregnancy where the fetus is considered to be at risk, to a scheme of management based on a precise mode of determining the physical and

metabolic status of the fetus, *who lies unborn, and at risk in the uterus* (Browne, 1969, p. 11; italics added).

The obstetrical pursuit of more and more knowledge about the fetal condition and life-style *in utero* is integral to the obstetrical claim to expertise in general. The desire for knowledge *preceded* the antenatal care revolution; as necessity is the mother of invention, so it has been only the technical *capacity* for knowledge that is truly new.

Lying prone

The reason why the woman in Figure 7.6 is lying down is because her fetus is having its heart monitored. It is, as one researcher has commented, most odd that, in view of the substantial evidence that 'the most unphysiologic thing one can do for either mother or baby is to lie mother flat on her back, it is a sobering thought that as we get more and more involved in . . . monitoring . . . the first thing we do is to lie mother flat on her back so that we can drape all our recording gear on her and baby' (Liley, 1976, p. 76). But if the new monitoring techniques do not strictly require physical passivity, they have certainly implied it ideologically. As the 'iron curtain' of the mother has been swept aside revealing the womb and its contents in their full glory, it has become no longer necessary to consult mothers about their attitudes. Accordingly, women have not been consulted, and almost none of the evaluations of the techniques described in this chapter have included an attempt to assess the attitudes of pregnant women. In their book *Birth Rites, Birth Rights* (1980) Judith Lumley and Jill Astbury point out that, out of more than 500 articles published on the fetal monitor in the preceding 10 years, only two considered women's attitudes (both these were written by women who were childbirth educators). A study in London by Wendy Farrant of women's responses to amniocentesis showed that, of the group of women routinely screened, a high proportion found the experience of waiting for the result of the test distressing. They developed symptoms of anxiety, some of which were severe (Farrant, 1980).

During the early years of obstetric ultrasound, the effect of this method of fetal surveillance on the fetus's mother (and thus on the fetus) was scarcely considered. Descriptions of the method were sometimes accompanied by allegations as to the patient's comfort, for example:

The frequency used for cephalometry is 2½ megacycles per second. The apparatus is portable on a trolley and is used at the bedside. For the patient the examination is simple and free from discomfort' (Willocks, et al., 1964, p. 13).

From the patient's point of view the examination must be reasonably brief. A woman with a large abdominal tumour or a gravid uterus does not tolerate a prolonged examination in the supine position, especially when the bladder may be filling rapidly as well (Donald, 1974b, p. 210).

— nor may she, of course, especially enjoy waiting for her ultrasound examination with a rapidly filling bladder. Finally, 'patient comfort' may be conceptualized as a brake on changes in the procedures:

The average time taken for each scan varies with the size of the patient and expanse required to be traversed but is usually from one to two minutes. The speed of the probe cannot be substantially increased or the patient will experience discomfort which is completely absent at the present speed (MacVicar and Donald, 1963, p. 388).

Beyond this matter of physical comfort during or before the procedure, there is the more complex question of pregnant women's attitudes to ultrasound examination, and the possible impact of the examination on the prenatal mother–child relationship. It may be alleged that to all concerned ultrasound scanning is a delightful experience: hence the following letter from two Glasgow obstetricians published recently in the *British Medical Journal*: 'In our experience all obstetricians provided with this service have found it most valuable; mothers have found fascinating and reassuring the sight of their fetuses moving on the real-time display' (Neilson and Whitfield, 1981, p. 94).

The pleasure obstetricians may gain from antenatal care, however deployed, is a matter that deserves serious attention, as is the parallel question of maternal satisfaction. To some extent the obstetrical pleasure is evidenced in the activities charted in this chapter: increased technical complexity has almost certainly boosted the zest with which many obstetricians are able to approach their antenatal clinics (which is one answer to the question, 'who enjoys antenatal care?' asked in the previous chapter). Maternal enjoyment of antenatal care, and particularly of such features as ultrasound, is more debatable. A recent attempt to evaluate one aspect of this issue divided pregnant women receiving ultrasound into two groups. The first 'high feedback' group were allowed to look at the screen and see the fetus, and were provided with 'verbal feedback as to fetal size, shape and movement'. The second 'low feedback' group were not; they were treated to 'a global evaluation of progress', that is, they were told that everything was all right. Results indicated that 'Women in the high-feedback group showed uniformly more positive attitudes toward the scan. There was no support for the view that scanning causes distress, although the emotional impact was influenced by the amount of feedback available' (Campbell, et al., 1982, p. 59).

One may conclude from this that pregnant women like being talked to by those providing them with antenatal care. This article also wins the prize for being the first published acknowledgement of the fact that while ultrasound enables obstetricians to see fetuses, 'It is now [24 years after the first published report on the obstetric uses of ultrasound] possible for a mother to see her fetus *in utero*' (p. 60).

What does this do to, or for, pregnant women? 'If such feedback enhances awareness of the fetus and influences compliance with health care recommendations such as stopping smoking and alcohol intake, then, as scanning accomplishes this at an earlier stage of pregnancy, there will be greater potential benefit to the fetus' (p. 60). According to this study, seeing the fetus does, indeed, encourage women to decrease their smoking and alcohol intake and go to the dentist more (Reading, et al., 1982). Ultrasound must, therefore, take its place in a long line of other well-used strategies for educating women to be good mothers. The opportunities are enormous:

When a mother undergoes ultrasound scanning of the fetus, this seems a great opportunity for her to meet her child socially and in this way, one hopes, to view him [sic] as a companion aboard rather than as a parasite . . . Doctors and technicians scanning mothers have a great opportunity to enable mothers to form an early affectionate bond to their child by demonstrating the child to the mother. This should help mothers to behave concernedly towards the fetus (Dewsbury, 1980, p. 481).

Antenatal care has finally discovered mother love. Along with postnatal bonding, prenatal bonding will now in future be added to the repertoire of reproductive activities named and controlled by obstetricians.

There is, of course, no evidence that mothers have ever regarded their fetuses as parasites, but it certainly seems possible that ultrasound changes the experience of pregnancy in ways of which we, as a society, are unaware. The following maternal viewpoint was published by the *New Yorker* (11 August 1980, pp. 21–2):

At first, it is hard to make sense of the swirling, unstable patterns of light and dark, but when the fetus is still, one can soon distinguish its head and then, a little less clearly, its torso. I . . . was unprepared to see that figure emerge from the initially unintelligible swirls, unprepared for the knowledge that I was looking at my baby specifically as it was at that very moment. The picture shocked me, as though I had broken a taboo, thrilled me for the extension of my powers, surprised me by its concrete actuality, frightened me by bringing me closer than I am accustomed to being to the nothingness out of which we all come.

8

Controlling Labour

For thousands of years the practice of obstetrics was almost exclusively in the hands of nonprofessional women. Induction of labour made its appearance when obstetrics became a part of medical science, and was freed from superstition and religious dogma.

Fields, et al., 1965, p. 13

As with the extent to which the condition of the fetus *in utero* may be known by obstetricians, technologies to control labour are an essential part of the argument about obstetrical expertise. Both the history of induction of labour and the history of intrauterine fetal surveillance are, in this sense, the history of 'a search for a technology of control and for the control of a technology' (Arney, 1982, p. 75). In clinical language, induction of labour is one of two methods (the other is caesarean section) of 'elective' delivery. 'Elective', meaning 'chosen', precisely represents the dominance of the obstetrical empire, since an elective delivery is one chosen by obstetricians and not by pregnant women. This chapter, then, looks briefly (and by no means comprehensively) at the rise and fall of some of the most important methods for controlling labour, and at their different articulations within clinical practice.

To begin in the middle, perhaps the most complete illustration of the importance of obstetrical control in the induction of labour is contained in an article entitled 'Elective Painless Rapid Childbirth Anticipating Labour' published in 1943. The article described 39 women in whom delivery was accomplished by giving spinal anaesthesia prior to the start of labour, and then manually dilating their cervices and delivering the babies with instruments. The time taken from the introduction of spinal anaesthesia to perineal repair (all the women had episiotomies) was never more than 30 minutes. The advantage to the mother was said to be that she was spared a single labour pain. The advantage to the obstetrician, aside from total control over the process of labour, was the impressive (albeit dangerous) ease with which cervices could be manually dilated and intravaginal manipulations carried out in the anaesthetized pelvis (Koster and Perrotta, 1943).

Understanding the uterus

Understanding the uterus belongs with visualizing the fetus as one of the main goals of twentieth-century research in obstetrics. As one doctor rightly observed in 1950:

> One of the most fascinating aspects of obstetrics is the fact that the uterus is almost completely inaccessible in so far as the direct study of its dynamics is concerned. If it were possible to observe the uterus in action we should be deprived of a huge and dramatic literature dealing with interpretations based upon isolated observations (Danforth, cited in Lash and Lash, 1950, p. 74).

Another locus of puzzlement, and hence of research activity, has been the way in which it is perceived that some uteruses do not contract efficiently enough to deliver their contents unaided, and some do so too early to deliver a fetus with a reasonable chance of survival.

Most of the early knowledge about how to induce labour was derived from techniques used to procure abortion, since the essential point to establish in either case was just which intervention would effectively stimulate uterine contractions (Baines, forthcoming). In medieval England, iris root was inserted into, or fumigated under, the womb in order to make a woman 'lose her child' (Rowland, 1981, p. 97). Alternatively, a plaster of artemisia 'from the navel to the privy members' would draw out a child, dead or alive, from the womb — but, if left there for too long would, unhappily, draw out the womb also (p. 137).

Strenuous exercise, putting foreign objects in the uterus, swallowing cathartics, and rupturing the membranes, have also all been used to procure abortion and induce labour. An interesting example of the migration of techniques from one field to the other is the practice of amniography (described in chapter 7). When injections of sodium and strontium iodide into the amniotic sac were found unfortunately to precipitate labour, it was decided to capitalize on this finding and use it deliberately to induce labour (Burke, 1935) — a technique hailed initially as safe, but not long after recognized as carrying a raised risk of fetal death.

Douglas Murphy, Assistant Professor of Obstetrics and Gynaecology at the University of Pennsylvania, recorded the contractions of 1,153 pregnant women in a book published in 1947. His object was to see if uterine inertia in labour could be predicted from patterns of uterine contractility in late pregnancy, and the inertia then successfully treated with small doses of oxytocic drugs. ('Oxytocic', a word that will crop up often in this chapter, comes from the Greek words 'oxy', meaning 'swift', and 'tocos', meaning 'birth'.) To study the nature of uterine contractions Murphy used an external measuring device developed in Germany in the mid-1930s and known as the Lorand tocograph. The apparatus rested on the woman's abdomen, and a movable rod, projecting from the bottom of the instrument and making contact with the abdominal wall, responded to uterine contractions by operating a level in the tocograph. The lever attached to an ink-containing pen drove the pen across a piece of paper and thus finally produced a readable recording.

There were lots of technical difficulties with the apparatus — the ink kept drying up and had to be replenished, the pen had to be dried out immediately after use, and the whole thing had to be cleaned frequently by a watch repairer. Nevertheless with its aid Murphy collected a total of 3,154 sets of observations, 1,936 before the onset of labour. He determined that pregnancy could be divided into three periods: (1) a period of 'relative quiescence' up to 34 weeks; (2) a period of 'non-rhythmic activity' from 35 to 38 weeks; and (3) a period of rhythmic activity at the end of pregnancy.

In settling upon the best instrument to use for recording contraction patterns, Murphy uncovered an uncomfortably colourful history of mechanical attempts to chart the subterranean activity of wombs. Two main methods had been used since the rise of what was called 'tokodynamometry' (Reynolds, et al., 1954) in the mid-nineteenth century. There were methods that involved inserting some measuring device actually into the uterus, and those that employed some external measuring technique.

The gentlemen (all men, and some not so gentle) who explored the field were nothing if not inventive in the strategies they tried. The first report on the characteristics of uterine contractions was published in 1861 by Kristeller in Germany. Kristeller wanted to improve the safety of obstetrical forceps by building into them some indicator of the amount of force being used by the accoucheur; thus, his delivery forceps incorporated into their handles a spring measuring device. Attempts to devise internal measures of the uterine state also date from the 1860s, and the first such improvised method was Schatz's balloon of 1872. Schatz who, like Kristeller, worked in Germany, introduced into the uterus a water-filled rubber bag of around 80 cc capacity. The pressure of the contracting uterus on the bag was then transmitted to two mercury manometers. This method was refined — if that is the correct word — by Poullet in 1880 who combined the intrauterine balloon with a rectal balloon, the logic being that one needed in addition to a measure of intrauterine pressure a measure of intra-abdominal pressure on the fetus.

An overwhelming disadvantage of internal measuring methods was that the presence of a large balloon in the uterus (or elsewhere internally) distorted results by creating an effect of its own. Furthermore, since the women experimented on were normal pregnant women in whom interruption of pregnancy was not desired, the inadvertent rupture of the membranes sometimes caused by the balloon counted against the method. Other variations of the internal monitoring method included bags in the bladder (Podleschka, 1932; Alvarez and Caldeyro, 1950), a combination of a blown-up condom in the uterus and one in the woman's stomach (Woodbury, Hamilton and Torpin, 1939), and the use of needles passed directly through the abdominal wall as early as the second month of pregnancy (Alvarez and Caldeyro, 1950). Figure 8.1 shows a pregnant woman attached to one of the tokodynamometers, incorporating a transabdominal needle, used by Alvarez and Caldeyro.[1]

As well as the transabdominal needle, Figure 9.1 shows seven external recording instruments. The resultant external mapping of the uterine territory is shown in Figure 8.2.

The uterus can also be mapped in terms of the way it responds to drugs. Investigations of drug effects on uterine behaviour began in the 1890s, when drugs such as morphine, ether and chloroform were found by intra-uterine measurement to alter the state of uteruses. In the twentieth century this work on drug effects has been extended, and by the mid 1960s it was established that the following agents, among others, could measurably alter uterine behaviour: local anaesthetics, general anaesthetics, sodium chloride, carbon dioxide, epinephrine and norepinephrine, ergot, sparteine sulphate, vasopressin, isoxuprine, relaxin, magnesium, meperidine (pethidine), promazine, dimenhydrinate (dramamine) and nicotine.

---

1. Apparently this research was started as a response to an extremely high (80 per cent) local caesarean section rate, and was an attempt to provide an understanding of the physiology of normal labour that could persuade clinicians to lower the section rate.

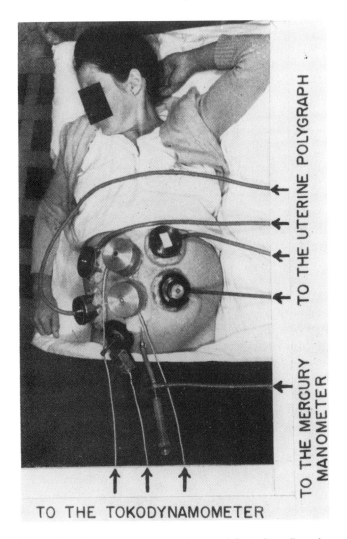

TO THE TOKODYNAMOMETER

Figure 8.1 Recording of intrauterine pressure by transabdominal needle and seven channel external recording of uterine activity
source: Reynolds, et al., *Clinical Measurement of Uterine Forces in Pregnancy and Later* 1954, p. 68, courtesy of CC Thomas, Publisher.

One major twentieth century development in understanding the uterus concerns the external method of monitoring. In 1931 Bode recorded the electrical activity of the pregnant human uterus in labour by means of an electrocardiograph with needle electrodes located on the abdominal wall at the level of the umbilicus. From the 1940s on, papers

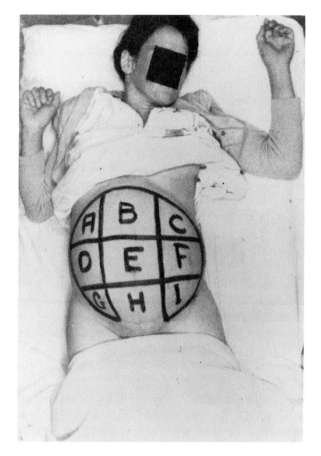

Figure 8.2 The nine areas used to identify the location of receptors in tokodynamometer
determinations
source: Reynolds, et al., 1954, p. 97, courtesy of CC Thomas, Publisher.

began to appear documenting the electrical activity of the uterus in true
and false labour and in progressive and unprogressive labour. The
resultant tracings were not easy to interpret. Indeed, the relevance to
clinical practice of graph-paper representations of uterine behaviour is
still not entirely clear today, and intra-observer variation in the interpretation of uterine contraction and fetal heart rate traces continues
to be something of a problem. It is significant that modern monitoring
equipment combines a tracing of uterine contractions with one of the
fetal heart rate: thus, it has been possible for obstetricians to see at one
glance both the condition of the uterus and the condition of the fetus
(but not the condition of the mother).

The 'incompetence' of the cervix

Another of the uterus's secrets was brought out into the open in 1950 in the form of the designation 'incompetent cervix'. This revealing phrase was used to describe those cervices which habitually dilate too early in pregnancy, thus precipitating a miscarriage or premature delivery, and was put before the world in an article entitled 'Habitual Abortion: the Incompetent Internal Os of the Cervix'. Its authors, A. F. and S. R. Lash, proposed that the offending os (cervical opening) could be one cause of recurrent abortion and suggested that the defect might be repaired between pregnancies. In 1953 Rubovits and his co-workers specified a method of diagnosing an incompetent cervix by putting balloons and cannulas in the uterus, injecting dye and taking five to six X-rays. In the same year V. N. Shirodkar, Professor of Obstetrics and Gynaecology in Bombay, added his name to obstetric terminology by describing a technique of using 'strips of fascia lata' to surround a weak cervical sphincter and give it strength. This type of cervical 'cerclage' is still used, along with another devised by McDonald (1957) which employs heavy silk or mersilene tape drawn up tightly like a purse string around the cervix. The effectiveness of cervical cerclage in preventing premature delivery is unproven, but the faith of obstetricians in the method is reflected in rates as high as 80 per 1,000 deliveries managed (Grant, et al., 1982).

The 'discovery' and mechanical treatment of the incompetent cervix was one move in the attempt to prevent the premature ejection of pregnancy by the uterus. As Anderson and Turnbull explain this motive behind obstetrical work:

> Death of a normally-formed fetus in association with spontaneous abortion or premature labour is particularly tragic when continuation of the pregnancy to term would have been likely to ensure survival. For this reason obstetricians have been anxious to find, and willing to use in clinical practice, therapies which appear to have a scientific basis for their action and which seem likely to be safe (Anderson and Turnbull, 1982, p. 163).

Most of the strategies used to this end have been drug treatments, with or without the addition of bedrest as a 'commonsense' approach to persuading the uterus into quiescence. Hormones — either natural or synthetic oestrogens and progestogens — were obvious candidates, and were first suggested in the 1930s. Progestogens were given to patients with recurrent spontaneous abortion, and from the 1960s to those at risk of preterm labour. Despite enormous local enthusiasm for these interventions, there was really no evidence of efficacy. The same is true of oestrogens, the most infamous of the oestrogen experiments being that of diethylstilboestrol (DES). DES was given to pregnant women mostly between 1940 and 1970, and mostly in the USA, with the aim of preventing miscarriage. It had the unexpected 'time bomb' effect of raising the risk of genital abnormalities, especially vaginal cancer, in people exposed *in utero* (Seaman and Seaman, 1978), and, additionally, appears to have raised the risk of cancer in the mothers themselves (Beral and Colwell, 1980).

In the 1980s, oestrogen and progestogen treatments designed to salvage high-risk pregnancy are still given. However, the major therapeutic intervention in the prevention of preterm delivery is now a group of drugs known as betamimetics. These are drugs which mimic certain actions of the sympathetic nervous system and do have an effect, not only on the muscles of the uterus, but on muscles throughout the body, including the heart. Lack of evidence, with these drugs too, as to the critical dual aim of effectiveness and safety, does not seem to have a substantial deterrent effect, with some 87 per cent of obstetricians in the UK being prepared to use betamimetics to try to arrest labour (Lewis, et al., 1980).

German corn and bougies, bladders and the OBE: inducing labour

Induction of labour with the aim of delivering a live fetus probably dates from the mid-eighteenth century. Denman's *An Introduction to the Practice of Midwifery* (1794) refers to the first case of a labour induced by artificial rupture of the membranes (ARM) and terminating in successful delivery, as occurring in 1756 in the wife of a London linen draper. (The indication for induction in this case was said to be contracted pelvis.) Yet midwives had been intervening in various ways to initiate labour for some time (Graham, 1950), and the stimulating action of herbal and other orally-administered agents on the uterus has long been recognized in many cultures, as have the oxytocic effect of breast stimulation, orgasm, and human semen (Mead and Newton, 1967).

One of the best known and most used of Nature's oxytocins is ergot, a fungous growth that is prone to appear on the heads of rye grain in wet, cold seasons. Ergot was used by wisewomen across Europe for centuries; they used five, seven, or nine (never an even number) of the black grains to start labour (Graham, 1950). Thus, the so-called discovery of ergot in 1808 by the US physician Stearns (1777–1848) belongs to the list of those technical landmarks in obstetrics which represent, rather, the relabelling by obstetricians of traditional midwifery expertise. In fact, it was from an immigrant German midwife that Stearns first learnt the wonderful properties of the 'new' drug (Wertz and Wertz, 1977). In the case of ergot, the renaming process was aided by the fact that ergot had been in disrepute for its toxic effects and use as an abortifacient; in Germany in the seventeenth and eighteenth centuries, the drug was actually outlawed.

Stearns was able to convince his medical peers that ergot could be used to speed labour without necessarily dire results: he reported 100 such cases (Fitzgerald, 1958). However, the early use of ergot by obstetricians to induce labour was accompanied by such a notable rise in stillbirths that in 1824 the Medical Society of New York carried out a special inquiry into the safety of the drug. During the course of this inquiry, ergot's title of 'pulvis [powder] ad partem' became, less charitably, 'pulvis ad mortem'.

None of the three main modern methods of inducing labour — ARM, drugs, and the mechanical dilatation of the cervix — are recent innovations. But, whereas the notion of inducing labour has been a consistent preoccupation among obstetricians, there has been much less consistency about how and whom to induce, and why. This variation in practice was, as we saw in chapter 4, already getting some prominence in medical journals by the 1930s, when obstetricians were taking a critical look at why antenatal care had not fulfilled its promise in substantially reducing obstetric mortality. As to methods, by this time obstetricians were also deeply engaged in the debate about the superiority of one technique over another. Writing in 1929, G. F. Gibberd of Guy's Hospital in London enthusiastically advocated the use of animal bladders and argued that this 'Continental' approach to induction of labour deserved to be used more often in England. Gibberd described the technique as follows:

The apparatus that has been found most satisfactory consists of a short piece of metal tube about one inch long to which is attached a piece of rubber tubing about six inches in length. Through this a long metal stylet is passed so that its point projects about five inches beyond the end of the metal tube . . . The animal bladders, which are obtainable ready sterilized in sealed glass tubes, are of two sizes — a large (pig's) bladder with a capacity of about 500 cubic cm and a small (sheep's) bladder with a capacity of about 200 cubic cm. The bladder is tied to the metal tube by means of a silk suture, and stretched by means of the stylet. It can thus be introduced through the cervical canal . . . and when it is completely within the uterine cavity the stylet is withdrawn and (in the case of a large bladder) about 200 cubic cm of pure sterile glycerin is injected into the bladder by means of a syringe. The rubber tubing is then clamped (Gibberd, 1929b, p. 617).

The women were given a general anaesthetic, and most had been subjected previously to unsuccessful attempts to induce labour with quinine and pituitary extract. Gibberd concluded that the hazards of animal bladders appeared to be no greater than those of any other instrument for inducing labour, and that the induction-labour interval was shorter. Gibberd's figures, based on 30 cases using animal bladders and 23 using stomach tubes or bougies, are given in table 8.1. (A 'bougie' is a term used to describe flexible instruments for dilating orifices.)

Table 8.1 Induction of labour at Guy's Hospital, 1929

| | *Method of induction used* | |
| | *Animal bladder** | *Stomach tube/bougie*** |
	%	%
Failures	10	9
Successes	90	91
Induction interval:		
less than 24 hrs	85	40
less than 12 hrs	63	20
less than 6 hrs	41	10
Puerperal morbidity***	15	11

* 30 cases
** 23 cases
***The BMA used a standard definition of a 'morbid puerperium' at the time, which hinged on the presence of a fever indicating infection.
source: adapted from Gibberd, G. F. The Results of Induction of Labour with Animal Bladders *British Medical Journal* 5 Oct. 1929, p. 617. With permission of the BMJ.

The easiest, cheapest and quite possibly oldest method of attempting induction is artificial rupture of the membranes, known as 'the English method', since it was mostly used in England until the late nineteenth century. Obstetricians in the USA were said to regard the method with disdain because it ignored the physiological importance of intact membranes to cervical dilatation in labour. But induction of labour using ARM constituted 'one of the notable trends in modern obstetrics' in the USA from the late 1920s onwards (Eastman, 1938, p. 721). As with many aspects of obstetric practice, its 'assumed benefits . . . in inducing labor, and particularly in augmenting labor, have not been proved' (Simkin, 1983, p. 112).

Other strategies for inducing labour attempted in the nineteenth and twentieth centuries have included electricity (1802), breast massage (1839), massage of the uterus (1820), vaginal tampons (1842), cervical plugs (1820), intrauterine injections of hot water (1846), or creosote and tar water (1884), seaweed in the vagina (the 1860s), toy balloons (the early 1900s), and, most of all, bougies. Bougies were popular from the mid-nineteenth century, though their popularity varied from place to place. In a study of 160 cases of bougie induction, published in 1930, D. G. Morton called the procedure successful in prompting progressive labour in 82.5 per cent of women. Two women in Morton's series died directly as a result of the procedure, one from a uterine infection and the other from a perforated uterus. Six babies also died as a consequence of cord prolapse. Morton used a 3 cm wide bougie, but pregnancy outcome with smaller bougies was not apparently much better; and even refinements such as X-raying to aid correct placement of the bougie could not obviate the dangers of infection and damage due to instrumental invasion of the uterus (Eastman, 1938). The use of both bougies and animal bladders continued throughout the 1950s and even into the 1960s on both sides of the Atlantic (Fields, et al., 1965).

Aside from ergot, an early and long-lived contender among nonmechanical inducers of labour was quinine, said to have been first described by Porak in 1878 as capable of galvanizing the pregnant uterus into action (Engström, 1959). It also had a considerable reputation as an abortifacient. From the early 1900s, quinine was fashionable for the elective induction of labour, often in combination with castor oil. In one Canadian practice in 1920, for example, women to be induced took 1 oz of castor oil followed two hours later by 10 grains of quinine in solution with 10 minims of hydrochloric acid. The dose was repeated two-hourly, up to a maximum of 30 grains. The doctor whose regime this was declared that the problem of safely inducing labour at term had thereby been solved. Around the same time at St Mary's Hospital, Manchester, up to 40 grains of quinine were given, though the drug was stopped when the patient complained of nausea and ringing in the ears.

In 1927, an American obstetrician, once himself a keen proponent of quinine induction, sounded the beginning of the end of the era of enthusiasm for it when he reported with alarm the death of a baby from a failed quinine induction two weeks before term (Gellhorn, 1927). His caution was underlined by findings the other side of the Atlantic, when a pharmacologist and a gynaecologist in Liverpool published 'A Preliminary Investigation of Foetal Deaths Following Quinine Induction'. Adding together figures from seven hospitals, including their own, they reported 'fourteen unaccountable stillbirths in 765 cases of [quinine] induction' (Dilling and Gemmell, 1929, p. 353). Apparently Porak, who had introduced quinine to the induction scene, had himself noted a higher incidence of meconium staining during labour and more neonatal jaundice afterwards.

By the 1940s, ardent inducers of labour were saved by the arrival of another substance — sparteine sulphate, an alkaloid related to ergot. A decade later, and especially in the USA, sparteine was in *its* turn being hailed as the completely safe induction agent, and as late as 1963 was regarded in some circles as the ideal induction drug (Plentl and Friedman, 1963). Embrey and Yates in Britain, who in 1964 carried out a 'tocographic' study of the impact of sparteine sulphate on the uterus, concluded with a caution about the unpredictable action of the drug, which not infrequently produced uterine tetany:

> It would be regrettable indeed, if these warnings went unheeded and sparteine continued to be regarded as the completely 'safe' and 'harmless' oxytocic. It is a matter of history that crude ergot was at one time thought 'safe' . . . It would be discreditable if once again history was repeated . . . As Kaminetsky puts it, there are 'no really safe biologically active drugs. There are only safe physicians' (Embrey and Yates, 1964, p. 35).

A good point.

The sequence of innovation, followed by enthusiasm, followed by, at first, isolated case-reports of untoward side-effects which then combine to produce a fall in the use of the said innovation, is a pattern found throughout medicine, and is described elsewhere in this book in relation to other antenatal procedures.

In the background to the seemingly perpetual discoveries of new pharmaceutical compounds for inducing labour were old faithfuls such as castor oil. Castor oil, sometime partner in the quinine debacle, was part of the OBE (oil, bath, enema) routine which generations of parturient women have had bestowed on them. The oxytocic properties of castor oil were recognized by the late eighteenth century.

In 1958 G. C. Nabors sent a questionnaire out to the heads of the Departments of Obstetrics in 50 USA medical schools: 32 returned the questionnaire, and half reported the use of castor oil to induce labour. Opinion differed dramatically as to its effectiveness. One professor termed it 'A dehydrating, debilitating, drastic drug' which 'should be used on machinery only' (Nabors, 1958, p. 38). A trial in 1959 with 60 women comparing the effects of castor oil, enema and hot bath, with each alone, and with another control group of 15 women, showed that use of the three methods together increased 'uterine contractile work' by 264 per cent, castor oil alone by 186 per cent, enemas by 95 per cent and hot baths not at all (Mathie and Dawson, 1959).

Inventing William

A persisting problem for would-be controllers of labour is the *individuality* of the pregnant uterus (reflecting the, at times, inconvenient individuality of the pregnant woman). Not all uteruses respond in the same way to the same intervention, or the same dosage of a drug. Indeed, in order to be adequately active, one uterus might require eight times the dose of oxytocin that would be sufficient for another (Turnbull and Anderson, 1967).

A major new advance in providing for uterine individuality was secured in the early 1960s with the development of the 'titration' method of delivering oxytocic drugs. The principle of this new method was described by its developers, A. C. Turnbull and Anne Anderson, then at Aberdeen Maternity Hospital: .

> We considered that an ideal regime for oxytocin administration would be to start with a low dose and increase the amount at short intervals until strong, regular uterine contractions were established. The optimum oxytocin dose would depend therefore on the strength and frequency of the uterine contractions produced and not on the amount of oxytocin being administered. In other words, oxytocin should be given in the form of a 'titration', the 'end-point' being optimal uterine activity (Turnbull and Anderson, 1968, p. 26).

The rate of infusion of the drug is thus automatically controlled, a solution to the task of inducing labour which appears to yield total control to the machine, but happily (or unhappily, depending on one's viewpoint), the machines are not 100 per cent reliable, and still need to be overseen by doctors and midwives. Indeed, an advantage of the new method, stressed by Turnbull and Anderson, was that it left medical and midwifery staff more time for the patient.

When the titration method of oxytocin infusion was first employed in Aberdeen, it was found particularly useful for patients who had experienced amniotomy, but had only ineffectually gone into labour. From

1960 to 1964 in Aberdeen Maternity Hospital, the percentage of patients having their labours accelerated rose nearly tenfold, from 1.1 to 10.4 per cent (Turnbull and Anderson, 1968, p. 33).

The original machine used for titrated oxytocin delivery was an infusion pump called a Continuous Slow Injector with a 12-speed gearbox. In 1970, the same research team published an account of a newly-automated piece of equipment which subsequently became known as the Cardiff Infusion Unit or, more significantly and affectionately, as 'William' (not 'Mary'; he was thus named by a female doctor) (Francis, et al., 1970). A picture of William is given in Figure 8.3.

William's invention solidified the achievements of an induction drug, oxytocin, whose own discovery marked a watershed in the history of induction. In 1906 Sir Henry Dale had reported an *in vitro* oxytocic effect of a substance called posterior pituitary extract. Dale later put pieces of the uteruses of virgin guinea pigs in dilute solutions of pituitary extract and watched them contract vigorously. In 1909 a paper was

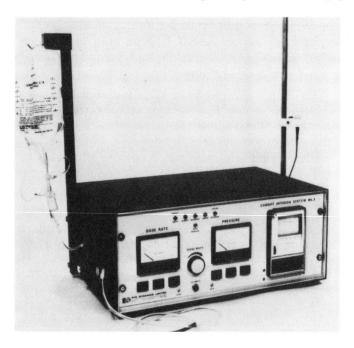

Figure 8.3 'William': The mechanical inducer of labour. (Cardiff infusion unit for control of oxytocin dose and intrauterine pressure.) (Photograph by courtesy of Pye Dynamics.)
source: Howie, P.W. Induction of Labour in Chard, T. and Richards, M. (eds.) *Benefits and Hazards of the New Obstetrics*, International Medical Publications, 1977, p. 83. With permission of the author.

published in the *British Medical Journal* by Blair Bell describing the application of this substance to the pregnant uterus. Reporting on its use in three cases, Bell came to the conclusion that 'in the future we shall rely on infundibular [pituitary] extract to produce contractions of the uterus in many serious obstetric complications and difficulties' (p. 1,611). In 1910 pituitary extract was used to accelerate labour in cases of uterine inertia, and in the next two years more than 100 publications appeared testifying to the 'outstanding acceptance of the new successful attack' on the slothful uterus (Hofbauer, 1955).

Bell administered pituitary extract intramuscularly, but evidence emerged that intramuscular injections did sometimes cause maternal death, so that eventually the preferred route became the intravenous one (Page, 1943). Before that the stuff was put in the mouth, up the nose, under the skin, and up the rectum — though some experiments were confined only to cats (Knaus, 1926). Indeed, pregnant women have been given induction drugs by almost every available biological route. Some drugs have been injected directly into the amniotic sac. One such was an iodine compound, Uroselectan B, which flourished as an induction agent in the 1930s. Reporting on its use in 115 cases at Queen Charlotte's Maternity Hospital and King's College Hospital, Playfair (1941) noted that 111 women were successfully induced and two babies died as a result of the method — a fetal mortality regarded at the time, interestingly, as acceptably low.

The advantages of the new intravenous method were said to be the approximation to a physiological effect, and the ability to interrupt the drip and thus the process of labour if fetus or mother appeared to be suffering unduly. Theobald, who pioneered the 'physiological' use of oxytocin in Bradford, reported in 1956 on over 1,000 inductions. The system used in St Luke's Maternity Hospital operated thus:

> the registrars decide on its use according to general instructions, and direct the house surgeons to set it [the drip] up. No special precautions are taken beyond seeing that the primary drip does not exceed a concentration of 1:5000 and that no untoward alteration in the rhythm or note of the foetal heart occurs during the first half hour (Theobald, et al., 1956, pp. 644–5).

This whole strategy rested on certain assumptions. For example, it was assumed that 'intact membranes during labour are a liability rather than an asset'; that 'every woman . . . should be nearing delivery after she has been in labour for 12 hours' and that all induced patients would receive morphine and other strong painkillers when in established labour. This was not all, however; individual patients also got eight-hourly intramuscular injections of penicillin and 10 mg of vitamin K orally — quite a package (both the penicillin and the vitamin K were given primarily, it was said, for the benefit of the infant).

Theobald's figures showed 6.5 per cent of Bradford births induced in 1952, of which 16.7 per cent had a pitocin [induction] drip. By 1954, the figures were 7.6 per cent and 28.3 per cent. As the use of pitocin rose, so did the incidence of caesarean section. As early as the mid-1950s a 'staggering' increase in the use of caesarean section was referred to in Britain and the USA.

The pituitary extract in use in the 1940s contained two hormones, vasopressin and oxytocin. The disadvantage of this was that vasopressin had an antidiuretic and blood pressure raising effect, and it was thus desirable to devise a way of separating the two hormones. This was achieved when in 1953–54 Vincent du Vigneaud and his co-workers developed a technique for isolating a highly purified form of the oxytocic fraction from pituitary extract and for manufacturing a synthetic version of oxytocin. Such experiments were merely of laboratory interest, how-ever, until it became possible to synthesize oxytocin on an industrial scale. This latter development, reported on by R. A. Boissonnas and co-workers in an article entitled 'Une nouvelle synthèse de l'oxytocine' in 1955, paved the way for the very considerable growth in the use of hormonal induction of labour that took place in many countries in the 1960s and early 1970s.

As with the fate of the whole pituitary extract in the 1920s, resear-chers were not content with trying only one route for oxytocin to the uterus. A few diehards of the transbuccal method were alive and well enough to have a go with 'linguets' in the mouth (Dillon, et al., 1962). N. E. Borglin from the Malmö General Hospital in Sweden put it up 96 women's noses: 'The solution was administered by a polyethylene tube . . . the patients were instructed to blow the entire dose into one of the nasal cavities' (Borglin, 1962, p. 241). Comparing results in these 96 women with those in 132 who received their oxytocin intravenously, Borglin found that 79 per cent of the 96 delivered as a result of one blow up the nose compared with 85 per cent of the 132 who got it intravenously.

Underlying these details of administrative technique, it was soon clear that oxytocin was far superior in terms of effecting the termination of pregnancy to the older methods of castor oil or quinine and castor oil. Most practitioners who used oxytocin combined it with ARM, though not necessarily simultaneously. As the practice developed, it became clear that another factor — the so-called 'ripeness' of the cervix — was involved in successful induction. In 1955 Bishop laid down the ground rule that for successful induction in multiparae the cervix should be soft, and admit one finger, and the presenting part of the fetus should have reached 1 cm above the spinal plane. Bishop's wisdom was formalized as the 'Bishop Pelvic Scoring System', known more familiarly as the Bishop score (Bishop, 1964). If the cervix was not ripe, it might sabotage the whole induction enterprise: figure 8.4 (originally drawn by someone called Cocks) shows cervical control over the efficiency of induction.

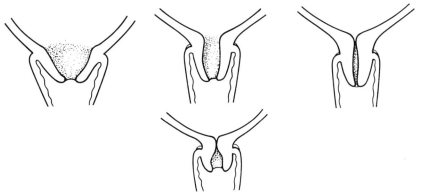

Figure 8.4 The relationship between the condition of the cervix and success rate of surgical induction
source: Llewellyn-Jones, 1969, p. 336, originally from Cocks, D. P. in *British Medical Journal*, 1955, With permission of the author.

Awareness of the role of a ripe versus unripe cervix led next, of course, to the pursuit of ways of artificially ripening it. These included the old favourite, quinine, and use of an intravenous oxytocin drip over a period of several days.

By 1969, it was said that 'although many drugs have been advocated for the initiation and augmentation of uterine action . . . only oxytocin enjoys the reputation of being relatively safe for the induction of labour' (Karim, et al., 1969, p. 769). Yet such is the nature of innovation in obstetrics, that the motive force which had produced oxytocin remained strongly harnessed to the goal of discovering the perfect drug, and by 1969 another group of drugs — the prostaglandins — had arrived on the induction scene. Strips of dead human pregnant uteruses contracted in response to prostaglandins in glass laboratory dishes from the early 1960s, and in 1968 ten women had their labours successfully induced at term with prostaglandin (Karim, et al., 1968). Prostaglandins were known to be present in human semen, thus providing a sophisticated pharmacological explanation for that natural method of labour induction practised in some small-scale societies. In the 1970s prostaglandins came to be used for ripening the cervix, for inducing labour and for securing induced abortion.

The 'active management of labour'

The synthesis of oxytocin and the later addition of prostaglandins to chemical techniques for controlling labour have enabled obstetricians to add a new concept to their professional vocabulary: the active management of labour. According to Kieran O'Driscoll, the Irish obstetrician whose name, more than anyone else's, is associated with this concept, under an 'active' regime, obstetricians are very closely involved in continuous management of all labours, both normal and abnormal. At the National Maternity Hospital in Dublin, where active management of labour is practised on all patients, rates of obstetrical intervention are relatively low, and the regime is combined with the principle of support in labour (every mother is guaranteed a personal nurse throughout her labour and delivery). The conjunction of the two principles is challenging: on the one hand, a clinically highly mangerial approach to labour and, on the other, the provision of a patient-sensitive social support system. Indeed, the Dublin scheme encapsulates the two contradictory directions in which obstetrics, including antenatal care, is now moving — towards a more social and user-sensitive agenda on the one hand, and in favour of mushrooming new technologies on the other.

O'Driscoll's agenda and its rationale are inflexible and dogmatic. Multigravidae and primigravidae are categorized as 'different biological species' and the multigravid cervix is said to be 'an entirely different organ' from the primigravid cervix (O'Driscoll and Meagher, 1980, p. 166, p. 187). The essence of active management is that no labour is allowed to last beyond 12 hours. (The graphs used for recording labour and delivery data in the National Maternity Hospital do not allow for recordings over more than a 12-hour period.) In primigravidae, active management of labour runs as follows: ARM is performed 1 hour after the initial diagnosis of labour 'unless dilatation of cervix is proceeding at a satisfactory rate' (p. 140). One hour after this unless the dilatation of the cervix has speeded up, oxytocin begins to be given intravenously:

> There is a standard procedure, applied in all circumstances and by every member of staff, as follows: 10 units of oxytocin in 1 litre of 5 per cent

dextrose solution is used, the rate of infusion starts at 10 drops and increases by 10 drops at intervals of 15 minutes to a maximum of 60 drops per minute. Neither the concentration, nor the rate, nor the volume can be exceeded so that it is not possible for a woman to receive more than 10 units of oxytocin or 1 litre of dextrose solution, or for treatment to last longer than 6 hours (O'Driscoll and Meagher, 1980, p. 142).

The notion of an actively managed labour — or the vision of all labours actively managed — summarizes the uncertainty of professional attenders of childbearing women in the face of a 'natural' process whose unknown laws undermine their would-be omniscient human expertise. Once more, the word 'active' refers to the obstetrician and not to the mother. However, very recently in Britain the 'Active Birth Movement', a coalescence of consumer and other maternity care groups, has set in motion a response to this assumption of obstetrical activity by arguing that it is the mother who should actively deliver her child.

Where have all the inductions gone?

Obstetricians have needed to develop safe and effective techniques for inducing labour in order to deal with obstetric abnormalities. Left to themselves, some 90 per cent of fetuses will be born between the 38th and 42nd week of pregnancy. Once these limits are transgressed, fetal chances of survival are increasingly compromised. A fetus that has died in late pregnancy or one known to be congenitally abnormal, or one whose mother is fatally ill, must be negotiated safely out of the womb, and 'Mother' Nature cannot be relied upon to complete this process successfully. Aside from this, safe and effective methods of controlling labour are needed for normal fetuses at risk of being born too soon or too late to survive in good health. Information about the dangers to the fetus of prolonged pregnancy has been especially important in expanding both the practice of induction and the search for new techniques. For example, the attention given, in the report of the 1958 Perinatal Mortality Survey in Britain to the raised perinatal mortality in post-term deliveries, was almost certainly responsible for a substantially increased use of induction subsequently in this group. The survey pointed, moreover, to long-term sequelae of staying in the uterus too long. The survey showed nearly the same percentage of poor readers in the group of babies born after 43 weeks of pregnancy as in those born before 37 weeks. Children who want to be good readers should therefore arrange to be born between 39 and 41 weeks (Butler and Alberman, 1969).

'What strikes one', said Munro Kerr in 1956, 'in reading the literature on this subject of the artificial termination of pregnancy, is the great difference of opinion expressed by obstetricians, especially the extreme position many of them take up with regard to the several indications, and how often apparent inconsistency is evidenced — extreme licence being allowed for one condition, and equally extreme restrictions being laid down for another' (Kerr, 1956, p. 625). In 1977 Iain Chalmers and Martin Richards called the picture with respect to rates of induction in different units, regions and countries, 'chaotic'. Their assessment applies retrospectively too: in the 1950s, for example, induction rates were 5.3 per cent in the Queen Victoria Hospital, Johannesburg (1952–55 data, van Dongen, 1956); 12.6 per cent in University College Hospital, London, (1952–56 data, Nixon and Smyth, 1959); and 21.9 per cent in Buffalo General Hospital in the USA (1955–56 data, Niswander, et al., 1960).

Obstetricians differ still as to the medical indications for induction of labour. Nevertheless, since the Second World War, improvements in techniques for inducing labour have functioned to make possible one immensely significant change: the invasion of obstetrics into the domain of normal midwifery. With an increase in the safety of pharmacologically-initiated labour in the period since the 1950s, it has been possible for obstetricians to broaden indications for induction to include many pregnancies which 50 or 20 years before would have been regarded as normal and inappropriate candidates for artificial induction.

Some indications for induction can only be considered 'social' rather than purely 'medical'. In her survey of induction in Britain in 1975, Cartwright found that more than half of the obstetricians questioned said they would agree to, or recommend, induction where there were staff shortages or restricted availability of anaesthetists to give epidurals. These dimensions of obstetric practice are reflected in the pattern of births by day of week, which shows a peak in the middle of the week and a trough at weekends, especially on Sundays (Macfarlane, 1978; Bjerkedal and Bakketeig, 1972). In the Cartwright survey of obstetricians, 46 per cent also said they would induce a woman having her first baby in whom obstetric conditions were favourable who wanted an induction three days before term, so that the baby could be born before her mother's return to Australia. Clearly, therefore, among the reasons for obstetricians' increased use of induction is some response to the stated needs of childbearing women. There is no doubt that some pregnant women have wanted, and do want, to have their labours induced (Cartwright, 1979; Oakley, unpublished data), just as it is equally obvious that unwarranted use of induction has formed a central motif of the consumer opposition to modern obstetrics (see chapter 10). From the late 1960s to the mid-1970s, induction of labour increased tremendously in Britain. From 12.7 per cent of total deliveries in England and Wales in 1966, the figure rose to 38.9 per cent in 1974 (Macfarlane, 1978). Thereafter, the documentation of the costs, as well as benefits of induction, combined with the consumer opposition to put the brakes on the advance or, rather, perhaps, to translate some of it into 'acceleration' of labour instead of 'induction' of labour.

Most of the evaluation of the effectiveness and safety of induction procedures has been in terms of maternal and perinatal mortality. The available evidence, including published trials of induction of labour, do not show a beneficial effect of induction of labour on perinatal mortality, though there is the important limitation that very large numbers would be needed to show either a clear positive or a negative effect. The possible hazards of induction of labour, even using the most up-to-date technologies, include iatrogenic prematurity, and increased use of other interventions (e.g. epidural analgesia), fetal distress (as a result of oxytocin stimulation), neonatal jaundice, greater labour pain and unhappiness in the mother resulting from her passive role in the delivery of her baby (Lumley, 1983).

Who likes induction?

As we have seen in this chapter, the pursuit of the perfect but elusive means of inducing labour has run in parallel with the growth of the profession of obstetrics. Busey in 1871 included the following opinion from the lips of a famous London obstetrician:

> The operation [of inducing labour] may be brought entirely within the control of the operator. *Instead of being the slave of circumstances, waiting anxiously for the response of nature to his provocations, he should be master of the position* (cited in Fields, et al., 1965, pp. 11–12, italics added).

Students of antenatal care may also recall the predictions of Ballantyne in 1906, peering into the hazy future of obstetrics. It was a crucial part of Ballantyne's vision that obstetricians would discover a 'tocophoric' serum that would give them control over the beginning and the end of labour — indeed, Ballantyne heralded this as the main revolutionary development in twentieth-century obstetrics.

It is as true of induction of labour as it is of the antenatal procedures described in chapter 7 that being at the receiving end of this obstetric innovation is a neglected research topic. In figure 8.5, which is taken from Fields, Greene and Smith's text of 1965, we do not see the individuality of the patient (nor even the whole of her head). The focus of attention of both the obstetrician and the nurse is on the captive womb and its mechanical appendages. The physical comfort or attitudes of pregnant women themselves are rarely referred to in the literature describing the development of induction technologies. Amongst the occasional reminders of their presence as people is the observation that around 25 per cent of women receiving quinine or pituitary extract experienced extreme nausea and vomiting (Vartan, 1962). In Cartwright's study, 81 per cent of the 2,378 surveyed mothers wanted to be able to exercise choice about the medical management of their pregnancies and labours. Seventy-eight per cent of women who had their labours induced, did not wish to repeat the experience, but 93 per cent who had their babies spontaneously would choose to do so again (Cartwright, 1979, p. 107).

In the same study, obstetricians were asked about the relationship between their own job satisfaction and induction; only 2 per cent

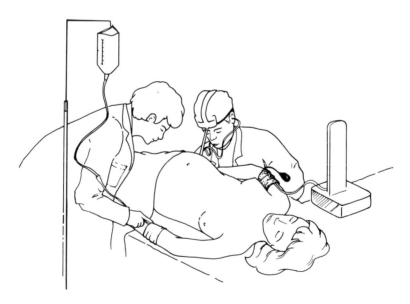

Figure 8.5 Constant observation during oxytocin administration
source: after Fields, H.; Greene, J.W. and Smith, K. *Induction of Labour*, 1965. With permission of the publisher Macmillan Publishing Company.

expressed the view that induction decreased their job satisfaction, while 23 per cent realized that it led to a deterioration in mothers' experiences of labour. Eight out of ten pointed to a lower perinatal mortality rate as a result of induction, despite the absence of relevant evidence. Much the same is apparently true of caesarean section as the other main mode of 'elective' delivery. A rise in caesarean section rates to the point at which from one in nine to one in five births are accomplished in this way must be due in part to 'the social structure of the medical profession': it cannot simply be a response to 'the medical needs of the individual woman' (Francome and Huntingford, 1980).

Modern methods for controlling labour rebound on, and follow from, many of the techniques of modern antenatal care examined in chapter 7. For example, safe induction of labour is facilitated by methods of surveying fetal condition *in utero*, because the state of the resulting baby can be known, not just intimated. But, in turn, the knowledge gleaned from fetal monitoring may increase the urgency for a safe induction technique: there is no point in knowing the fetus is in trouble if there is no way of getting the uterus safely to let it out. The technique of inducing labour with oxytocic drugs has also directly spurned the need for new or improved labour technologies, for instance, the development of electronic fetal heart rate monitoring. But two, perhaps less visible, accompaniments of the rise of modern methods of induction have been the decreasingly autonomous role of midwives and the increasing concentration of births in hospital. These developments are looked at in the next chapter.

Part III
Unsolved Problems of Antenatal Care

9

No Place Like Home

The important thing is to define who is at risk. The problem of maternal mortality has been largely overcome — pregnancy and labour are no longer a risk to the mother. It is the problem of the fetus that concerns us at the moment, because the quality of the fetus is our investment for the future in the family and for the country.

Beard, 1977, p. 251

When antenatal care began, a few per cent of pregnant women were regarded as 'at risk' of their own or their fetuses' mortality and morbidity. The task of antenatal care was to screen a population of basically normal pregnant women in order to pick up the few who were at risk of disease or death. Today the situation is reversed, and the object of antenatal care is to screen a population suffering from the pathology of pregnancy for the few women who are normal enough to give birth with the minimum of midwifery attention. Increasingly, this issue of risk has centred on the matching of medical condition with place of birth.

Home or hospital: 'the unresolvable dilemma'

The *British Medical Journal* in 1979 published some reflections by a rural GP, W. J. Reilly, on the experience of GP obstetrics in the 1960s. 'Undiagnosed premature twins, breech deliveries, and postpartum haemorrhages' were part of the job:

I remember delivering a woman of her 13th baby in a cottage bedroom. The fleas were jumping all over the place and sterility was non-existent. A drawer from a chest acted as the baby's cot. Such an event must be unheard of nowadays.

If we took such episodes in our stride it wasn't with any sense of complacency, and I used to approach each domiciliary confinement with

some apprehension. What finally turned me against the whole business
was a bad postpartum haemorrhage (Reilly, 1979, p. 1077).

Today for most GPs a postpartum haemorrhage is no unresolvable
dilemma: the answer is plain. But not all agree, and, indeed, the *British
Medical Journal* published a year after W. J. Reilly's piece the views of
another GP who wrote with nostalgia of home deliveries in rural Suffolk
in the 1940s; of successful pregnancies in appalling social conditions,
and of the sense of 'the communion of a miracle' entered into by
midwife, nurse and doctor (Kuenssberg, 1980).

The home versus hospital controversy is one that, in the 1980s,
generates much heat. It would be too simple to describe it as a polariz-
ation of opinion: doctors versus patients. Many women value the 'security' of hospital, and some doctors are brave enough to take the
responsibility for overseeing the delivery of babies at home. Nevertheless, it is no longer the woman who wants to have her baby in hospital
who has to fight, but the woman who wants a home birth. When the
majority of babies are born in hospital, and when hospital is seen as the
only real place of safety, the demand for home delivery is bound to
sound like anachronistic 'back to nature faddism'. Going a step further
is a home delivery in the hands of no one more (or less) qualified than
the baby's father. Two recent cases of men who performed this role
raised the hackles of the midwifery authorities to the point at which the
fathers were taken to court for illegal midwifery (*Sunday Times*, 13 June
1982; *Guardian*, 8 September 1982). In Wolverhampton, where Brian
Radley delivered his son, aptly named Sunny after a sunny day, the
District Nursing Officer, Mrs Winifred Andrews, said he couldn't be
allowed to get away with it because other couples might try it. Figure
A.6, p. 299, shows the rise in institutional births from the early 1950s as a
line that almost merges with that for total births in the late 1970s.

The emergence of this situation, in which a mere 1 per cent of British
babies are born at home, is a story of piecemeal evolution guided by
unevidenced assumptions and unwavering faiths of various kinds, not to
mention the strong hand of powerful interest groups.

The potential importance of place of delivery was first recognized by
the British Registrar-General in 1927, when his Statistical Review
contained an 'incidental' tabulation of institutional deliveries. In that
year, the figure stood at 15 per cent of all live births, divided into 11.7
per cent in hospitals, maternity homes, etc., and 3.3 per cent in Poor
Law Institutions. The Registrar-General thought institutional deliveries
were due to lack of home facilities rather than predisposition to institu-

tional treatment, but, observing a trend over the period 1920–27 for legitimate births to occur increasingly in Poor Law Institutions, he acknowledged that the growth in institutional confinement might be due either 'to national policy or increasing individual recognition of the superiority of institutional treatment' (Registrar-General, 1929, p. 112, 125).

By 1932 (24 per cent of births in institutions) the Registrar-General's Statistical Review could afford to be somewhat more definite on the reasons behind the move to hospital. Of course it was partly a response to more beds, but it was also

> partly assignable to changes, both economic and sentimental, in the outlook of expectant mothers. The reluctance shown in the past to enter certain classes of institutions is being gradually overcome, and this, together with the superiority of much institutional practice, the unsuitability of many present-day dwellings for maternity patients, and the general economic depression, probably account for the changes which are so rapidly taking place (Registrar-General, 1935, p. 144).

The trend towards 100 per cent hospital delivery is, unlike the trend towards 100 per cent antenatal care, not found in all industrialized countries. In Britain the gradient of the increase in hospital deliveries has not been stable. The proportion of deliveries in hospital was 63.7 per cent in 1954, and only slightly more, 64.7 per cent in 1960. In 1954 the *British Medical Journal* was still prepared to arbitrate decisively that 'the proper place for the confinement is the patient's own home' (24 April 1954), and many doctors were willing to make this possible, though some complained about their working conditions: 'These are the days of divan beds', reflected F. J. Browne, 'and it is most unwise to attempt the delivery of a baby on a bed of this design' (Browne, 1955, p. 53).

The biggest growth in hospital delivery took place between 1963 and 1972, when the rate leapt up from 68.2 per cent to 91.4 per cent. The Cranbrook Committee reporting in 1959 had recommended a 70 per cent hospital confinement rate. The Committee had reached its target figure on a number of grounds, including the apparent eagerness of many women to get into hospital, and the home location of a significant proportion of 'avoidable' maternal deaths. Undoubtedly one factor behind Cranbrook's selection of the 70 per cent figure was that it was close to the rate already prevailing (the institutional confinement rate in England and Wales in 1959 was 64.2 per cent): thus the new target would soon be achieved, and another bigger and better target could be set. There was enormous geographical variation in hospital confinement rates. The highest rate was in London and the South East, where 58.6 per cent of babies were born in hospital, as against 27.1 per cent in the neighbouring Southern Counties of Hampshire, Berkshire, and Dorset (Butler and Bonham, 1963, p. 58). The Cranbrook Committee took this variation as proof that 'the proportion of hospital to domiciliary confinements had not been determined on medical grounds alone, but partly by long standing custom and partly by the availability of beds' (p. 20).

In a speech to the Annual Conference of the National Association for Maternal and Child Welfare in 1959, the Earl of Cranbrook discussed the evidence on place of delivery which his Committee had taken:

> I do not think it an unfair summmary of the evidence we received from, on the one side, those responsible for the hospital maternity service, and, on the other side, those responsible for the domiciliary maternity service, that the first were of the opinion that none of the second should be allowed anywhere near any woman between the age of puberty and the menopause, and the second were equally satisfied that no consultant obstetrician should ever look at a woman when there was a possibility of her bearing a child.

The Earl went on to comment on the relevance of 'evidence' to policy:

> I was told by my grandmother, my mother, by my wife, and now by my daughters that every mother loses a tooth for every child, and it was that, I presume, which gave rise to the setting up of the priority dental service. We could, however, find no scientific evidence that if a woman had triplets she lost three of her teeth (NAMCW, Report of the *Annual Conference*, July 1959, pp. 66–71).

In other words, the modern equivalent of old wives' tales are young doctors' tales.

A desire to 'nail down the coffin of home delivery' is rumoured to be among the motives for the setting up of the 1958 Perinatal Mortality Survey. In the 1950s, it was common to find the view expressed in medical circles that the decline in maternal mortality and stillbirth were hardly coincidentally linked to the growth in hospital confinement; in one memorable letter to the *British Medical Journal*, Dugald Baird, of Aberdeen fame, made this very observation, at the same time as reminiscing that he had enjoyed the home births of all four of his own children, 'incidentally made more comfortable and enjoyable for all concerned by the presence of a cook, housemaid, and resident midwife' (*British Medical Journal* 7 June 1952, p. 1246).

Following Cranbrook, and the impact of the 1958 Perinatal Mortality Survey, came the Peel Report of 1970. The brief of the Peel Committee was to look at the domiciliary midwifery service and the hospital maternity bed situation, bearing in mind the falling birth-rate and the increasing fashion for hospital birth. On the matter of hospital confinement in the future, the Peel Report said that

> It was unanimously agreed that the upward trend in hospital confinement would continue . . . There seems to be a gradually increasing appreciation in the profession and amongst the general public that confinement in hospital is the safest arrangement, irrespective of considerations of finance or convenience (Peel Report, 1970, pp. 39–40).

Further,

> We consider that the greater safety of hospital confinement for mother and child justifies the objective of providing hospital facilities for every woman who desires or needs to have a hospital confinement. Even without specific policy direction, the institutional confinement rate has risen from 64.6 per cent in 1957 to 80.7 per cent in 1968 and shows every sign of continuing to rise, so that discussion of the advantages and disadvantages of home or hospital confinement is in one sense academic (p. 54).

Academic it may have been, but it was, significantly, a discussion in which the Committee did not engage in its Report, save for a few observations about the high perinatal mortality rates of women booked for home delivery but transferred to hospital. Thus the main ground for the Report's highly influential recommendation of 100 per cent hospital confinement was that the rate was already moving in that direction. The question of bed availability and occupancy was also relevant. The birth-rate had been falling from 1964, and the total number of births per available hospital bed had therefore fallen, with the result that, as the Report put it, '*a special stimulus may be needed if the proportion of births in hospital is to continue to rise as it has done recently*' (Peel Report, 1970, p. 123; italics added). In support of this move, the Report argued, too, that the providers of care whose opinions had been tapped in evidence had said that hospital confinement was safer and therefore better for all mothers. The relationship between the written evidence taken by the Committee and the recommendations is, at best, tangential: for instance only 77 of the 134 questionnaires sent out to Local Medical Committees were completed (an unimpressive 58 per cent response rate) and only 15 per cent of these responses actually came out against the continuation of domiciliary midwifery.

The Peel Committee attempted a sophisticated economic forecast of maternity bed needs, but some of the statistics it presented carried a relatively simple message, for example, the 26 per cent rise in the number of consultant obstetricians in the nine years between 1959 and 1968. Obstetrical enthusiasm for higher hospital delivery rates took the form of a 70 per cent rate recommended by the Royal College of Obstetricians and Gynaecologists in 1944, 15 years before Cranbrook; and as early as 1964 the RCOG had also anticipated Peel by talking of a desirable 95 per cent hospital delivery rate (RCOG, 1944; Lewis, 1964). Consultant obstetricians had begun to infiltrate local authority antenatal care in the late 1950s. The upward trend in consultant unit beds shown in the Peel Report ran virtually parallel with the increase in total maternity beds between 1955 and 1970. In figure A.9, p. 303, the decline in women attending community antenatal clinics occurs at the same time as the increase in first attendances at consultant obstetric clinics. Figure A.7, p. 301, shows that the rise in GP maternity unit beds from the early 1960s to the early 1970s is neatly paralleled by a rise in consultant obstetric unit beds. Neither of these developments can be understood without taking into account the data used to compile figure A.14, p. 306 — a steady rise in the numbers of consultants in obstetrics and gynaecology over the 30 years from 1950.

Since 1970 the DHSS has continued to base its maternity service policy on the canons of the Peel Report. The latest official report to examine place of birth, the Short Report on *Perinatal and Neonatal Mortality* published in 1980, updated Peel by recommending 'that an increasing number of mothers be delivered in large units . . . and that home delivery is phased out further' (p. 27). Here, once again, is a recommendation based on a *fait accompli*; there were, in 1978, only 15 units left in the whole of England with less than 50 obstetric or GP maternity beds. From 1973 to 1978 in Britain there was a 25 per cent fall in the number of maternity units with less than 500 births a year.

The phrase 'an unresolvable dilemma' is taken from the Short Report and refers to the fact that 'the understandable preferences of mothers in regard to place of delivery may not be compatible with the requirements for the maximum lowering of perinatal and neonatal mortalilty' (Short Report, 1980, p. 27). Such circumlocutions cannot deny the great personal *angst* undergone by mothers who not only want a home birth but are convinced that this is actually safer for themselves and their babies. Nor are they able to deny the historical background to the present situation of confrontation. 'The main argument', said the Peel Committee a decade before, 'hinges on the safety of hospital delivery on the one hand and the emotional security for the patient and her other children in home delivery on the other', and it 'is not easily resolved' (p. 10).

What was not 'easily resolved' in 1970 had become 'unresolvable' by 1980. Some obstetricians would go further than this: the President of the American College of Obstetricians and Gynecologists referred in a sonorous and terrifying phrase to home delivery as 'the earliest form of child abuse' (Stone, 1979). It is said that paediatricians in the USA have, indeed, reported couples achieving home births to State authorities, on charges of child abuse (Minerva, *British Medical Journal*, 11 November, p. 1377).

A preference for one's own habitation?

Of all the pronouncements on the subject of what mothers really want in government reports on the maternity services, the Short Committee's attaches least value in terms of deciding maternity care policy to maternal preferences. Of course, over the years, women have been credited with a variety of views about place of delivery, most of which have not been based on a systematic sampling of their experiences. In 1819 Augustus Granville at the Westminster General Dispensary in London, wrote, 'however distressed the poor mother may be, she will always prefer her own habitations and the unbought, soothing cares of her own family during her hour of trial' (Granville, 1819, p. 19).

More recently, when the preferences of women as to place of delivery have been surveyed, the proportion who would like to have a baby at home is always higher than the proportion so booked (Macintyre, 1977). The preference for home delivery appears to rise with parity, and also with the *experience* of home delivery, as in Goldthorpe and Richman's study of unintended home delivery due to a strike by hospital ancillary staff. In addition to the psychological costs paid by women for what they may regard as inappropriate forms of care, there are the economic costs. One analysis of the relative costs of home and hospital delivery showed that the public sector costs of consultant unit antenatal, delivery and postpartum care are higher than those of GP care, which are, in turn, higher than those of home care. But, of the three types of care, the family costs of GP delivery are lowest and they are highest for consultant care (Stilwell, 1979).

Predicting risk

The pathway from the sensitivity to women's preferences evidenced in
the official reports of the 1920s and 1930s, to the Short Report's
dismissal in 1980 of women's preferences as irrelevant to policy formu-
lation, takes us through two interrelated policy developments. Firstly,
there is the emergence of antenatal care as a screening or risk-
prediction exercise with respect to place of birth (the beginnings of
which were noted in chapter 6). Secondly, there is the general labelling
within medicine of 'consumer' preferences as lying outside the arena of
medical decision-making. What women want, once seen as an all-
important force shaping maternity care, comes from the 1950s on, to be
seen as some kind of luxury 'extra', incompatible with the medical
determination of risk.

The beginnings of this process can be detected in the pages of the
1932 Report on *Maternal Mortality*, which declared that an institutional
booking should be made; 'where ante-natal examination has revealed
abnormalities to require caesarean section, induction of labour or difficult forceps delivery. The admission of primigravidae for confinement,
even when no complications are expected', the Report continued, 'is a
precautionary measure favoured by some experienced obstetricians'
(Departmental Committee, 1932, p. 38). The Cranbrook Committee in
1959 could not afford to be entirely cavalier towards women's attitudes,
since the dilemma the Committee faced was one in which the demand
for maternity beds outstripped the supply. Their recommended policy
was that beds should be filled on the basis of (1) obstetric reasons; and
(2) adverse social conditions — and (1) should not necessarily include all
primigravidae. Eleven years later, the Peel Report did not discuss
medical indications for hospital confinement at all, for the good reason
that the indications are considered by then to refer to all childbearing
women. However it, like other reports (some more equanimously than
others) does put the view that mothers who chose home confinements
should have their choice respected provided 'there are no medical or
social contra-indications' (Peel Report, p. 54).

The exercise of what is known by clinicians as 'risk-assessment' or
'risk-prediction' has entailed the use of many different scoring systems
according to which a pregnant women is given a score on the basis of her
obstetric and medical history, present pregnancy condition, and social
factors such as single or married motherhood and educational level: the
combined figure is then supposed to predict the degree of risk she runs

of such adverse pregnancy outcomes as a low birthweight baby. The proportion of the childbearing population falling into low- and high-risk groups goes from 12 to 55 per cent, depending on the population and the scoring system used (Lesinski, 1975). The overwhelming disadvantage of all such systems is that they are not very successful in correctly identifying pregnant women and fetuses who actually turn out to be 'at risk', and in *not* identifying as at risk those who do *not* turn out to be (Newcombe and Chalmers, 1981). One of the most commonly-used systems, that of Hobel and his co-workers, correctly picks up only 59 per cent of women who experience a bad outcome and only 48 per cent of those who do not (Hobel, 1978; Selwyn, 1982).

The 1958 Perinatal Mortality Survey certainly did show the difficulty of correctly selecting, antenatally, those patients who could safely be delivered at home. Some 14 per cent of women booked for home delivery, and some 12 per cent of those booked for delivery in GP Units were eventually transferred to hospital, with perinatal mortality rates more than three times the average. This finding was subsequently used to justify the demand for more specialist obstetric care, although its statistical basis is flimsy, and the subject of prolonged debate still in the 1980s (see p. 147).

'Shared' antenatal care and the logic of centralization

Behind policy and practice on place of birth in the post-war years is the logic of centralization. This was anticipated in the 1924 Report on *Maternal Mortality* which referred to the new Ministry of Health's policy encouraging local health authorities to provide small maternity homes:

> This policy of the Ministry has not passed without criticism . . . as it has been said that the science and art of obstetrics would be far better served by the establishment of a few large, well-equipped hospitals, with full facilities for teaching as well as for treatment, than by a much larger number of small and comparatively expensive homes, with partial facilities, where first-rate midwifery would be difficult to secure (Ministry of Health, 1924, p. 78).

It has been said, of course, that the total centralization of all maternity care in large hospitals (or even just hospitals) is most unlikely ever to be achieved — unless obstetricians are prepared to exercise that degree of total control over the process of labour stumbled on in the process of expanding the scientific armamentarium of obstetrics which is described in the last chapter: even then there would be women who would deliver prematurely outside hospital. Such practical considerations do not mean that the obstetrical gaze is prepared to relinquish its vision of every birth a hospital birth; in Norway at the present time it is policy to accommodate mothers living in isolated rural areas in hotels adjacent to maternity hospitals in order to ensure a correctly-located delivery every time (Bakketeig and Bergsjø, 1977).

Centralization of delivery care is not the sole factor shaping the degree of centralization in antenatal care, but it is an important one. The antenatal care of a woman booked for hospital delivery may be 'shared' with a GP or community midwife or local authority medical officer, but there is no uncertainty about who is doing the sharing: 'Many obstetricians', said the Annual Report of the Chief Medical Officer of Health for 1963 (p. 2) 'refer patients to their own doctors for interim antenatal care, which relieves pressure in crowded antenatal clinics'. Table 9.1 shows antenatal care provision by status of the provider and whether or not care was 'shared' or 'exclusive' in the 1970 British Births survey. Thirty-six per cent of women had exclusive antenatal care, two-thirds of

Table 9.1 Antenatal care
British Births Survey, 1970

Exclusive	%
Hospital medical staff	22.7
LHAMO*	0.4
GP	11.2
Hospital midwife	0.2
GP unit midwife	0.5
Domiciliary midwife	0.5
Other	0.0
Shared	
Hospital + GP	38.7
Hospital + LHAMO*	1.5
Hospital + midwife	0.7
GP + LHAMO*	1.2
GP + midwife	21.1
LHAMO* + midwife	0.2
Midwife + midwife	0.2
Insufficient information	1.0
Total	100.1

* Local health authority medical officer.
source: Chamberlain, et al., British Births, 1970 vol. 2 in
Obstetric Care 1978, p. 10. With permission of the
publisher William Heinemann Medical Books Ltd.

these from hospital medical staff. Of those who had shared care, the most common partnership was between hospital and GP followed by GP and midwife.

According to one doctor, in 1961, the maternity services had become 'primarily a battleground for GPs and consultant obstetricians in their struggle for power', so that the safety of mother and child had become 'of secondary importance' (Patterson, 1961). Whether or not the safety of mother and child suffered, the allegation of a power struggle was certainly correct. Buried in the Cranbrook Committee's recommendation of a 70 per cent hospital confinement rate is a less well-known fact — the proposal that the extra beds required to achieve this level should be GP beds. In 1970 the Peel Report recorded a rise in GP maternity beds of 82.8 per cent since 1958, as compared with a rise of 4.3 per cent in consultant beds; GP beds then made up about 21 per cent of the total. The triumph of the GP was shortlived, as the perinatal mortality surveys rated GP unit delivery care as scarcely superior to home. By the mid-1970s, although GPs were still delivering babies, their care of childbearing women was showing marked signs of segmentation, and the issue instead centred on whether or not GPs should continue to be involved in antenatal and postnatal care. In 1977, about a third of maternity service payments to GPs were for partial antenatal care without delivery care, and another third were for partial antenatal and partial postnatal care ('office obstetrics'). Figure A.13, p. 305, shows GP claims for both total and partial care over 20 years from the early 1960s, and the gap between the two is by 1982 quite striking.

Whether or not GPs were responsible for delivery care, nobody could deny (or has been able to since) the GP's signally important role as women's first point of contact with the maternity services. 'The family doctor is a law unto himself [sic]. This is a precious and prized heritage which often acts for the common good, but which, like other privileges, is open to abuse' (O'Brien, 1963, p. 571). Underlying GPs' choice of maternity care for their patients is the economic motive of the level of payment for maternity services. A GP in Britain not on the Obstetric List is currently paid £45.30 for complete obstetric care — in pregnancy, during labour and delivery and in the postpartum period: if on the Obstetric List, the fee is £77.65. There is clearly not a fortune to be made out of doing complete obstetric care, but, on the other hand, a considerable part of the fee — £26.45 or £45.30 on the Obstetric List — is payable for antenatal care alone. GPs are able to claim full payment for antenatal care only if it is begun before sixteen weeks of pregnancy; financial inducement to early antenatal care is thus built into conditions of service provision, even if not yet into those of service use (see pp. 272–3).

Despite the trends marked by the statistics of GP maternity services claims, in 1981 a reinvigorated defence of the 'full part' GPs can and should play in providing 'a high standard of humane care to mothers and their babies' was put together by a Joint Working Party of the Royal College of Obstetricians and Gynaecologists and Royal College of General Practitioners. The first reason advanced in the Report as to why GPs should be active in obstetrics was the 'views of patients' — 'keen to see a return to personal care given by one individual'. A good indicator of the complexity of antenatal care in the 1980s is contained in Appendix II of the Report which sets out 'Training objectives' for GPs' role in antenatal care:

The doctor should:
1 appreciate the preventive role, and understand the significance of all routine procedures used in modern antenatal care
2 have a thorough understanding of the epidemiology of maternal and perinatal morbidity and mortality
3 be able to undertake the initial management of common and life threatening emergencies in early pregnancy
4 know when pregnant women require referral for specialist opinion or care and which are suitable for shared care or full care by the general practitioner
5 understand the principles of counselling women faced with possible or real problems of fetal malformation
6 know the methods by which congenital malformation of the fetus may be detected
7 be aware of the methods of, and provision for education for pregnancy, childbirth and care of the newborn
8 understand the importance of social and emotional factors in pregnancy and childbirth
9 understand their own role and that of different members of the health team in this field
10 understand the management of common conditions for which pregnant women are admitted to hospital e.g., premature labour, preeclampsia, multiple pregnancy, fetal growth retardation, antepartum haemorrhage, maternal disease, etc.
11 be able to recognise the signs and symptoms of onset of labour
12 understand the principles and methods of the current management of labour
13 understand the importance of accurate and detailed records in all aspects of obstetric care and recognise the value of such records in clinical audit

14 be able to carry out routine examination of the newborn infant
15 understand the normal development of the newborn
16 recognise common diseases arising in the newborn
17 recognise congenital abnormalities in the newborn
18 understand how breast feeding is established and maintained
19 recognise and understand the management of physical and psychological problems of the mother in the postnatal period e.g., puerperal depression
20 understand the normal involutional processes in the post partum period
21 understand the indications for maternal immunization with anti D and rubella vaccine and the importance of confirming their efficacy
22 be able to advise and provide suitable methods of family planning (RCOG and RCGP, 1981, p. 19).

Of all these requirements, the first two must surely be the most demanding, not only for GPs but for all who have looked at and wondered about antenatal care.

Reports on the maternity services from the 1960s on are spattered with references to the need for more efficient co-operation and communication between, not only providers and users of maternity care, but also between the three branches of the maternity services themselves. The introduction of the maternity co-operation card for women having shared care was a step in the right direction, but by 1970 it had still not been universally adopted, nor had national agreement been reached between the hospital authorities and GPs about the ideal form of the card. It could be said that the centralization of antenatal and delivery care in hospital represents one of the three available simple solutions to the enduring lacunae of the tripartite structure. The other two simple solutions, GP and local authority care, would both necessitate the placement of maternity care squarely within the community, a resolution argued for by some groups of users and providers, but going unremittingly against the grain of twentieth-century specialization.

The trend out of community-based care and into hospital consultant care has naturally had an enormous impact on the work of midwives. 'It does not seem to be sufficiently appreciated', observes the Short Report with rare acumen, 'that midwives are a dying species' (p. 71). This epidemic of mortality is laid at the door of the obstetricians' invasion into the domain of 'normal' cases — a development endorsed by the Committee. When they asked a representative of the Royal College of Midwives whether the job description of midwives needed to be rewritten, she replied in the negative, but added that midwives ought to be allowed to fulfil their job description.

The continuity of care it was possible for midwives to provide before the NHS either in women's own homes or the local authority clinic was, as we observed in chapter 6, immediately threatened by the GPs' new role within the NHS as the pregnant woman's first point of contact with the health care system. Nevertheless, midwives went on providing antenatal care in every kind of setting; even in hospital clinics in the 1950s they worked alongside their obstetrician colleagues, in some places holding their own clinics. By the 1960s and 1970s this relatively independent antenatal practice of midwives was challenged by the move away from home delivery and towards hospital antenatal care for hospital-booked women. The resulting move of midwives out of community and into hospital practice is reflected in the statistics of contracting community midwifery: a 23 per cent fall in the number of community midwives between 1977 and 1979 (Short Report, p. 73).

Table 9.2 is taken from the study done at Chelsea College in London, of midwives' work. It shows that midwives play a very important role in hospital antenatal care, and an even more important role in community antenatal care. However, this same study reveals midwives' dependence on medical authority: 90 per cent or more of simple examinations for oedema, or of the pregnant abdomen, are done by midwives and repeated by doctors, or are done by doctors only. This bizarre duplication of midwives' work is less common in community antenatal care, where only about half of these two examinations are done by midwives first, then repeated by doctors. Like GPs, many midwives in the community find themselves doing solely antenatal and postnatal care, and in particular the aftercare of mothers discharged from hospital a few hours or days after birth. Midwives have been increasingly concerned with this

Table 9.2 Proportion of midwives undertaking tasks in antenatal care

Task	Hospital midwives (N = 634)		Community midwives (N = 1159)	
	%	No.	%	No.
History taking	84.1	533	78.3	907
Abdominal examination	79.3	503	89.4	1036
Examination for oedema	81.2	515	91.3	1058
Taking blood pressure	90.9	576	94.0	1090
Weighing	76.0	482	92.1	1068
Testing urine	72.9	462	92.0	1066
Taking venous blood	66.4	421	61.5	713

source: Robinson et al., The role of the midwife in the provision of antenatal care in Enkin, M. and Chalmers, I. (eds.) *Effectiveness and Satisfaction in Antenatal Care* 1982, p. 240. Crown copyright, 1982. Reproduced with permission of the DHSS.

last function, as the average length of mothers' postnatal hospital stay in England and Wales has, since the mid-1950s, fallen considerably, and this is illustrated dramatically in figure A.12, which shows the almost insignificant role played by community midwives doing home deliveries compared to their share of the market in supervising early hospital-discharge cases.

Brief (and not so brief) encounters

One observational study of antenatal care carried out by the author in a London maternity hospital in the mid-1970s captured the style of some 878 encounters between doctors and pregnant women. Two of these are reproduced below. Both doctors are junior housemen; the first patient is a hairdresser, ten weeks pregnant, attending for her first antenatal visit, and the second is a briefer exchange with a patient who works as a waitress. The clinic works on the 'assembly line' principle of six curtained cubicles in one large room with the patients prepared for the doctors' examinations by the clinic midwives who check the urine, weight and blood pressure.

(1) D: Hallo, have you been seen?
P: No.
D: Mrs Wilson?[1]
P: Yes.
D: You're twenty-one, and this is your first baby, your last period was 7 July, have you had any bleeding since then?
P: No.
D: That was an absolutely normal period?
P: Yes.
D: And before that your periods were regular?
P: Yes, I was on the pill.
D: You came off the pill in May, so you must have had one or two since then.
P: Yes. They were normal.
D: Have you had any operations?
P: Only my tonsils out.
D: Any serious illnesses — TB, diabetes, rheumatic fever, jaundice?
P: No.
D: Has anyone in the family had diabetes?
P: No.

---

1. The patient's name in this and other case-material cited in the text is a pseudonym.

D: Any kidney disease in the family?
P: No.
D: You've had some vomiting in this pregnancy?
P: Yes, and I've fainted twice.
D: Do you find debendox helps?
P: Yes, but I've only taken them a couple of times.
D: When do you vomit?
P: When I've had a rich meal, or I've eaten too much.
D: Well, you know the answer to that don't you!
P: Yes.

[D examines breasts, and teeth.]

D: Are you going to breastfeed?
P: Yes.

[D examines ankles and legs.]

D: No varicose veins?
P: No.
D: Fine, I want to do an internal examination and do a smear; have you had one before?
P: Yes.
D: How long ago?
P: The year before last November.
D: Put your knees up [examines] fine [uses speculum] okay, all finished. Fine, everything's absolutely normal, you're about right for dates, and there are no problems at all, we'd like to see you in a month. Is there anything you want to ask me?
P: No.

(6.25 minutes)

The doctor is very efficient in his questioning, examination, and in declaring there to be absolutely no problems in the pregnancy. The patient is mostly monosyllabic, and does what the doctor asks her to.

(2) D: Hallo. Mrs Donelly?
    P: Yes, doctor.
    D: Thirty weeks pregnant?
    P: Yes, doctor.
    D: Where've you been the last two times?
    P: I had to bury my father in Ireland.
    D: Oh, I'm sorry to hear that [palpates]. Baby moving a lot it seems?
    P: Yes, the baby's very active, doctor.
    D: Very low. It's rather low.

P: It's driving me . . .
D: Potty?
P: Yes.
D: Are you taking your iron tablets?
P: Yes, doctor.
D: We'll need to do a blood test this week.
P: I didn't think I'd get away without that.

(1.38 minutes)

This more abrupt conversation is characteristic of those in middle trimester of pregnancy, when the doctor's role is often little more than a ritual 'laying on of hands'.

In this series of antenatal encounters, the average length of time doctors and pregnant women spent together was 3.9 minutes. Time spent by consultants was highest at 4.3 minutes on average; house officers came next at 3.9 minutes and registrars at 3.5 minutes. Booking visits, such as the first example above, were longest — average 8.2 minutes. About a third of the questions asked by patients of doctors in the antenatal clinic concerned antenatal tests of one sort or another — for example ultrasound or blood tests: 20 per cent of questions concerned the size, position or condition of the baby, and a further 20 per cent the physiology of pregnancy and birth in general. There was a statistically significant tendency for middle-class women to ask more questions of doctors than working-class women, which would seem to reiterate Cartwright's (1979) findings (see p. 245).

Some data on clinical examinations and tasks as part of hospital and GP antenatal care over the last 20 years were given in chapter 6. In some ways it is probably true that GP care has changed less than hospital care — but in other ways more. In one rural practice in Gloucestershire, England, an unusually efficient style of record-keeping has made it possible to look at the GP's work in maternity care, especially antenatal care, over the whole period from 1946–80. Some parameters are picked out in table 9.3. While a few have remained fairly constant, for example the use of vaginal examinations in pregnancy, others have altered, for instance the number of drug prescriptions written for pregnant women went up markedly between the late 1960s and the late 1970s (and home deliveries, as one would expect, went down).

Case-records at this particular practice drawn from recent years convey exactly that brand of 'family' doctoring advertised as the selling point of GP maternity care over the years by those who have defended GP obstetrics. Margaret Mitchell had her second pregnancy in 1978:

The Captured Womb

Table 9.3 GP Antenatal Care in Gloucestershire 1946–1980[2]

	1946–50	1956–60	1966–70	1976–80
First visit				
(weeks pregnant)	17.9	15.7	11.5	9.2
Number of visits	4.2	5.1	8.4	10.7
Blood pressure				
measurements	1.8	3.1	4.3	6.8
Blood tests	0.1	1.2	2.1	4.2
Drugs prescribed*	1.3	1.9	1.8	5.8
Vaginal examinations	0.5	1.9	0.4	0.8
Laboratory pregnancy				
tests (per cent				
of women)	1.3	5.0	22.5	38.8
Home deliveries				
(per cent of women)	71.3	31.3	35.0	1.3
Number of case-notes				
in series	80	80	80	80

* Includes iron and vitamin supplements

15 March	Below par. Hoping to conceive. Recurrent throat and upper resp. infections. Has stopped Eugynon. Wanting another pregnancy. Blood picture. Fersamel 5 ml. t. d. s. Son has threadworms. Pripsen sachets.
16	*Blood report*: — Hb. 12.8. ESR. 18 Latex test for Glandular fever — Negative. Occasional atypical mononuclear cells seen.
1 April	T. Cons. Now pregnant. TCI.
30	LMP about 15.4.78 EDD 22.1.78 Urine Nad.Bp 115/60 Fundus possibly high for dates. Cert. for welfare foods. Refer Querns [the local maternity home].
11 May	Rubella contact but has had rubella so reassured. I don't see any reason to worry about her recent mild attack of glandular fever either. Now feels entirely well. Some general chat about pregnancy.
15 June	*Blood report*: No atypical antibodies detected. VDRL test negative. Hb 12.1. Alpha-fetoprotein 46.
25	AN Well. Chest and heart NAD. Abdo. — foetal movements felt. Uterus 16–18 weeks size. 19 weeks by dates. Bp 110/60. Severe introital itching. Gynodaktarin. Crem. Timodine. Caps. Fefol 90.
22 July	AN Well. 22 weeks size and dates, Bp 115/60 Introital itching cured.

2. Data provided by Dr Edgar Hope-Simpson. Since the data are taken from GP records, they contain only partial information about the extent of hospital or other forms of antenatal care.

31 August	*Blood report*: Hb.11.3.
17 September	Well. AN 30½ weeks date and size. Bp 100/40. Urine NAD. Wt. 10.2.To double iron. Caps Fefol 2 daily — 90 days. Advised girdle for pelvic pain. Form Mat. BI.
October 5	*Blood report*: Hb.12.2.
15	Usual relaxed self. Bp 120/60 Urine NAD Wt. 10.7 More comfortable with girdle. 35 weeks, fixed. ROA.FHH. Wishes for 48 hour discharge.
9 November	AN Bp 120/60 Urine NAD Wt. 11.0 Uterus = dates = 38 weeks. Vertex engaged. FHH. Probable fracture right minimus foot. Now settling. Strapped.
12	*Blood report*: Hb.12.5.
16	Feels very well. Bp 140/85 (taken on three occasions). Wt. 71K 500 grms, which is a gain of 14 Kgs in one week. Says she felt her rings tighten and her boots a little difficult to get on. Urine NAD. No oedema palpable. Uterus 39 weeks, equivalent to dates. Head deeply engaged. *PM* Bp has remained at 140/85. Admit Querns for bedrest.

Margaret Mitchell had her labour induced with ARM and syntocinon at the Maternity Hospital to which she was referred from the Maternity Home and she gave birth to a daughter weighing 2,980 g. Two days later she was transferred back to the Maternity Home, and four days later the GP visited and found the patient her 'usual calm composed self'.

Clinical antenatal care, more heavily dependent in 1978 on laboratory investigations and specialist referrals than it was 20 years before, is here combined with family health care ('son has threadworms'), with observations about the pregnant woman's general wellbeing ('usual relaxed self') and with an overall advisory role ('general chat about pregnancy').

The football team of perinatal medicine: its fourth goal

The analogy between the work of perinatal medicine and the game of football was first made by obstetrician Melville Kerr in 1975. Kerr argued that, when either a football team or the perinatal medical services find themselves at an embarrassingly low position in the international league table, the response is to spend large amounts of money in an attempt to improve ratings. But more expensive facilities and expertise cannot cure underlying problems. More doesn't necessarily mean better.

Although never completely absent from the ideological chorus, the theme equating medical care in pregnancy with national wellbeing and international status experienced a new lease of life in the 1970s. The government health document *Reducing the Risk: safer pregnancy and childbirth (1977)* was precise about the invidiousness of the comparison:

> In 1960 the infant mortality rate in France was 22% above that in the U.K., but by 1982 the French rate was 10% lower. In 1960 the rates in England and Wales and in Finland were the same, but in 1972 the Finnish rate was 30% lower ... Although infant mortality has been falling steadily in Britain for a long time, our rate today is no better than the Scandinavian rate of 10 years ago (DHSS, 1977, p. 12).

Scandinavia figures prominently as the perinatal paradise, much as it did when pregnancy first became a matter for government and medical scrutiny in Britain during the First World War. It seems that, whatever the British maternity services have done, it is never enough, because the Scandinavians have done it better (and sooner). On the graph included in *Reducing the Risk* the Swedish infant mortality rate takes a downward plunge actually below the horizontal axis. The main point about such representations of national reproductive performance is, as always, that childbearing is too important to be left to women. Even if it is shown that the international league position of England and Wales' perinatal mortality rate improved over the period from 1955 to 1972 (Lambert, 1976) the main thrust of the argument is left untouched. The main thrust of the argument is about the importance of women and childbearing, not about the precise condition of the perinatal (or infant) mortality rate. Thus what befell infant mortality in the midst of the infant mortality clamour of the early 1900s has also befallen the perinatal mortality rate, which began a mysterious sustained decline at just about the peak of the public outcry (Macfarlane, 1979).

Among the conclusions drawn in this most recent exercise of inter-national comparisons, two themes — one old, one new — have dominated policy-making: the idea that medical care has not improved mortality because pregnant women have not used it enough, and the idea that the same is true because babies have not used it enough. Although the quality of medical care provided for normal weight babies does form an issue within this debate (indeed, differences in outcome among such babies may be an especially sensitive indicator of differences in the quality of medical care) it is the destiny of the low birthweight (< 2,500 g) baby on which the spotlight now falls. Low birthweight is important because perinatal deaths are concentrated in this group: 7.2 per cent of all births in England and Wales in 1980 were of infants weighing 2,500 g or less, and perinatal deaths were 25 times higher in low birthweight infants than in their heavier peers. Clearly, therefore, if a greater proportion of low birthweight babies can be persuaded to survive, the perinatal mortality rate overall is likely to improve markedly. In addition, since some two-thirds of low birthweight babies have fathers in manual occupations, a higher survival rate might be expected to make some difference to another important issue in perinatal care: the unequal life-chances of babies in different social classes.

There is no doubt that paediatricians are making more strenuous efforts to keep alive a greater proportion of low birthweight infants and are having greater success than previously. In 1978 the *British Medical Journal* (21 October, p. 1105) reported improved neonatal survival rates in babies of very low birthweight, following the introduction of intensive care facilities in a number of centres. In 'good units' survival rates of babies weighing 750–1,000 g and 1,001–1,500 g at birth were 50 per cent and over 70 per cent respectively. This appears to be a world-wide phenomenon in developed countries, dating from around 1960 (Stewart, et al., 1981). There is some doubt, however, about the quality of life among small babies who survive. Do they decrease their country's perinatal mortality at personal cost to themselves in terms of physical or mental impairment through life? It seems that increased survival among low birthweight babies may be correlated with an increased incidence of cerebral palsy (Paneth, et al., 1981) and there are documented iatrogenic hazards of neonatal intensive care (Yu, et al., 1979). But there are simply no data on childhood morbidity and handicap which can be used to examine the true impact of the increased survival associated with intensive paediatric care.

The absence of adequate data has not, however, prevented a campaign by both professionals and some lay maternity pressure groups to raise the status, provision and financing of neonatal intensive care, any more than the absence of good statistical data impeded any of the other campaigns that have characterized the growth of maternity care in its various epochs. The neonatal intensive care campaign began on the basis of the Short Committee's decision that 'the total number of babies who unnecessarily die or suffer permanent handicap in the perinatal and neonatal period is at least 8–10,000' a year (p. 158). The figure of 8–10,000 was made up of 3–5,000 'avoidable deaths' plus 'at least 5,000' children surviving with 'important handicaps' (p. 158). These inspired calculations provoked such media headlines as 'Lack of cash puts 6,000 babies at risk' (*Guardian* 3 December 1982); '5,000 babies need not die' (*Daily Mail* 17 July 1980); and 'Babies dying in cots' shortage' (*Times Health Supplement* 30 October 1981) — an appeal, accompanied by a photograph with the erroneous, but not inappropriate, caption: 'A nurse checks a baby's condition in the *antenatal* intensive care unit'.

As part of this battle to improve life for Britain's babies, the Spastics Society began its 'Save a Baby' campaign and sponsored publications referring to 'the scandal of avoidable death and handicap amongst Britain's newborn babies' (Spastics Society, 1981, p. 31). Many lay groups organized around this battlecry, and one such, an organization called BLISS ('Baby Life Support Systems') marched to 10 Downing Street pushing a newborn baby in an incubator. In the last five years the focus of attention has thus moved from human to man-made wombs. Many more babies are now placed in the second sort of womb: one in 20 British babies went into special-care cots in 1964; one in five in 1977 (Richards, 1980). By the end of the 1970s the demand among neonatal paediatricians and consumer pressure groups was not for special care but for intensive care, and the Short Committee noted that neonatal intensive care cots had sprung up 'in an uncontrolled way' all over the country.

The fact that attention is focused on the technological medical care of small babies concentrates the mind wonderfully on more intensive medical surveillance of pregnancy itself. Obstetricians must deliver to paediatricians good quality obstetrical products. Yet another way in which the new perinatal medicine is potentially relevant to antenatal care concerns the tricky business of looking at outcomes other than death, in order to measure the effectiveness and safety of medical care, or the health of nations. 'Morbidity' in the case of babies has to include both mental and physical handicap, because the second may be expressed in terms of the first. A slightly different meaning of morbidity has recently been put forward as the 'fourth goal of perinatal medicine': failure of the early relationship between mother and baby (Ounsted, et al., 1982). Satisfactory measures of this relationship have not been developed, but all would agree that a sign of its failure is child abuse. Contrary to the contention of the President of the American College of Obstetricians and Gynaecologists cited earlier, home delivery does not seem to equate with child abuse. On the contrary, child abuse is more often preceded by hospital delivery and particularly by difficult deliveries with high levels of medical intervention followed by a period of separation for mother and baby (Lynch, 1975). Difficult social conditions at home do not promote easy parent-child relationships either. The prevalence of child abuse, only the tip of the iceberg of such problems, has been estimated at around 6 per 1,000 live births, a little below the 'best' perinatal mortality rates. Possibly one of the most surprising aspects of the place of birth debate is the way in which it has singled out place of birth, as opposed to place, and way, of life, as the chief consideration affecting the survival and health of mothers and babies, and has, at the same time, adopted a narrow definition — the mere avoidance of mortality — of successful medical risk-prediction. Adding new goals to the serious game of perinatal medicine can only mean a substantial widening of the field on which it is played.

10

Consumers' Revolt

What a pity it is that childbirth, that most creative and joyous of events, should have become in the last few years a battle-ground, to be fought over by opposing factions whose only common characteristic, seemingly, and yet the one which divides them most deeply, is a sincere desire to do what is right. Should childbirth be 'done' this way or that way; who knows best; can we afford it; is it necessary; who do they think they are? Wherever health care is mentioned, there in the front rank of controversy is childbirth; they know best because they know obstetrics/ administration/psychology/money; we know best, because we know ourselves. They are coldly clinical, they won't listen to us; we are emotional, we won't listen to them. So what do we do now?

Association for Improvements in the Maternity Services Newsletter, October 1978, p. 1

The brave new world of hospital-dominated obstetrical technology described in the last 3 chapters has generated a new historical response: the consumer[1] revolt. Women using the maternity services in Britain (and many other countries experiencing similar patterns of development) have joined together in formal organizations in order to make their voices heard. Consumer dissatisfaction with antenatal care has always existed, as earlier parts of this book have shown, but the health care and wider political climate of the 1960s and 1970s has allowed the dissatisfaction an organizational voice of its own.

The deception of childbearing women

In 1975 Suzanne Arms, an American journalist and mother, published a book catchily entitled *Immaculate Deception*. The book claimed to be a new look at women and childbirth in America, and Suzanne Arms's

---

1. Not a wholly appropriate term. See Logan, et al., 1971; Stacey, 1976, for a critique.

motive in writing it had been her own bad birth experience. Anticipating a 'natural' birth, she had, in the event, received caudal anaesthesia, acceleration of labour with pitocin, and an instrumental delivery resulting in a torn cervix: 'I came out of delivery numb from the waist to the knees, dry and sour in the mouth, flat on my back, and strapped to a metal table four feet off the ground'. In the brief account of her own experience which prefaces the main text of *Immaculate Deception* Arms doesn't mention the fate of her child; indeed, she remarks instead that 'I was only a child at the birth of my own baby' (Arms 1977 edition, p. xiii). The deception of which Arms speaks is the deception — the unattainable ideal — of the no-risk birth. In order to reduce risk obstetricians, says Arms, have redefined the natural process of childbearing as unnatural, and have thereby provoked an exponential rise in the *actual* risks of childbirth by insisting on hospital and medical interference as the rule for all births. Women are deceived in assenting to this technological system of childbirth management by believing that only thus will they safely achieve motherhood.

Arms' book was one of a species that began to appear from the mid-1960s. This literature, which took up the theme of the 'new obstetrics' and how women feel about it, was not always written by women; it includes, for example, Frederick Leboyer's *Birth Without Violence* (1975), a moving invective against the crying and dangling-upside-down of babies at birth, which struck a chord in the hearts of many thousands of women — and this despite its habit of referring to the mother (from the supposed viewpoint of the baby) as 'the enemy', a 'monster', and a 'hated prison'. Advocacy, whether male or female, of more natural forms of childbirth opposed to interventionist obstetrics was not, of course, new. Appeals to nature as a corrective to the unbalanced mechanistic tendencies of obstetricians appear as soon as obstetrics starts to enter its technological mode in the eighteenth century (Donnison, 1977). Sheila Kitzinger, the doyenne of natural childbirth education in Britain, wisely observes in one of her own first statements on the subject, *The Experience of Childbirth* (1962), that just where the modern natural childbirth movement came from is a matter of dispute. Like the antenatal movement, the natural childbirth movement has always possessed an international character. Neither would it be correct to equate the modern natural childbirth movement entirely with a resistance on the

2. The development of the consumer revolt in North America appears to have been somewhat different, in that the attack on unnecessary technology was intrinsic to even the earliest complaints. See Haire, 1972.

part of pregnant women and their advocates to high technology and hospital-based childbirth. The *ideological* roots of the movement are to be found in an attack on that age-old curse of childbearing women — the pain of labour and delivery. This was the initial focus of the National Childbirth Trust (NCT) founded (at first as the Natural Childbirth Association) in Britain in 1956; its initial goal was the improvement of women's knowledge about childbirth and the promotion of classes in relaxation and breathing for labour, on the premise that removing fear and inspiring confidence was essential to the successful handling of pain, and successful handling of pain by women rather than obstetricians was the key to a good experience of childbirth (for women).

In proposing this, advocates of natural childbirth succeeded in putting forward an important alternative model of birth from the prevailing medical one. In this alternative model, a good birth is one achieved without drugs, without interventions and in which, most of all, the mother retains control of herself, her body and her baby. Childbirth becomes a social event: 'successful' childbirth means the delivery and subsequent incorporation of the baby into a network of thriving social relationships. This alternative model of childbirth, with its emphasis on a different set of indices for measuring successful birth from the more narrowly-conceived medical ones, was then available to be taken up and used by other consumer organizations in the maternity care field, whose objectives were not necessarily to be those of 'natural' childbirth itself.[2]

The focus of the alternative model proposed by the natural childbirth movement was the time of labour and delivery, not the antenatal period. Some of the early 'consumer revolt' literature took an exceptionally naive view of the benefits about medical antenatal care — that is, compared to their developed scepticism of medical intranatal care. For example, Suzanne Arms attributes much of the blame for the USA's poor infant mortality record to poor prenatal care: 'Time and time again it has been proved that prenatal care is a key to lowering risks for poverty mothers and for paving the way for normal births and healthy children for all pregnant women' (Arms, 1975, p. 51). There is an uneasy balance to be struck here between a dependence on medical authority and the need to trust one's own knowledge of one's body. 'Remember', admonishes a guide to *Naturebirth*, 'that you probably know as much about you in relation to pregnancy and the fetus in relation to you as anyone, and that you are going to the medical profession because they are trained to try to define the relation of you and the fetus to mortality' (Brook, 1976, pp. 169–70). It is not clear how defining this confers the obligation to ignore the subjective expertise of the consumer, or how consumers may not themselves have intimations of mortality from time to time.

Societies for the prevention of cruelty to pregnant women

The problem was that antenatal care as it existed in the early 1960s, in both Britain and the USA, did not encourage pregnant women's confidence in themselves. The Association for Improvements in the Maternity Services (AIMS, founded 1960), one of the largest consumer organizations of its kind in Britain, was based from the start on problems reported by women with antenatal care. AIMS's founder, Sally Willmington, spent six weeks of her own pregnancy in an antenatal ward. She did not enjoy the experience, wrote to the national press about it, and a letter by her published in the *Observer* newspaper provoked a flood of other such letters. The letter-writers met and decided to form a pressure group to bring about improvements in maternity care, whose name would be the Society for the Prevention of Cruelty to Pregnant Women — shortly afterwards changed to the more saccharine AIMS. The objectives of SPCPW/AIMS in 1960 went as follows:

(1) *More money*: A greater proportion of the national income to be spent on the NHS, especially on the maternity services and especially on hospital provision.
(2) *Midwives*: A recruitment drive for more midwives; improvement of midwives' conditions of work, training and pay.
(3) *Home helps*: More home helps especially for home deliveries.
(4) *Loneliness in labour*. It should be mandatory for no woman in established labour to be left alone against her will.
(5) *Research and training of doctors and midwives*: More research into relief of pain in childbirth and into psychological aspects of childbearing — the latter to be incorporated into the training of doctors and midwives.

In 1981 its current Chairperson, Beverley Beech, commented that this list looked very much like the 1981 objectives (Beech, 1981). As an Aims Newsletter the previous year had observed in relation to antenatal care:

We still receive reports from women of antenatal clinics described as cattle-markets, of block-booked appointments and long sordid waits for a brief prod by a stranger (different each visit) who is hostile to women's questions about their own bodies; where women who ask what is their temperature or blood pressure or dilatation are told to mind their own business; where women's tentative choices are treated with contempt . . . AND THIS IS 1980. (AIMS Newsletter, Summer, 1980, p. 1).

Jo Garcia's 1982 survey of the literature on consumer opinions of antenatal care shows how the same topics appear over and over again: the conveyor-belt syndrome, unsatisfactory staff–patient communication, badly-worked appointments systems, overcrowded clinics with no facilities for older children, lack of explanation and advice for the special personal labour of growing a baby. The experiences of pregnant women, often described by clinicians and policy-makers as 'anecdotes', juxtapose the subjectivity of the care-user to that of the care-provider, more usually termed 'clinical experience'.

AIMS is an association composed of voluntary workers — as indeed are most consumer organizations in this field. It has local groups scattered all over the country and actively maintains close contact with other groups, including some NCT groups and some focused on home births, such as the Society to Support Home Confinements set up by Margaret Whyte in Durham in mid-1974. During AIMS's early years, years of campaigning for the current interpretation of 'freedom of choice' in maternity care — more hospital beds — the Association tended to welcome the new technical developments in intranatal and antenatal and postnatal care. However this initial enthusiasm was quickly replaced by an awareness of the price that often had to be paid by mothers and babies for the use of the new techniques. By 1981, the objectives of the Association were reformulated to focus on 'the right of the mother to experience normal physiological childbirth without interference unless she wants it or there are clear indications that it is needed' — a reversion to the core doctrine of the natural childbirth model, a sign that the underlying conflict between users and providers of care *was* precisely centred on this dispute about the ideology and statistics of normality versus pathology.

What AIMS came to say was that its members, and the unaffiliated for whom the Association also spoke, would have preferred obstetrics to have developed as an activity designed to maximize the chances of normal childbearing, whereas it had in fact evolved in the opposite mould, as an exercise based on the principle of probable abnormality. The conflict between the two definitions of obstetric care runs throughout the whole period of pregnancy, delivery and the postpartum. Thus AIMS's 1981 list of objectives recognized the need to normalize antenatal as well as intranatal and postnatal care, and to locate it decisively within the social domain. Goals outlined for antenatal care in 1981 included:

> Antenatal care, delivery and postnatal care for all low-risk women to be organized and controlled by midwives.

> Immediate provision of antenatal care for low-risk women to be community or GP based.

Antenatal checks to include an investigation into the mother's eating habits and adequate dietary service provided about fetal growth.

A system introduced to offer nutritional assistance for those mothers-to-be suffering from an inadequate diet.

All pregnant women to receive the maternity grant as a right. The maternity grant to be increased to £100, without pre-conditions
(AIMS newsletter, Spring 1981, p. 2).

While the objectives of more midwife-controlled and community-based antenatal care, and an increase in the maternity grant, seem eminently reasonable, given existing evidence, the requirement of dietary surveillance is somewhat Orwellian in tone. Is eating to be a new area of the state's intrusion into the privacy of its citizens and citizens-to-be? (See chapter 12.)

Human relations?

A final objective of the 1981 AIMS agenda relates to a document with an important place in the history of the consumer movement in maternity care — a document entitled 'Human Relations in Obstetrics'.

'Human Relations in Obstetrics' began life as a lecture by Norman Morris, Professor of Obstetrics and Gynaecology at Charing Cross Hospital Medical School on the occasion of the opening of the new obstetric unit in February, 1960. It was published in the *Lancet* (23 April 1961, p. 913–15), and subsequently lent its title to a document published by the then Ministry of Health in 1961 (Central Health Services Council, 1961). Morris referred in his lecture to the increasing safety of childbearing and asked the leading question 'But are we to measure success simply in terms of life and death?' Drawing on his own observations, as well as extracts from several hundreds of letters sent to a women's magazine, Morris presented a case against the prevailing hospital system. The central idea was that within this system, women's 'feeling of personal achievement is lost, drowned in a sea of inhumanity.' About antenatal clinics, he said:

Women attend these clinics regularly, often as many as fourteen times. The clinic is usually drab and colourless, painted in bottle green, brown, or dirty cream. There are rows of uncomfortable benches. There is an atmosphere of coldness, unfriendliness, and severity more in keeping with the spirit of an income-tax office. The clinic is often very overcrowded, and at best a crude appointment system is in operation. Despite this, women often wait 1–3 hours. The interview itself is usually extremely brief, and under such conditions there is little encouragement for the patient to ask questions or relieve herself of any nagging fears or doubts. Therefore she often remains in gross ignorance of what is happening to her. The doctors and nurses also remain virtual strangers since she rarely sees the same one at each visit (Morris, *Lancet*, 23 April 1961, p. 913).

This common antenatal scenario is, notes Morris, also dissatisfying to hospital staff. In recommending how the situation might be improved, he pleads for hospital staff to recognize the vulnerability and sensitivity of pregnant women, to realize that we are all human beings together, and maternity units should 'reflect joy rather than sorrow, hope rather than gloom, life rather than death' (p. 915).

It is difficult to imagine how anyone could disagree (now or then) with such fine sentiments, and it is significant that seeing the consumer revolt in terms of a demand for better psychological care poses no threat to the current corporate structure of maternity care provision. The super-structure of psychological services to the consumer can be improved, whilst the basic structure of medical services and format of clinical care remain unchanged. Indeed, this seems to be what has happened with those aspects of intranatal and postnatal care identified as negative in 'Human Relations in Obstetrics'. The psychosocial side of birth and the postnatal period has been modified with the admission of fathers to the delivery room; there is a new enthusiasm for postnatal bonding of mother and baby, and flexibility of birth positions in some hospitals for suitably selected 'low-risk' women. There has also been some reconsideration of the need for such routine practices as pre-delivery enemas and pubic hair shaving. The emotional impact of childbirth upon the family, and (to some extent) the advantage of a woman feeling herself to be the active agent at delivery, have been conceded. But the story with antenatal care is another matter. Either the conception of the consumer revolt in terms of the psychological superstructure has not yet brought about change in the antenatal care domain, or there is some-thing inherently misleading about this conception itself.

But what do women really want?

Nobody, of course, is in a position to answer this question, since women do not form a homogenous group. It is often asserted that, behind all the modern fuss about inhumane obstetrics, most women are satisfied: the articulate minority has merely succeeded in creating a false impression of mass discontent. As Minerva in the *British Medical Journal* protested:

> The middle class women who seem to have little good to say about British obstetrics might reflect that with all the technological changes that they deplore perinatal mortality in mothers from the professional class is now down to twelve or thereabouts — very near to Scandinavian levels (Minerva, *British Medical Journal*, 16 December 1978, p. 1722).[3]

Even if it were true that only a few women complain about their care, it is, as Riley (1977) points out, incorrect to assume that the disappointments of a minority may with impunity be ignored. What is a minority and why are its sufferings unimportant? The basic methodological question here is one about the equation of silence with satisfaction: the woman who does not complain about her antenatal care is assumed to be satisfied with it. The assumption of the satisfactory meaning of silence is to be found not only in obstetrics but in many other fields; indeed, it is generally characteristic of the ideological stance of dominant groups towards oppressed minorities. Thus the middle classes deem the working classes satisfied with their lot, white people conjure up the image of the happy slave, and men point to the contented housewife in order to defuse the explosive potential of women's liberation.

In 1971 the Consumers' Association (CA) published in its magazine *Which?* its own survey of CA members' experience of antenatal care, and included the results of interviewing two further samples of non-CA members. Table 10.1 compares the findings. In all three samples, hospital antenatal care gets the blackest mark.

Social scientists have come into their own in the last ten years to fill the hiatus created by obstetricians' pronouncements and consumer organization surveys. Tables 10.2 and 10.3 are taken from the national sample of pregnancies and births covered by the Institute of Social Studies in Medical Care's survey of induction of labour in 1975. The study showed, overall, that women liked antenatal care better when it was provided by GPs rather than in hospital. In particular, 'treatment as a person' was considered superior in the hands of GPs. Two in five mothers did not regard their medical and nursing care provided in hospital as very good, nearly half found the hospital treatment impersonal, more than half did not feel the hospital staff were good about explaining things, and two out of five did not feel able to discuss their questions with hospital staff. Table 10.2 establishes that continuity of

---

3. The Scandinavian reference is in the tradition of the early invidious comparisons of the British obstetric record with those of other countries in the 1920s and 1930s (see pp. 76–7).

The Captured Womb

Table 10.1 Antenatal care, 1971

	No. of mothers	Average waiting time minutes	Waiting over an hour %	Complaining of lack of privacy %	Satisfied overall %
CA mothers					
GP	2,646	14	2	4	86
Hospital	1,868	42	20	18	73
LA Clinic	448	22	5	16	83
Private	167	10	—	2	91
non-CA mothers — Midland City					
GP	153	28	7	12	90
Hospital	132	87	64	20	84
non-CA mothers — Southern County					
GP	109	13	2	6	93
Hospital	96	45	27	9	84

source: *Which?*, June 1971, p. 166. With permission of the Consumers Association.

Table 10.2 Women's attitudes to care by whether cared for by the same or different people each time

Views about aspect of care	Hospital		GP	
	Care from one or two people	Care from different people each time	Care from one or two people	Care from different people each time
Medical and nursing care 'very good'	75%	57%	72%	50%
Treatment as a person 'very good'	68%	48%	80%	49%
'Very good' about explaining things	58%	37%	62%	35%
Felt able to discuss things	76%	52%	82%	60%
Number of women (= 100%)	561	836	1622	109

source: O'Brien and Smith, Women's Experience of Antenatal Care, *Practitioner* 225 1981, p. 125. With permission of the publisher Morgan–Grampian Ltd.

care helps to override the disadvantages of hospital treatment: both in hospital and in the GP's surgery antenatal care provided by one or two people is much more satisfactory to the user than care involving different people each time. In table 10.3, visibility is given to one practical consideration which can shift the balance of satisfaction; the average amount of women's time absorbed by hospital antental care is more than twice that taken up by a visit to the GP — 157 as against 70 minutes.

Table 10.3 Time spent on antenatal visits to the hospital and general
practitioner

| | Average time (in minutes) at: | |
	Hospital	GP
Time spent travelling to and from place where care received	57	30
Time spent waiting	62	22
Time spent being examined and having tests	37	17
Time spent on whole visit (from time left home or work to time got back)	156	69
Number of women (= 100%)	1589	1774

source: O'Brien and Smith, 1981, p. 124

Table 10.4 addresses more centrally the question of the attitudes of
the inarticulate majority. It may be that working-class mothers do not
ask questions in antenatal clinics, but they most clearly have a greater
unsatisfied need for information. This unmet need may be set in the
context of the findings of two other studies carried out in Yorkshire in
the mid-1970s by Hilary Graham and Lorna McKee, and in Aberdeen
in the early 1980s by Sally Macintyre. In the first of these two studies
(table 10.5) three-quarters of the women learnt nothing from their
antenatal checkups; in the second (table 10.6) only about one in ten
women described their booking visit to an antenatal clinic as useful and

Table 10.4 Social class and desire for more information

Social class	Average number of items would have liked more information about	Number of mothers (= 100%)
I Professional	3.3	195
II Intermediate	3.9	369
III Skilled {Non-manual	4.4	239
{Manual	4.7	856
IV Semi-skilled	4.6	311
V Unskilled	5.5	114
Unclassified	4.1	94
All mothers	4.4	2178

source: Cartwright, A. *The Dignity of Labour? A Story of Child-bearing and Induction* 1979, p. 101. With permission of the publisher Tavistock Publications.

Table 10.5 Women's attitudes to antenatal care

	Enjoyed check-ups %	Learnt from check-ups %
Yes	37	25
No	47	73
Don't know/mixed	17	3

source: Adapted from Graham, H. and McKee, L. *The First Months of Motherhood*, 1979, p. 42. Reproduced by kind permission of the Health Education Council.

Table 10.6 Mothers' views of the value of routine antenatal care

Antenatal care described as:	Booking visit %	At 34 weeks %
Useful	12	0
Reassurance only	39	71
Mixed/uncertain	37	4
Useless	10	11
Not stated	2	13

source: Adapted from Macintyre, S. *Expectations and Experiences of First Pregnancy*. Occasional Paper 5, 1981, p. 149. With permission of the Institute of Medical Sociology, Aberdeen University.

none considered the 34-week visit useful. A similar proportion described each of these two visits unequivocally as 'useless'. Around a third at the booking visit and two-thirds at the 34-week visit attached importance to antenatal care only for its reassurance value.

According to table 10.5 slightly more than a third of women enjoy their antenatal care. In a recent case which attracted a good deal of attention in the British media, a couple appeared in court charged with the delivery of the baby without having called for professional help. The mother explained that she had chosen not to have 'professional' care for this pregnancy because in a previous pregnancy she had tried antenatal care but had not enjoyed it. The judge reprimanded her to the effect that antenatal care is not meant to be enjoyed. In this most decisive legalistic manner antenatal care is identified in 1982 as an exercise that now runs counter to women's interests. (It would hardly have been thus described in 1922.) The extent and meaning of this change in definition is a theme taken up in the next chapter: we turn meanwhile to the broader social context within which the consumer revolt in maternity care was born.

Changing and unchanging relations

Over the last 20 years in many industrialized countries there has emerged a self-help health-care movement which has attempted to remove some of the responsibility for health from health care professionals, and reclaim it as the responsibility of the individual. This new concern with personal health has spawned a multitude of self-help groups. It has generated the holistic health movement: 'a remarkably diverse challenge to orthodox medicine', which includes healing methods such as

> meditation and biofeedback, polarity therapy ('balancing life energy') iridology ('interprets the neural-optic reflexes in the sensitive tissue of the iris'), guided imagery, nutritional therapies, movement or dance therapy, rolfing ('a technique for reordering the body'), massage, and various healing methods adopted from naturopathy, homeopathy, and Native American and Eastern traditions (Crawford, 1980, p. 366).

In the domain of perinatal care, alternative services to those officially provided have developed widely in Europe and North America. These alternative perinatal services (in some countries linked to the feminist movement and in others not) are an extremely important manifestation of consumer dissatisfaction. Not only is the consumer revolt expressed in the form of consumer organizations, but in the move towards alternative forms of care, some of which are provided by the consumer herself (Houd and Oakley, 1983). In the USA lay midwifery developed as a response to dissatisfaction with the official maternity services and embodied a holistic approach to childbirth. Techniques common in the holistic health movement (massage, yoga, etc.) are used, and the clinical surveillance is but a small strand in a social caretaking sensitive to the individual needs of pregnant women.

What was happening — has happened — in the 1950s and 1960s to fertilize the soil of the consumer revolt and the setting up of alternative services? In the first place, in Britain, the immediate post-war belief in the ability of the NHS to confer not only equal health care but equal health on all segments of the population came to flounder in the 1950s on the rock-like reality of a society critically divided both economically and socially. Medicine, even nationalized medicine, confronted its own limits and own limited conception of itself in the face of these enduring class divisions. Social class differences in infant mortality, for example, identified by Richard Titmuss, before the NHS, in 1943, were still found in a 1955 analysis. 'There has been no narrowing of the social gap in infant mortality', reported the authors of this analysis, J. N. Morris and J. A. Heady: 'if anything it may have widened slightly. This finding was unexpected. At any rate, something different was hoped for'. Morris and Heady noted that this phenomenon was not confined to infant mortality:

> In all the major conditions from which adult men [sic] in social class v had a higher death rate in 1930–32 than social class I, the gap was as big in 1950 as twenty years before — and if anything slightly wider. In trying to understand the recent social history of infant mortality, therefore, regard should also be paid to the more general phenomenon. The persistence of the gap between the social classes in infant mortality is unlikely to be entirely explained by factors concerned only with childbearing (Morris and Heady, 1955, pp. 556–7).

Since 1955 the social class difference in risks of mortality, including perinatal mortality has remained the statistical backdrop against which antenatal care, along with other preventive health programmes, strives to produce better health.

The other inequality that has persisted, despite the NHS, is the differential social class use of medical care. In their *The Cost of the National Health Service* (1956), Titmuss and Abel-Smith drew attention to 'excessive' middle-class demands on the health services. In 1980 the Black Report (Townsend and Davidson, 1982) summarized much of the subsequent evidence, and concluded (which is interesting from the point of view of antenatal care) that under-utilization of medical care among the working classes is greatest in relation to the preventive services.

But evidence as to the apparently immovable substratum of social class differences in health, and the uptake of health care, does not mean that medical professionals are about to relinquish their hard-won claims to expertise. Instead, the medical profession has reacted by digging its heels into the ground and reasserting its power to heal in a new and unequivocally technological mode. What is claimed is both less and much more than before. Of course the internal conflict between general and specialist branches of medicine contained in the format of the NHS has served to enhace this territorial response, and the right to control this or that aspect of health care has been disputed not only between medicine and society but within medicine itself.

By the mid-1950s, professional pundits were saying that patients had changed as well as doctors. The average patient was said to be 'aware that his [sic] doctor now knows relatively much less about medicine as a whole than he did a few years ago' (Clark-Kennedy, 1955, p. 619) —

and the cause of this altered consciousness was said to be the impact of the media, better education, the result of public health campaigns designed precisely to make the public health- and health-care conscious. In the childbirth field, media publicity was undeniably important in shaping the consciousness of the consumer: 'Machines, technology and interference with nature are currently fashionable in obstetrics', wrote Oliver and Louise Gillie in what transpired to be an epoch-making article called 'The childbirth revolution' in the *Sunday Times* (13 October 1974): 'Obstetricians are not much interested in the woman with a normal pregnancy who wants to have her baby naturally. The needs of the normal woman and her baby are often lost among the clinical bustle.' The Gillies did not mention antenatal care, espoused somewhat uncritically Leboyer's 'gentle ritual of love', and argued that epidurals should be given on demand. They succeeded, nevertheless, in focusing the public (and medical) awareness on the alternative claim of the consumer to a physiological experience of childbirth untrammelled by routine technological practices — the natural childbirth model.

In this way obstetricians and doctors in general have become targets for criticism. Consumer demands have not been — are not being — met. One solution to the problem is the co-option of the consumer revolt by the medical profession. The Maternity Alliance, founded in 1980 on the initiative of the Spastics Society, the National Council for One Parent Families, and the Child Poverty Action Group, describes itself as a 'non-partisan' forum for 'any group, individual or specialist organization' involved in providing better services for Britain's mothers and babies. What is 'non-partisan' about the Maternity Alliance is precisely the location under the same label of medical and non-medical interests. In the same way, the Active Birth Movement, founded in Britain in 1982, puts itself forward as an alliance of consumers and care-providers.

With these recent exceptions, the consumer revolt has fought, and continues to fight, against prevailing medical definitions of pregnancy and antenatal care for the very sound reason that what pregnant women have complained about is the capturing of the womb by medical professionals. The consumers' focus has been the reduction of the social and personal experience of pregnancy, and the individuality of pregnant women, to the mechanical image of the womb housed in the body of either a reluctant or compliant patient, and processed on the principle that a no-risk birth is only to be achieved by exposing all wombs and their owners to an identical all-risk monitoring process.

11
Women, the State and the Medical Profession

It is instructive to observe that the proposals now made, and accepted as necessary, imply a paternal — or ought I to say maternal? — interest by the State in the wellbeing of motherhood, which is an admirable example of modern collective humanism.

Newman, 1930, p. 149

The modelling of the body produces a knowledge of the individual ... and the acquisition of skills is inextricably linked with the establishment of power relations.

Foucault, 1977, pp. 294–5

The consumer movement in obstetrics discussed in the last chapter represents a new historical response to the medical surveillance of pregnancy. It suggests some antagonism between women as the social group using antenatal care on the one hand, and the State and the medical profession as the providers and policy-makers in antenatal care, on the other. This gives prominence to a central and important theme of this book, namely the function of antenatal care as a strategy for the social control of women. The present chapter explores this theme further, and attempts in the process to draw together some of the main arguments of the book as a whole.

What is antenatal care?

Before understanding how antenatal care might control women, we must first understand what antenatal care is. As previous chapters have amply illustrated, antenatal care is what different people and social groups over the years have said it is; it is what some people have done, what others have had done to them, what some have eulogized and others have complained about. Countless official documents and personal and professional exchanges have proclaimed or debated its meaning; and under the apparently consistent heading of antenatal care, a complex and variegated admixture of practices have been located at different times and in different places. It is significant that, in explaining and justifying the practice of antenatal care, its purveyors have been uniformly more interested in spelling out its benefits and objectives, and in decreeing what it *ought* to be, than in defining what it actually is. Thus, we receive such alternative messages as: antenatal care promises the abolition of toxaemia, is the answer to maternal mortality, will produce future generations of mothers educated properly in the hygiene of parenting. Antenatal care ought to be done by medical specialists, or by general practitioners, or by midwives: the surveillance of mothers' home environments is important, or is a distraction from the principal business of clinical care. Antenatal care is an art demanding skills in human relations; or, it is a science, erected and practised on a rational, physicalist basis.

Munro Kerr in 1933 was not alone in objecting that the protagonists of antenatalism had lost sight of the wood for the trees. No committee, he said, had ever really yet defined what adequate antenatal care might consist of. 'Let us be perfectly explicit on the point', continued Kerr confidently, 'it [antenatal care] implies efficient and constant supervision of the pregnant woman from the commencement of pregnancy, the correction of any dyscrasia [abnormality] whenever it occurs, and the transference to an institution of every patient who cannot be suitably treated and nursed in her own home' (Kerr, 1933, p. 176). Kerr's certainty must have been an inspiration to some of his fellow antenatalists, but in 1980 a Government Committee still could not define antenatal care. A 'great deal of both opinion and factual evidence' on this point was presented to the Social Services Committee reporting on Perinatal and Neonatal Mortality chaired by Renée Short MP, and the Committee found itself 'unhesitatingly' able to accept 'the often reiterated claim of antenatal care as a means of reducing perinatal and neonatal mortality'. Yet 'what exactly antenatal care consists of and how it works', said the Committee, 'has been less clear to us' (Short Report, 1980, p. 21). Even more recently that august institution, the RCOG, was strikingly able to produce a report on 'Antenatal and Intrapartum Care' which in the course of its 51 pages did not define the concept or objectives of antenatal care at all (RCOG 1982a).

Renée Short's committee identified the cause of the problem of defining antenatal care as the lack of a consensus definition of antenatal care within the medical profession itself. Though views and practices of antenatal care have altered in kaleidoscopic fashion over the decades, some unilinear evolution is present to reassure us of the (limited) value of the Darwinian paradigm. From the wonderful optimism of the early years in which antenatal care was the cure for almost every gestational malady, we move to more guarded claims about antenatal care being principally concerned with the management of detectable disease (Chamberlain, 1976). But, within this view, the ineffectiveness of antenatal care as an overall screening programme not only renders it less than it was claimed to be; it does not even then say what it is.

The antenatal control of women

In these shifting sands of antenatal care's perceived potential, we may, however, detect a lurking skeleton of its essential definition. Antenatal care has involved some kind of relationship between three elements in society: women, the state and the medical profession. Antenatal care is something that is done to women. It represents an attempt to control the behaviour of women's bodies. Of course this is obvious. Pregnancy is a condition only experienced by women. But the obviousness of this point does not make it uninteresting, indeed, on the contrary, it raises the essential and provocative question of how far it is possible to separate the ideology and practice of antenatal care from the ideology and practice of womanhood.

Since antenatal care is an exercise done to women, it must involve some element of controlling women. The term for antenatal care in some languages is, even, as noted earlier, antenatal 'control'. In a sense, any activity targeted at a particular social group has these overtones of social control, less well-developed when participation is voluntary (e.g. anti-smoking campaigns), more so when it is not (e.g. imprisonment). As Michel Foucault has observed of systems of social control in general, no history of the body can be written without considering the body's location in a political field. Given the intimate relation between the economic and political structure, and the way in which 'knowledge' about the body is constituted, we need to abandon the tradition 'that allows us to imagine that knowledge can exist only where the power relations are suspended and that knowledge can develop only outside its injunctions, its demands and its interests' (Foucault, 1977, p. 27). Because of the covert social control function of antenatal care, there is a dialectical relationship within the philosophy and practice of antenatal care over the years between what is happening to antenatal care and what is happening to women. It is not simply that, as antenatal care acquires the status of a commandment, the power of women declines: indeed, if anything, the reverse is the case, and the greater enfranchisement of women has been accompanied by a vigorous renewal of the commandment of antenatal care.

Some aspects of the relationship between women's situation and the practice of antenatal care have already been discussed; for examine the continuing high rate of maternal mortality in the 1920s and early 1930s focused the attention of antenatalists — of both the state and the medical profession — more and more sharply on the *mother's* condition. Conversely, as the risks encountered by women in childbearing became less in the 1950s, mothers gradually began to acquire within the medical perspective a new guise as containers of fetuses. The economic poverty of women's lives in the family before and after the First World War nurtured a holistic approach to pregnancy care, and urged a medico-political awareness of the need for a national health service. Since the promotion of childbearing cannot be separated from its prevention, the inability of women over most of the period covered by this book to obtain free and safe abortion and contraception has hedged the health-promoting potential of antenatal care with limits not of its own making (and represents the investment of not only the state but the Church in women's reproductive role).

There are many other examples of links between the domain of antenatal care and the position of women, and among these the relationship between feminism and antenatal care is probably the most complex. Antenatal care was born almost at the moment the woman's movement died, and it has lived through the birth, youth and middle-age of another woman's movement. As antenatal care's mentor, J. W. Ballantyne, once said (1914, p. 104), 'the vote can't compensate women for loss of motherhood, but nor, on the other hand, was it ever intended to.' Political investment in women's health care between the wars was an obvious and much-needed direction for ex-suffragettes to take, and as Jane Lewis shows in her historical analysis of *The Politics of Motherhood* (1980), they were joined by many women activitists who would not have allied themselves with feminism at all. It was possible in those days to defend the interests of women and not be called (or call oneself) a feminist, just as it has always been possible to defend the interests of men without being known as a masculinist.

In the twentieth century's second wave of feminism, the promotion of motherhood did not at first loom large. Feminist ideology in the early 1970s was an ideology of women's liberation from the burden of reproduction: the ideological platform included free abortion on demand, free and easily-available contraception and sterilization, and twenty-four-hour-a-day childcare. The feminists were not demanding natural childbirth, or the rights of women as patients, or the need for self-determination in the achievement of motherhood; motherhood itself was viewed as an obstacle to the goal of sex equality. The battles of women in antenatal clinics to have their voices heard and their interests as individuals considered were strictly offlimits to feminism. There were good reasons for this initial location of feminist health care interests outside the sphere of maternity; the long evolution of an equal rights (women-must-become-equal-to-men) philosophy, the childless background of the first women's liberationists in the late 1960s and early 1970s. Indeed, it could be said with some justification that it was as these early liberationists themselves embarked on motherhood that motherhood became of interest to the women's movement as a whole.

Yet almost in order to make up for this feminist lack of interest in maternity care, obstetricians have tended to equate the protesting consumer with the ardent feminist. A wealth of epithets and caricatures of 'women's liberationists', the 'vocal minority', etc, abounds in debates about the consumer point of view, and there is supporting evidence to suggest that obstetrics and gynaecology may be a particularly misogynist medical specialty (see, for example, Scully, 1980). Its misogynism springs, in part, from its masculinity: in 1982 four out of five NHS doctors working in obstetrics and gynaecology in Britain were men. Men have figured prominently, too, in the technical and institutional history of obstetrics, as we have seen countless times in the pages of this book. Divisions within medicine — obstetrics, gynaecology, paediatrics, neonatal paediatrics, fetal medicine, reproductive medicine — have segmented women's bodies into competing professional charters and domains of medical work; womanhood and motherhood have become a battlefield for not only patriarchal but professional supremacy; the medical profession has been able to harness paternal/patriarchal assumptions about women's personality and role to the service of its own ascent to professionalization.

The motive of professionalization and professional dominance as an explanation of changes in medical care should never be underrated (Freidson, 1972). New antenatal technologies, for example, are scarcely welcome merely in themselves, but rather as items in the medical armamentarium — witness the placing of lay female self-help groups under police surveillance in the United States in the early 1970s (Ruzek, 1979). The anthropologist Margaret Mead, a long-time commentator on the habits of the so-called civilized world, made the acute observation that 'men began taking over obstetrics and they invented a tool [the vaginal speculum] that allowed them to look inside women. You could call this progress, except that when women tried to look inside themselves, this was called practising medicine without a license' (Mead, 1974, p. 6).

The social position of the medical profession is such as to ward off all lay attacks on its ideology and practice. For, as Brian Harrison observes in his commentary on 'Women's Health and the Women's Movement in Britain 1840–1940':

> A profession of any kind is in some respects antithetical to the popular pressure group, for it is by definition concerned with exclusion, whereas the popular agitator seeks comprehensiveness. The profession fears the layman [sic] who is the agitator's main asset; the profession fraternizes with those in authority, whose unpopularity fuels the reformer's fire; the profession defends an interest, whereas altruism is the popular agitator's proudest boast (Harrison, 1981, p. 34).

It is not hard to see this dialectic in the words of medical professionals about burning issues raised by consumers of maternity care. Thus, a *British Medical Journal* editorial on episiotomy in 1982 (23 January 1982, p. 220) referred to the 'increasing insistence' with which 'individual women, and sometimes well-organized groups, are asking whether some procedure is manifestly to the advantage of mother and baby or amounts to unnecessary interference by doctors . . . It would . . . be a pity', the editorial concludes, 'if clinical practice were changed on insufficient evidence because of a patient-led protest. *The answers should come from clinical research*' (italics added).

Medicine and the agency of the state

The state too has its misogynist policies. For example, the economic dependency of wives and mothers has been an assumption behind state welfare schemes ever since the state first began to take some responsibility for the wellbeing of its members; this assumption has always been profoundly contradicted by the realities of family life and the sexual division of labour under capitalism (Lewis, 1983). Yet the misogynies of the state and the medical profession do not merely parallel or mutually reinforce one another. The medical sociologist Eliot Freid-

son has described the alliance between the state and the medical profession in the following terms:

> The foundation of medicine's control over its work is thus clearly political
> in character, involving the aid of the state in establishing and maintaining
> the profession's preeminence. The occupation itself has formal repre-
> sentatives, organizational or individual, which attempt to direct the efforts
> of the state toward policies desired by the occupational group . . . it is by
> the interaction between formal agents or agencies of the occupation and
> officials of the state that the occupation's control over its work is estab-
> lished and shaped. The most strategic and treasured characteristic of the
> profession — its autonomy — is therefore owed to its relationship to the
> sovereign state (Freidson, 1972, pp. 23–4).

Ultimately, therefore, the medical profession is not autonomous and the
state is. Indeed, the extent to which the health sector, together with its
relevant professions, is embedded in the state's corporate power has
grown in recent years. The allocation of health care resources has
increasingly been perceived in Western capitalist societies as a public
responsibility, and increasingly funded out of the public purse (though
the state also has an interest in fostering private sector care). The
organization of medicine builds upon the class relations of capitalist
state social organization, both practically and ideologically.[1] Social policy and health policy are, from this point of view, indistinguishable
(McKinlay, 1979). Though the state's intervention in political, social,
economic and medical life has multiplied, in practice, so far as medicine
is concerned, the state exercises control over the social and economic
organization of medical work, but leaves the profession control over the
technological side. Significantly, the state does not supervise or intervene in the process of medical–technological development or evaluation.
Since medicine has technical autonomy, and since medical work has
become increasingly technological, medical hegemony over the lives of
patients is substantial. We have seen how this is manifested in antenatal
care in the period since the Second World War. And more generally, of
course, charting the history of antenatal care since its beginnings has
provided an exercise in the exact articulation between the process of
medical professionalization on the one hand, and the infiltration of state
power into citizens' lives, on the other.

---

1. See Navarro, 1976, for one exposition of the relationship between the capitalist state and the
medical profession.

A new discovery calls for a new commandment: antenatal care and the control of women

Ballantyne's edict, 'A new discovery calls for a new commandment' (1914, p. 1) likened the birth of antenatal care to the invention of motor cars. Just as the latter had produced new laws and regulations governing safety on the road, so the former necessitated the obedience of women to new sets of laws regarding pregnancy hygiene. Although Ballantyne admitted the then imperfect state of medical knowledge concerning life before birth, he insisted that mothers' obedience to the laws of 'gestational therapeutics' should possess all the urgency of a biological imperative. Doctors might not know very much, but women must consult them. Always fond of metaphors, Ballantyne compared doctors to potters and fetuses to the vessels on the potter's wheel:

> When the potter . . . fashions a vessel upon the wheel he may find his work marred not only by reason of some inherent defect in the clay from which he makes it, but also on account of faults of handling, of turning, of drying, of firing, of glazing, and of decorating; the expert workman may do much even with an inferior material, whilst in the hands of the bungler the finest substance may be fatally spoiled (Ballantyne, 1914, p. 810).

Ballantyne's enthusiasm for the laws of antenatal hygiene was, of course, in part a protest against the eugenicists' argument that unhealthy parents bred unhealthy babies and both were best eliminated by natural selection. His view was that, on the contrary, both parents and doctors might have to contend with inferior biological material, yet a proper alliance between them would be able to save many infants 'from many evils which are in no sense hereditary'.

In this purported alliance between mothers and doctors, the main imperative for mothers was to solicit, and pay attention to, medical advice. It was recognized in the 1920s and 1930s, and even later, that uneven enthusiasm among doctors for antenatal care meant that on occasions mothers would have to demand it — but the major problem was nevertheless perceived as an educational one. Women had to be educated in two ways. First they had to see the need for medical antenatal care. Second, this aspect of anticipated motherhood had to be set in the broader context of 'mothercraft', a necessary skill in women that could only be produced by education.

In chapters 2 and 3 we saw how the medical and social movement for maternal and child welfare developed in the early years of this century in

Britain in response to a concern with the quality and quantity of the population. High infant death-rates, combined with deficiences in Britain's military personnel, focused attention on women as the reproducers of the nation. Cynics might have said, along with women's health campaigner Margery Spring Rice in 1939 (pp. 18–19) that 'the woman comes onto the map of the public conscience only when she is performing the bodily function of producing a child'; there were certainly important social and ideological divisions throughout the 1920s, 1930s and 1940s between those who wanted improvements in the health of *mothers*, and those who pursued the wider goal of improving the health of *women*. What the ex-President of the local Government Board Herbert Samuel referred to as 'the woman's claim for help for her own sake' (Hope, 1917, p. 1) would not have been on the lips of most maternity service policy-makers. Most of them approached the problem from the other direction — not by asking what an improved standard of health among women would achieve, but by asking why not enough children were born and lived, and by declaring themselves in possession of the knowledge that maternal ignorance was indubitably the cause of low birth- and survival-rates.

Since the invention of antenatal care invoked the new commandment of using it, what is perceived by the providers and protagonists of antenatal care as the struggle to overcome maternal ignorance of its value is thus one absolutely central motivating force of the antenatal movement. On what was the assumption of maternal ignorance based? As we saw in chapter 2, thinking about public health moved from emphasizing the environment to emphasizing the individual in the early years of this century, and the exigency of living in insanitary conditions came to be identified more narrowly as the responsibility of the individual: this provides part of the answer. The disadvantaged social conditions in which many mothers lived need not be translated into reproductive mortality and illness if only mothers could be taught to make the best of things. The assumption of ignorance among mothers also logically followed from the fact that antenatal care was not an invention dreamed up by mothers themselves. Since other people had designed it, it was assumed that mothers would not know about it.

Wherever the idea of ignorance among mothers had come from, it was not based on evidence. In the 1920s and 1930s the attitudes and practices of women concerning motherhood were not actually surveyed. This absence of data made no difference to three developments. Firstly, the education of mothers did not mean education by other mothers within the community; it meant education by voluntary workers of superordinate social status, or by health-care professionals. Secondly, the educational side of antenatal work evolved integrally with medical antenatal care, and has only since the 1960s split off from this as a recognizably different exercise. Thirdly, as antenatal care has developed, the vocabulary of mothers' assumed ignorance has increasingly been translated into the more exact invective of 'why don't women attend for antenatal care?' It is within this invective, some of which was traced earlier in this book, that the motive of controlling women is most nakedly revealed.

Educating the educated

It was Dr Haig Ferguson, remembered for his early promotion of antenatal care, who commented in 1912 on the following paradox: a certain school Board passed, on the same day, two resolutions, one of which recommended the purchase of full-sized dolls to teach schoolgirls the elements of infant care, the other of which forbade mothers to keep their elder daughters at home to help them when their younger siblings were born. Ferguson preferred the latter domestic instruction, albeit for self-confessedly chauvinistic reasons (the proper place for all females is the home). But the school Board needed to initiate a new mode of learning about motherhood in which the correct way to mother was taught within the formal educational system. This strategy, brought about by the new official philosophy of population improvement, provoked a direct clash with the informal community education system. Women were involved in a continual process of educating one another. They talked to one another about childbearing and childrearing, and they gave one another advice. They chose to depend on the experienced but untrained midwife, rather than on her professionally-trained colleague. This alternative educational system was potentially subversive of the new educational ideology of motherhood from the start, and references to it abound in official reports and obstetric textbooks.

In the very early days of Schools for Mothers, babies were not brought for weighing, although voluntary workers distributed leaflets admonishing mothers to 'Bring your baby to be weighed.' After the first such leafleting campaign only four babies materialized: a 'superstition' prevailed among mothers that weighing a baby brought bad luck. Coming up against the same tradition of community advice, the 1910 Annual Report of the Board of Education bemoaned the 'apparently invincible prejudice' of women in favour of advice given by untrained or older midwives (one can only suppose that the combination of age and lack of training must have been particularly explosive). By 1932, the year of the Departmental Committee on Maternal Mortality and Morbidity's Final Report, this had become an injunction to 'the husband, relatives, friends — in fact, the general public' to 'understand that the pregnant woman requires more skilled advice than can be obtained in her own family or drawn from her own experience' (p. 31). 'Propaganda' was again the term used by the Departmental Committee to describe the strategies necessary to counter the family influence. Some 20 years further on, F. J. Browne's 1955 edition of *Antenatal Care* identifies most patients' information about childbearing as 'acquired from conversations with relatives and friends, or from books and periodicals, or in these days even from the cinema and theatre'. In this situation 'the duty of the doctor is to ascertain what ideas the patient already has ... [and to explain] what is probably a more normal state of affairs as it exists in reality ... it is believed that this aspect of antenatal work is of great importance' (Browne, 1955, pp. 54–5).

This cancelling out of one sort of education by another is one of the great continuities in the history of antenatal care, though like the proverbial leopard it is liable to change its spots along with changes in the scenery. There is nothing especially new about the admonitions of Gordon Bourne in his advice book for women, *Pregnancy*, to discount the 'cartload of rubbish' represented by old wives' tales and ignore the information yielded by 'wicked women with their malicious lying tongues' (Bourne, 1975, pp. 6–7). But by this time, as we shall see later in this chapter, it had become necessary to counteract female community influences on pregnant patients' attitudes to a novel aspect of maternity care: technological surveillance.

An equally important function: the place of education in antenatal care

During the first half of its lifetime, from 1915 to about 1950, the educational aspect of antenatal care received almost equal emphasis with its clinical aspect. Doctors, midwives and health visitors providing antenatal care were urged to remember their educational role *vis-à-vis* the expectant mother: as a Ministry of Health circular put it in 1924, 'Antenatal supervision is required primarily to detect and provide timely treatment for abnormal conditions, but it has an almost equally important function — namely, the education of the expectant mother in the care of her own health and in the proper management of her baby when it is born' (quoted in Departmental Committee, 1930, p. 89).

This definition of antenatal care, if that is what one can call it, was a direct successor to the philosophy expressed by the Local Government Board some years earlier, when it reduced the problem of infant mortality to the 'problems of maternity or "mothercraft", which in their turn are fundamentally problems of education' (Local Government Board, 1913, p. 330). As Sidney and Beatrice Webb remark in *The State and the Doctor* (1910), this educational intervention in mothers' lives represented the earliest form of midwifery provision made by the public health authorities in Britain, and of course it owed a good deal to the relative underdevelopment of the *clinical* side of antenatal care. The physiology of normal pregnancy was still in many ways a mystery, there was as yet no reliable way for clinicians to diagnose early pregnancy, and the treatment of obstetric disasters such as eclampsia and haemorrhage had not improved since the nineteenth century. The setting up of a structure and system of antenatal care meant that something more than this minimal clinical work had to be done.

Until the 1950s official policy on antenatal care retained some emphasis on the integrated character of educational and clinical work — integrated in the sense that both were said to be important, although a division of responsibility between local authority and hospital maternity services accounted for a certain uneasy segmentation in practice. 'Both types [of services]' said J. S. Fairbairn in the 1944 edition of Browne's *Antenatal and Postnatal Care*, 'have become experts in different aspects of the work without one learning from the other' (p. 104).

Nevertheless, in its 1946 Report 'A Complete Maternity Service', Political and Economic Planning was still able to say that, 'Education in all matters relating to the health of the mother and the care of the baby is an integral part of the maternity services and closely associated with every phase of that work.' As the Report acknowledged, this integration was made possible by the key linkage role of the health visitor who performed her educational work in the home, in the clinic, in the form of individual advice, or as 'lectures, classes and exhibitions' (PEP Report, 1946, p. 8).

The PEP Report did, however, comment on one new development in antenatal education work, namely that midwives were beginning to take over such work. As a municipal midwifery service got off the ground, midwives became educational agents as well, taking official formulae for a healthy life into the home as well as adding it to their clinic midwifery care. This trend away from education provided by the health visitor accelerated in the 1950s as the hospital confinement rate rose. With increased hospitalization, problems were in turn posed for the concentration of antenatal education in the local authority sector. Witnesses who gave evidence to the Cranbrook Committee on the Maternity Services in 1959 were agreed that the local health authority remained the best location for this side of antenatal care, but Cranbrook reported conflicting evidence 'that women receiving all their antenatal care in hospital would not wish to attend a separate clinic for health and mothercraft instruction' (p. 44).

In Britain in the 1980s local health authorities continue to provide antenatal classes, and these have also become a prominent development in the private sector, but hospital-provided antenatal classes have indeed materialized, as part of the general trend towards hospitalization. At first sight, it would seem that this provides even more of an integrated service than was possible before — most women will, after all, have the opportunity to attend hospital antenatal clinics and hospital antenatal classes as well. They no longer have to get their clinical treatment in one locale and their information and advice in another. Yet the reality is less benign, for there is plenty of evidence to suggest that curricula of hospital-provided antenatal education have the narrow objective of transmitting prevailing obstetrical policies to women rather than enlightening them in any more general way about the social or biological hygiene of motherhood (see Oakley, 1980). The result is certainly an integrated service of a kind, but it is one in which the broader agenda of educating mothers has been entirely subsumed within a specific programming of information about hospital policy. The motive of education which, in the early stages of the antenatal movement provided some sort of link between mother's medical care and their social environments, thus passes over the years into an increasingly narrow educational format, and is finally transmogrified into an ideological programming of women for hospital care.

Something of the flavour of the new hospital-based 'education' of pregnant women may be gleaned by quoting the words of one obstetrician, speaking in the late 1970s to the effect that 'Antenatal care should now involve a fair amount of education. Modern women are intelligent and want to take an active part in their pregnancy and labour. It is unwise to introduce a woman into a labour ward and attach her to a machine without telling her what it's all about' (Beard, 1977, p. 252–3).

In the high technology obstetrics of the 1970s and 1980s the education of mothers has thus acquired a new element, namely education in the advantages of technology. The 1980 Report of the Social Services Committee on Perinatal and Neonatal Mortality expresses a general concern with the need for antenatal health education as a 'thread' running right through their enquiry, but also identifies the specific concern of getting women to use and accept technological approaches to maternity care. Women 'must . . . be told that to make maximum use of innovations in medical care they need to be aware of such preventive programmes as rubella immunization . . . and prenatal screening for fetal disease which are only possible where there is early attendance for antenatal care.' Pregnant women also 'should be told about any procedure they are likely to encounter when they come to hospital, such as epidural anaesthesia and fetal monitoring' and this information 'should be an important part of their care through the medium of antenatal classes and discussion when they attend the clinics' (Short Report, 1980, pp. 127–8, p. 92).

Introducing mothers to the machines is not [yet] an explicit goal of hospital antenatal classes. Williams and Booth's *Antenatal Education: guidelines for teachers* (1974) gives the following 'aims' for antenatal education:

(1) To give a woman more confidence.
(2) To help her to have a healthy, happy pregnancy and a speedy rehabilitation afterwards.
(3) To prepare her for the reality of labour.
(4) To integrate her into a group having similar problems to her own.
(5) To begin to prepare her to care for her baby (Williams and Booth 1974, p. 157).

It is easy to see how introduction to the policies and types of technological surveillance and intervention practised in individual hospitals could be fitted into this agenda, since, for a start, the 'reality of labour' is a concept capable of multiple interpretations. There is now a whole industry of antenatal educational aids to facilitate the preparation of pregnant women, from plastic pelves, to plastic fetuses which come complete with placenta and cord, to patterns for knitted uteruses and films with such insufficiently intriguing titles as 'Ready for Baby' and 'Changing Baby's Nappie' (sic). In the first of these two films, various members of one hospital's staff are shown instructing a group of Irish mothers in preparation for childbirth. Several mothers are filmed in labour: 'one mother is delivered on her side, another on her back, with a drip in her arm. In each case the baby is filmed from the mother's angle and is joyfully welcomed. No fathers are present' (Williams and Booth, 1974, p. 167).

Hospital antenatal classes are also vehicles for teaching women particular relaxation and breathing techniques which, it is thought, may help them to cope with labour and delivery. This incorporation into the domain of hospital antenatal care of 'psychological' preparation for childbirth began in the 1950s and is now widespread, although as Chamberlain (1976, p. 29) observes, this is an enterprise which tends to elicit more 'lip service' than 'real work'. One explicit aim of psychoprophylactic methods of childbirth preparation is the reduction of maternal anxiety, an aim entirely synchronistic with the ideological roots of the antenatal movement, and no doubt inflating its attractiveness to hospital antenatal educators.

It is, predictably, J. W. Ballantyne who is supposed to have said that 'The removal of anxiety and dread from the minds of expectant, parturient and puerperal patients' is the primary objective of antenatal care (Browne, 1956, p. 13). Whether he used thest exact words, or truly put anxiety-removal first on the list, the idea that women are worried about childbearing has always absorbed the sympathies of their professional care-providers, and has provided one seemingly unpatronizing rationale for the enterprise of antenatal education. In Ian Donald's bestselling *Practical Obstetric Problems* (1979, p. 15), antenatal classes 'all have the primary objective of fighting ignorance and fear based on ignorance . . . The confidence and trust engendered and the personal contacts established make a great difference to morale.' John Clark MD, 173 years earlier, phrased it thus:

> Labour in women is . . . liable to be affected by the operation of the mind, in which they differ from animals; and it is well-known that fear and want of confidence will disturb and retard, just as confidence and hope will facilitate, labour. Much will depend upon the skill of the practitioner in regulating the passions of the mind of his [sic] patient, so that their undue influence may not interfere with the regular process of parturition (Clarke, 1806, p. 15).

The need to dispel the 'undue influence' of negative 'passions of the mind' is not so much because women's general well-being is thus improved, but because anxiety impairs the mechanics of reproductive performance.

It is for this reason that antenatal education came to possess another agenda: question-answering. 'Time given to talks and discussion about the many trifles that occupy her mind is never in vain', decreed Fairbairn in Browne's *Antenatal and Postnatal Care* (1955 edition, p. 51); 'No question asked by the patient, however stupid it may appear', added A. J. Wrigley, 'should ever be turned down lightly. It is probable that the doubt has been a source of worry for some time, and a full explanation must be given as to why her fears were needless' (p. 55). Antenatal classes rather than clinics become the proper place for question-asking, because the latter give no time for developing the communication between staff and patient.

Controlling women has thus been and remains, in these several ways, an intrinsic part of antenatal care. In order for antenatal care to 'succeed', education for motherhood has had to be removed from the female community; it has had to be relocated and rephrased as expert advice, requiring one commandment above all others: doing what the doctor says. The educational side of antenatal care in reality depends, as much as does any educational system or curriculum, on an exact philosophy and methodology of indoctrination. The motives and content of education do not materialize from, or exist in, a vacuum; education is always education of one social group by another with some particular objective in mind (Althusser, 1971).

However, not much has yet been said about the main manifestation and motif of antenatal care's character as social control — that recurrent theme in the history of the antenatal movement, 'Why don't women attend for antenatal care?'

The phenomenon of non-attendance; or how to resist control

As Donald has aptly put it, 'there is an old English saying that a bird must first be caught before salt can be put on its tail' (Donald, 1979, p. 94). For this reason urging women to present themselves for antenatal care was necessary pragmatism in the early years of the antenatal movement. Yet policy-makers and practitioners of maternity care have continued to inquire repeatedly into women's motives for underusing both antenatal classes and clinical antenatal care, and they have done so over a period in which the statistics of antenatal attendance have risen from 0 to 100 per cent.

Some example of the phrasing of these inquiries in official reports from 1922–49 were given in chapter 3. In the 1950s the Annual Reports of the Chief Medical Officer of the Ministry of Health began to refer constantly to the spectre of the antenatal 'defaulter' (a concept that makes its appearance at least as early as 1935 in the Scottish Report on Maternal Mortality and Morbidity). During the 1950s the CMO's Reports preached the need for an efficient system to round up defaulting patients: in 1958 it was reported that 21 local Health Authorities now possessed such schemes (Annual Report of the CMO for 1958). The reasons why pursuing the defaulter was important seemed self-evident, since over this period the results of confidential inquiries into maternal deaths continued to be published within the pages of the CMO's Report, and always contained a figure for the number of mothers who died having previously had no antenatal care. The first Report of the 1958 British Perinatal Mortality Survey added its own weight: 'The importance of early prenatal care cannot be overemphasized.' The authors of the Report regarded it as a serious indictment of 'present standards of prenatal care' that only 48.8 per cent of mothers in the survey had begun antenatal care before 16 weeks (Butler and Bonham, 1963, p. 62). The following year the Cranbrook Committee returned to the defaulter theme and, in attempting to unravel the problems of who should do what within the complex tripartite structure of the maternity services, brightly suggested that the local health authorities could help out the hospitals by chasing up their antenatal defaulters for them.

In the 1960s follow-up of defaulters was still needed, and there were policy-makers who departed from the orthodoxy that under-use of antenatal care was a cause of mortality. In the USA a sophisticated analysis by Collver and his colleagues found that patterns of antenatal attendance could be predicted from knowledge of patients' background variables (age, education, etc.) — it was not necessary to be acquainted with the patient's *attitude* at all (Collver, et al., 1967). Discussing 'foetal access to medical care' round about the same time Britain's Alwyn Smith, Professor of Social and Preventive Medicine at the University of Manchester, did not agree and cited a 'poor attitude' to antenatal care as a principal reason for delayed and infrequent attendance (Smith, 1970, p. 19). Inadequate take-up of antenatal care may not have been especially in the limelight in the 1960s, yet the Queen Charlotte's textbook of obstetrics (1970 edition) was able to reassert the issue in language reminiscent of much earlier official pronouncements on the theme: 'Unfortunately the importance of antenatal supervision is not properly realized even at the present time, and our first task is to convince women of the value of consulting their doctor at an early stage and at intervals afterwards to make sure that all is right' (p. 73).

By this time the apparent paradox of least antenatal care among those in greatest 'need' was readily acknowledged. The renowned General John Frederick Maurice had referred to this syndrome in 1903 in his 'National Health: A Soldier's Study'; he recounted a story concerning a teacher sent by Surrey County Council to a small village with the aim of instructing the women of the village in 'domestic cottage cookery' — or how to make economical use of the food they bought:

> The teaching was in every way appropriate and excellent . . . All the ladies of the place eagerly attended the lessons. I think I am right in saying that no single woman of the labouring class would be induced even to put in an appearance. The greatest difficulty in dealing with ignorance is that it has no idea that there is anything it does not know' (Maurice, 1903, p. 52).

Maurice's anecdote was to be repeated a thousand times in the history of antenatal education. Once systematic studies begin to be done of the proportion of women availing themselves of the opportunity to be educated antenatally, it seemed that half or less were enthusiastic enough to do so, and that the unenthusiastic were concentrated at the lower end of the social class spectrum. In 1958, two GPs surveying general practice antenatal work in Scotland reported that about half the surveyed patients were provided with mothercraft instruction (Kuenssberg and Sklaroff, 1958). In a hospital study carried out in 1968–69, some 57 per cent of primiparae attended antenatal classes; the figure was 30 per cent in a similar study elsewhere in England in 1972–73, and 58 per cent in a Scottish survey reported in 1980 (Mandelstam, 1971; Gillett, 1976; Reid and McIlwaine, 1980). Geoffrey Chamberlain's survey of Queen Charlotte's Hospital in 1975 showed a 48 per cent take-up rate for all mothers (Chamberlain, 1975).

In the 1970 British Births Survey, Chamberlain and his co-authors investigated antenatal preparation in some detail, obtaining the 'disappointing' answer that some three-quarters of mothers had not exposed themselves to this influence at all. Table 11.1 and Figures 11.1

Table 11.1 Source of antenatal preparation — singletons only

Site of instruction	No.	% of women attending instruction	% of women in survey
Independent instruction	637	14.3	3.8
Local Authority-run classes	2,152	48.4	12.8
Hospital-based classes	1,312	29.5	7.8
Combinations of the above	97	2.2	0.6
Other	245	5.5	1.5
Total known attenders	4,443	99.9	26.5

source: Chamberlain, et al., 1978, p. 35. With permission.

and 11.2 are taken from *British Births*. These show the sources of antenatal preparation used by the quarter of the survey women who did attend classes (table 11.1), the concentration of class-attenders in parities 1, 2 and 3 (not unreasonably 93 per cent of those having their fourth or later baby did not bother to attend), (figure 11.1), and the social class gradient in class attendance (figure 11.2).

The social class picture was, of course, completely consistent with that for use of clinical antenatal care. Non-attendance, late attendance and irregular attendance were all more likely among working-class women who in turn, ran a higher risk of unsuccessful pregnancy outcome. A new characteristic of non-attenders as 'late bookers' arose as the statistics of use of antenatal care became gradually unable to support the argument of non-attendance pure and simple, and attempts were

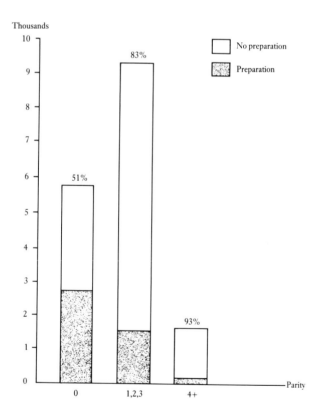

Figure 11.1 Antenatal preparation by parity
source: Chamberlain, et al., 1978, p. 34. With permission.

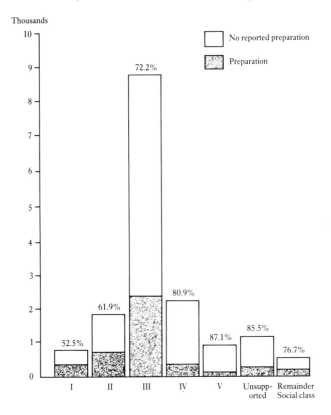

Figure 11.2 Antenatal preparation by social class
source: Chamberlain, et al., 1978, p. 37. With permission.

made more fully to describe 'late bookers' as those who were too afraid, ignorant or prejudiced to use the maternity and child welfare services, and who had invariably left school and married young husbands with a tendency to be unemployed.

By the 1960s social scientists had joined the 'why don't women attend? debate and began to tackle the problem of the seeming irrationality of women's behaviour. An early contribution was Raymond Illsley's exposition of one significant reason for delayed antenatal attendance: illegitimate pregnancy. 'Much of the late attendance occurs because women who conceive prenuptially delay attendance until they are married' reported Illsley. 'This seems inevitable in a society where it is conventional for conception to occur within wedlock', he ventured. In his conclusion Illsley acknowledged the attractiveness of the proposition that 'every effort should be made to secure earlier attendance.' However, he went on to say that

> the easier fruits of health education have already been gathered and it is doubtful whether mere intensification of propaganda would induce earlier attendance among primigravidae waiting for marriage or among the mothers of illegitimate children or whether with increasing parity (and increasing familiarity with the process of pregnancy) multigravidae can or should be persuaded to maintain the attendance habits of their first pregnancies (Illsley, 1956, p. 111).

In other words, once the irrationality imputed to women's behaviour could be persuaded to make way for an investigation of their real motives, non-attendance could be interpreted quite differently. Since Illsley's study there have been many other social–scientific surveys of women's attitudes to antenatal care which have uncovered a wealth of respectable reasons for non-attendance. As well as those he found, there are many disincentives associated with the organization of antenatal care itself, as we saw in chapter 10. Many clinics are crowded, appointment systems do not work efficiently, there is hardly any continuity of care, little provision for a mother's other children, and attending clinics can be expensive, especially as small maternity units and community antenatal clinics increasingly give way to centralized antenatal care in large hospitals (Garcia, 1982). The influence of the lay female community which may, at times, see little purpose in antenatal care is still with us (McKinlay, 1970; Hubert, 1974) and, to add insult to injury, some of women's late attendance is actually due to inefficient communication between GPs and hospitals (Heward and Clarke, 1976; Simpson and Walker, 1980; Lewis, 1982). Much the same can be said about antenatal education, which seems redundant to women still versed in the art of teaching one another about motherhood, is poorly organized to allow for women's other social responsibilities, and in fact may not even be *offered* to pregnant women: 28 per cent of the 687 mothers questioned by Perkins in her 1977 study said that they had not even been told about the existence of antenatal classes in their district (Perkins, 1980).

In the face of what is known about how many antenatal clinics work the appropriate question, it has been suggested (McIlwaine, 1980) is not 'why don't women attend?' but 'why *do* they?'. Since no researcher has asked this question we do not know the answer, though it would be reasonable to surmise from the evidence that women seek antenatal care when they consider that the benefits of antenatal care outweigh any possible personal disadvantages associated with its use. In a Nottinghamshire study of antenatal care attendance, three distinct groups of non-attenders were found within the 0.5 per cent of the pregnant population who availed themselves of either no, or minimal, antenatal care. The largest group was 'frightened teenagers' — young single women, like those described by Illsley in Aberdeen in the 1950s, who had good social reasons for concealing pregnancy. The second group of non-attenders in the Nottinghamshire study were 'competent childbearers' — women whose previous experience of childbearing led them to dismiss the need for medical help. The smallest group were those with poor obstetric histories combined with massive social problems (Parsons and Perkins, 1980). In other words, it would be fair to say that not attending for antenatal care, or for antenatal education, or deviating from the officially recommended pattern of antenatal behaviour in some other way, is a form of resistance on the part of women to the social control function of antenatal care.

This 'voting with one's feet' may be viewed as passive rather than active resistance. Women's behaviour tends to be socially interpreted in terms of passivity, although women themselves may see it differently, as active manipulation of the system.[2] Such, indeed, would seem to be the case with antenatal care. Women who do not attend early or regularly may not necessarily be indifferent to the potential value of antenatal care, nor are they all passive victims of unfortunate circumstances. Experience of antenatal care may be the mother of its rejection. Non-use of the system can be an active choice. In addition, a view of women as lacking an autonomous identity encourages another unhelpful habit of thinking, namely that organizational problems (in employment and antenatal care) may be attributed to women rather than to their surroundings. This 'social problem of women' perspective has enjoyed a long life, despite the accumulating evidence that (so far as antenatal care is concerned) the problems identified of care-provision and use are at least partly problems in the services themselves rather than problems somehow located within women (Graham, 1978).

Money or militancy?: the final solution

In 1981 an editorial in the *Lancet* reported a novel means of inducing

---

2. See Fiona McNally's study of women's office work (1979), where she makes a similar point in a different context.

women to use antenatal care. The British Army in Hong Kong, consisting mainly of Gurkhas from Nepal, had instituted an order which said that 'Any family failing to report a pregnancy during the first three months, will be sent back to Nepal 60 days after the birth of the child. Such families will never be allowed back into family lines. Severe disciplinary action will be taken against the soldier' (*Lancet*, 19 September 1981, p. 620; Rasor, 1981).

The dual penalities of being sent home and being subject to 'severe' disciplinary action are harsh, but unusual only in their selection of fathers as targets of control. Otherwise the Gurkhas' solution is the latest in a series of punitive manoeuvres designed or suggested to secure higher antenatal attendance rates. In the 1920s, the Australians used the police force; but it has been more customary to employ existing health care personnel to persuade mothers into antenatal care. In 1980 'commando' groups of these health personnel were suggested by the Social Services Committee.

A commonly suggested carrot has been money. Midwives were paid in some areas in the early years of British antenatal care to notify pregnancy and thus bring potential antenatal attenders to official attention (see chapter 2). The idea of paying pregnant women themselves was first floated in 1917 (Hope, 1917) and has been discussed in almost every report on the maternity services since then, as well as consistently in the medical press. 'It is felt that to secure her co-operation', determined the Departmental Committee on Maternal Mortality and Morbidity in 1930 (p. 92), 'it may . . . be found advisable to offer some financial inducement'; 'It is for consideration', ventured the 1935 Scottish Report on the same subject (p. 27), 'whether it is practicable to make the obtaining of adequate antenatal care an essential condition of payment of maternity benefit.'

'Minerva' in the *British Medical Journal* (23 September 1978, p. 899) fastened on to a theme exposed by many others: 'In France, where social security payments are linked with early reporting for antenatal care, 96 per cent of women attend before the 15th week . . . the DHSS has given priority to finding ways of ensuring booking before the 15th week. Surely the answer is plain!' This splendid example of the French solution is somewhat marred by the fact that it was introduced around 30 years ago (before any benefit in lowered perinatal mortality could possibly be argued); that in France the *maternal* mortality rate is twice as high as in England and Wales; that the average number of antenatal visits is lower in France than in Britain; and the French themselves do not see any intimate connection between the social security–antenatal care linkage and measures of pregnancy outcome (Blondel, et al., 1982; Chalmers, 1979). Nonetheless, such well-documented reservations did not deter the Social Services Committee in 1980 from giving the financial inducement argument the usual serious consideration. There seems to be something enduringly attractive about the financial solution to the perceived problem of inadequate antenatal attendance. Perhaps its simplicity? As sociologist Margot Jefferys observed at a DHSS/Child Poverty Action Group Conference in 1978, the implications for the medical care system in general of paying would-be patients to utilize medical care can only be considered profound (Jefferys, 1978) — and clearly more, rather than less, so in an economic climate in which money is actually being taken away from the services themselves. Yet this is only one of many manifestations of that curious habit of thought which singles out maternity care/antenatal care as a unique exercise rather than as an exemplar of the broader struggle to treat problems of health and illness with medical care.

And, in turn, we may see this singling out of antenatal care as an exact illustration of its thesis, that antenatal care is nothing if women cannot be controlled. There have been two main periods in the history of antenatal care — the first 20 years and the last 10 — in which, for a mixture of political reasons, invidious comparisons have been made between the obstetric mortality rates of Britain and those of other countries. In both these periods there have been orchestrations of the 'why don't women attend?' theme. Though the theme died down in the 1960s and early 1970s, by the mid-1970s it was being played more loudly than ever, and the 1977 Health Department's policy document *Reducing the Risk: safer pregnancy and childbirth* allowed itself no caution in asserting the major risk-reducing pathway to lie with early antenatal care (perhaps with some kind of financial inducement thrown in as well?). Between these two periods in which Britain comes off 'badly' in international league table comparisons of obstetric mortality, and in which the irresistible appeal of motivating women's antenatal attendance rates takes command of the field, the proportion of women attending for antenatal care rose from almost none to everyone — with, by no means all, but very many, women in the latter period experiencing new forms of technological surveillance such as ultrasound scanning, in addition to the standard 'package' of antenatal visits and examinations. This is a decisive argument for the contextual nature of women's purported error in neglecting antenatal care. The primary need is not to secure 100 per cent attendance rates before 12 or 10 weeks' gestation or whatever, the primary need is to control the biological behaviour of women by negotiating them all into an identical pattern of social behaviour. In this sense, an important context for understanding the official and medical emphasis on the non-attendance phenomenon is the parallel attempt within obstetrics to control the processes of conception, gestation, labour and delivery. The development of modes of visualizing the interior events of the womb, and of techniques for controlling the delivery by obstetricians of healthy fetuses from it, imitates the superficial rationality of the official response to the spectre of women resisting antenatal care: 'but *why* don't they attend?' on the one hand, and 'mothers are merely containers of fetuses' on the other.

Certainly there are some deaths and illnesses among pregnant and newly-delivered women and their fetuses/babies in Britain that are preventable, and in the battle to prevent every fatality that is conceivably preventable, medical antenatal care must be counted as an essential ally. But we delude ourselves about the character of antenatal care, the position of women, the standing of the medical profession, and the nature of the state's interest in reproduction if we think that's all there is to it.

12

Tomorrow's World

A tool exploited for its own sake is no better than a saw given to a small boy for cutting wood who must presently look around the home for suitable objects of furniture inviting amputation.

Donald, 1980, p. 2.

The evolution of antenatal care charted in the pages of this book provides a case-study of how one society over a given period of time has defined one area of biological behaviour. Since this area of behaviour is reserved for women, looking at antenatal care has also meant looking at women. But the focus on antenatal care in its own terms, and as an exercise in controlling women, must not be allowed to detract from the task of seeing it in a broader context. The rise of antenatal care is part of the medicalization of life. It thus participates in the same morality and logic as this broader transformation of life in the twentieth century. Many other human conditions and events besides pregnancy have become encapsulated within a medical terminology.

Existence transitions; and what doctors have done to them

The medicalization of everyday life is a phenomenon described in many radical and liberal critiques of medicine, but most notably in the words of Ivan Illich:

The medicalization of life appears as the encroachment of health-care on the budget, the dependence on professional care, and as the addiction to medical drugs; it also takes form in iatrogenic labelling of the ages of man [sic]. This labelling becomes part of a culture when laymen [sic] accept it as a trivial verity that people require routine medical ministrations for the simple fact that they are unborn, newborn, infants, in their climacteric, or old . . . The doctor's grasp over life starts with the monthly prenatal checkup when he [sic] decides if and how the fetus shall be born; it ends with his decision to abandon further resuscitation. The environment comes to be seen as a mechanical womb and the health professional as the bureaucrat who assigns each to his proper corner (Illich, 1975, pp. 44–5).

Pregnancy and birth, like death, are bodily experiences which have different 'negotiated realities' in different cultures. In pre-modern cultures, for example, the process of dying was accompanied by a low level of medical technology, late detection of potentially fatal conditions, a high incidence of acute causes of death, and a somewhat 'fatalistic passivity' towards dying people (Lofland, 1976). Likewise, before the modern era, pregnancy and birth were more prone to be unpredictably fatal conditions, and their social monitoring occurred without technological overlay. For both birth and death normal signs have become neon lights flagging risks which demand and validate medical intervention. In the case of death, the heroic use of medical technologies interrupts a 'terminal' state. In the case of impending birth, electronically-evoked fetal heart signals enable a baby who could have entered the world through the untechnological vagina to do so, instead, courtesy of the surgeon–obstetrician's instruments and technical prowess.

The medicalization of 'existence transitions' (Devries, 1981) redefines control of birth and death as the property of institutions and doctors who, even on a pragmatic level, prepare for public viewing those who have given birth, are born, or have died. The technological aspect — the expanded potency of machines to sustain life — increasingly provokes ethical dilemmas about who should live, under what circumstances, and who should decide. It has also, over a period of time, and in the dialectic of 'alternative' health movements, generated one partly spurious answer to its own problems: the spectre of a 'natural' way to be born or to die. The 'natural' alternative is spurious because all ways of birth and death are cultural accretions. In fact, of course, the alignment is not nature versus medicine, but the birthers and die-ers within their own lay community versus the medical technicians in their socially sterile hospital or clinic.

This particular dialetic of consumer protest and medical control is clearly present within antenatal care. Thus, when we consider what the future of antenatal care might look like, we see two possible scenarios. Like sitting in a room watching the landscape from two windows pointing in two different directions, it is a matter of which way your head is turned. Out of one window there is accelerated technological growth and a further dehumanization, or de-socialization, of pregnancy. From the other we see, instead, the re-instatement of antenatal care as a social concern, sensitive to the psychosocial needs of mothers, fathers and babies, and recognizing that parents possess a wisdom at least equal to that of machines. Intrinsic to this second vision are programmes for evaluating antenatal care's costs, benefits and effectiveness which include an appraisal of its technological components. But let us turn our heads the other way first and look at the implications for the future of antenatal care of what Richard Taylor in his *Medicine Out of Control* (1979) has dubbed 'science fiction medicine'.

Test-tube babies?

The spirit of today's science-fiction medicine is captured in the cartoons reproduced as figure 12.1: a delivery delayed because the computer is unable to function, and two care-providers (or machine-attendants) admitting to confusion in a sea of computer print-out. Perhaps predictably, science-fiction obstetrics has already enlisted the aid of micro-computers in the antenatal clinic. A 'feasibility study' of computerized history-taking was reported by Lilford and Chard in the *British Medical Journal* in 1981. The computer proved somewhat slower than the conventional human system (20 minutes versus 15 for recording the medical history of a woman with one previous pregnancy). One advantage was that the computer could issue various built-in reminders to the clinicians, for instance that women over thirty-seven should be considered for amniocentesis. A computerized system also allows for the standardization of a process of data-collection which is at the moment very variable: the total number of items asked for in the 1982 obstetric case-notes of 41 UK teaching hospitals ranged from 29 to 136 (Fawdry, 1982). Sometimes patients are apparently prepared to tell a computer what they would not tell a person, though others may worry about the threat to medical secrecy. The biggest problem with computerized antenatal records is said to be technical breakdown. Yet this does not prevent their being seen as 'a conventional and uncontroversial' part of every antenatal clinic by the end of the century (Lilford and Chard, 1981).

Microcomputers as history-takers are an easier answer than the subtle difficulties of interpersonal communication. The history of antenatal care has been marked by a search for easy answers, though in this respect it is hardly unique. One recent example of the 'easy answer' phenomenon concerns the causes and treatment of toxaemia of pregnancy. In the 1920s, toxaemia was regarded as a nut that antenatal care

K

would crack. To date it has not done so, although the condition appears to be less common; treatment has improved vastly, but aetiology remains obscure. In early 1983 scientists in the USA claimed to have found the

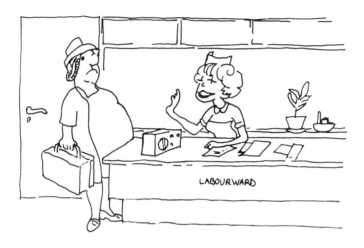

'Sorry Mrs. Smith, you can't have your baby this week — the computer is in for service.'

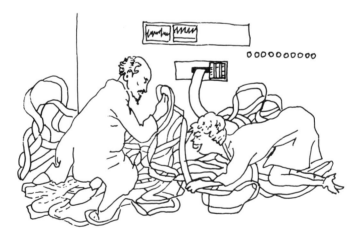

'With a bit of luck she will have delivered by the time we analyse this lot.'

Figure 12.1 Science-fiction obstetrics
source: Klopper and Farr, n.d.

answer — a worm. It was about one-sixteenth of an inch long, and they named it *hydatoxi lualba* (Lueck, et al., 1983). But the worm unhappily turned out to be a figment of the laboratory microscope, an artefact of scientific technique. In reality the worm was an empty space (Gau, et al., 1983).

As chapters 7 and 8 demonstrated, direct visualization and prenatal sampling of the fetus, rather than fictional placental worms, have for long constituted important clinical motivations in antenatal care, and in the last two decades especially have been translated into concrete technical achievements. Prenatal chromosome analysis is now available in most obstetric departments in this country and others, as is visualization of pregnancy with ultrasound. Since 1981, a new technique for fetal visualization has emerged to compete with ultrasound. The technique is nuclear magnetic resonance (NMR) imaging. NMR subjects the body placed in a magnetic field to short pulses of radiowaves and permits assessment of tissue biochemistry. It is a technique which has migrated into obstetrics from other areas of medical work. In 1983 a Report from the Department of Nuclear Medicine at Aberdeen Royal Infirmary compared its value in early pregnancy with that of ultrasound. At ten weeks the 'products of conception' were demonstrable with NMR, and fetal biparietal measurements and placental localization were said to be comparable with ultrasound results. NMR displayed the fetus in greater detail than ultrasound. The report concluded that 'NMR imaging has now been in clinical use for over two years and there is no evidence that it is mutagenic . . . we believe that it will prove to be safe and . . . will [have] . . . wide application in obstetric practice' (Smith, et al., 1983). It is worth noting that despite these new ways of seeing fetuses the old ways persist: in 1976 some 30 per cent of fetuses in a group of British hospitals were still being X-rayed (Carmichael and Berry, 1976). For the detection of disorders which cannot be diagnosed (or cannot be diagnosed sufficiently early) with either ultrasound or amniocentesis, access to the womb for direct sampling of pregnancy material is now also increasingly being tried. A case report in the *Lancet* in 1983 described the sexing at eight weeks in a chorion biopsy of a fetus at risk for Duchenne muscular dystrophy (*Lancet*, 3 September 1983, pp. 568–9). Another report, the same year, recounted details of a new 'direct vision technique' for sampling first trimester chorionic tissue. Thirty-three women who were going to have their pregnancies terminated had 150 ml of a saline drip inserted into their uteruses and a specimen of placental tissue taken. 'On reaching the internal orifice [of the cervical canal], the extra-amniotic space is already distended by the continuously instilled saline, and the ovum is instantly and clearly visualized . . . the specimens are examined immediately under a dissecting microscope in the operating room' (Gustavii, 1983, p. 508). Later in prenatal life the biopsy technique is applied to specific fetal organs, for example the fetal liver, in order to detect biochemical abnormalities where these are suspected from the family history (Rodeck, et al., 1982). Such biopsies can be done early enough (mid-second trimester) to allow termination of affected pregnancies. An increasing multitude of fetal anatomical and biochemical abnormalities are now being picked up by the new sampling techniques, and frequent letters to the medical journals are appearing reporting the first antenatal diagnosis of this or that abnormality (see Royal College of Obstetricians, 1984).

Much of this work is, of course, still experimental. Nonetheless, it adds up to an accelerated technical mode within obstetrics. It has also been cause and product of a movement towards further technical specialization of professionals within obstetrics and gynaecology. A Working Party Report of the Royal College of Obstetricians and Gynaecologists on this very topic aptly summarized the main dilemma thus:

> During the past 15 years there has been a massive accumulation of new knowledge in fetal physiology and pathology. Therefore, as in other branches of medicine, it has become impossible for the individual obstetrician–gynaecologist to master [sic] in depth all, or even most, areas of his [sic] specialty (RCOG Report, 1982b, p. 4).

The Report argues the case for further specialization within obstetrics and gynaecology along the lines of similar developments in medicine and surgery, but rejects the seemingly logical solution of dividing the obstetrics from the gynaecology, because such a rupture would too much disturb the traditional career pattern. Instead, a division is proposed in obstetrics between 'reproductive' and 'fetal' medicine, with the former covering gynaecological endocrinology and infertility (and including 'ovulation induction', artificial insemination, tubal microsurgery, and *in vitro* fertilization), and the latter having 'as its focus the recognition, assessment and management of the high risk fetus.' This infant specialty of fetal medicine would run from preconception 'through antenatal diagnosis and antepartum monitoring, to the merging of fetal and neonatal intensive care at delivery'. It would combine 'technology and clinical skills . . . intrauterine diagnosis and treatment', and involve close teamwork with other disciplines 'including medical genetics, perinatal pathology, biochemistry, bio-engineering and neonatal paediatrics' (RCOG Report, 1982b, p. 27).

Fetal medicine is to be the largest of the subspecialties with a national target of 45–50 appointments; a few such appointments have already been made. The chief role of the 'fetal medicine specialist' as the antenatalist of the future is to provide a consistent policy for the use of technological monitoring methods, including cardiotocography and ultrasound. The fetal medicine specialist should be an expert in the use of ultrasound to detect fetal abnormalities and patterns of intrauterine growth. He should ideally have under his command a small day unit to provide a fetal assessment service using all available monitoring techniques. A main reason why a fetal medicine subspecialty needs to be instituted within obstetrics could perhaps be guessed from certain proven historical continuities in antenatal care: it is said, unsurprisingly, to be because of Britain's 'persistently' high perinatal mortality. Fetal medicine is also, significantly, the obstetricians' answer to the paediatricians' colonization of the immediate post-birth period with the subspecialty of neonatal paediatrics. Whether inside its mother's womb or not, the fetus–neonate is the subject of intra-professional rivalry. The moment of birth has become a line in a demarcation dispute.

Each of these science-fiction aspects of today's and tomorrow's antenatal care does, however, pale into insignificance beside the most fictional, and yet now real, scientific scenario of all: the advent of artificial reproduction. Louise Brown, the world's first 'test-tube baby', was born by caesarean section on 25 July 1978. Her conception was engineered by Drs Steptoe and Edwards in the laboratory on 10 November 1977, and the fertilised egg that became Louise Brown was implanted at eight-cell stage into the maternal uterus two and a half days later (Steptoe and Edwards, 1978). A subsequent report by paediatricians (Hilson, et al., 1978) attempted to allay fears that *in vitro* fertilization might result in congenital morbidity: the baby seemed normal. Since 1978 others have taken up the technique and more artificially conceived infants have been born world-wide, offering hope to those women whose infertility is due to tubal blockage. The technique has a high natural abortion and ectopic pregnancy rate, and Louise Brown's normality has been followed by other reports of abnormality (see Trounson and Conti, 1982). It is also the subject of heated ethical debate (Walters and Singer, 1982), as are variations on the technique, such as that somewhat clumsily described as 'non-surgical transfer of *in vitro* fertilised donated ova' (Buster, et al., 1983). In this procedure, sperm from an infertile woman's husband is used to inseminate a fertile woman; the fertilized ovum is then retrieved and implanted into the infertile woman's uterus. The baby that is born is the child of its legal father but not of its legal

282 *The Captured Womb*

mother — or rather it is hers in the singular sense that her womb housed it antenatally although her ovaries did not produce the original ovum.

There is a whole new world of scientifically-engineered parenthood here — more variations on the theme, perhaps, than have been anticipated in that genre called science fiction. Somewhere on the horizon of this new world is the revolutionary prospect of male (abdominal) pregnancy (he, like the infertile woman above, would have to borrow an egg), but nowhere, quite yet, is the spectre of an entirely laboratory-made human pregnancy. Beginning with the glass dish and ending with the neonatal intensive care unit, getting on for half the total span of human pregnancy can now be accomplished outside the female body. We may, however, confidently say that the intensive care provided by the human uterus will continue for some time in the antenatal world of the future to provide a sanctuary for the fetus which is technically superior to that of any man-made (sic) substitute.

Artificial reproduction raises important questions about the value of antenatal technology, and about the limits of medicine in controlling reproduction and women. In the first place, is it a good thing? Obviously it is a good thing for infertile women to have their chances of motherhood increased, but there are other, possibly more sinister, rationales for this new interpretation of antenatal 'care', including genetic experimentation and research, sex preselection of fetuses, and the final resolution of that old masculine dilemma, Am I really the father of my child? (Hanmer, 1980). In these other agendas, laboratory-based techniques have the potential radically to alter social arrangements. It seems, for example, that if sex preselection ever became a routine part of antenatal practice, this would be most likely to result in a marked shift in the sex ratio in favour of males and in favour of a male dominance among first-born children (Williamson, 1976; Steinbacher, 1981). More men in relation to women, and substantially more male than female first-borns would (given what is known about the effect of family position on personality and life chances) considerably strengthen what is already a structural inequality in life chances between the sexes.

Quite clearly, the extent to which these techniques may alter the sexual division of labour in society cannot be determined by looking at the techniques themselves. The absolute removal of pregnancy from women's uteruses to laboratories could either be liberating or oppressive for women. Some have argued that women as a species will thereby become obsolescent — though it is reasonable to suppose that their personhood may still be of some value. To counter this, others might point out that frozen sperm and artificial insemination requiring a non-specialist technology has already achieved the theoretical redundancy of men (Feminist Self-Insemination Group, 1980). But men have not become redundant, and this is understandable, in view of their ascendancy in social, economic and political power structures. The bottom line is power. One of the central questions about the new reproductive technology is, Who controls it? The control of the new reproductive technologies by a male-dominated medical profession, with essentially conservative paternalistic interests, is well-illustrated in the recent RCOG's Report of the Ethics Committee on *in vitro* fertilization and embryo replacement or transfer (RCOG, 1983b). In considering whether or not doctors are obliged to treat everyone who wants the new technique, the Committee voices 'grave reservations' about use in circumstances that are not those of a 'stable heterosexual "marriage"'. Such techniques, says the Committee, put extra strain on doctors, who are not only acting as 'enablers', but 'are taking part in the formation of the embryo itself', a role which brings 'a special sense of responsibility for the welfare of the child thus conceived'. Translated into practice, this responsibility means that the medical enabling of artificial conception should be restricted to 'natural' family environments (RCOG, 1983b, p. 6).

The patriarchal note in medical ideology has finally burst into the canon of obstetrical fatherhood — obstetricians are to determine in this, as well as other ways, which women are to become mothers. As a matter of fact, there has been a surreptitious spreading of obstetrical fatherhood for some time in the vogue for using medical sperm in AID. Preferred donors for artificial insemination are English, middle-class, medical students (Snowden and Mitchell, 1983); it is said (without evidence) that an acceptable level of intelligence, a stable personality, and character as a good 'all-rounder' is thereby assured (Philipp, 1975). Commenting on the idea that this is a sociobiological strategy for the distribution of 'superior' genes, Minerva in the *British Medical Journal* (10 November 1979) noted that lawyers would probably pick legal sperm. Professional dominance combined with a dangerously misleading faith in genes are powerful motives for populating women's wombs with this or that particular brand of sperm.

Evaluating the practice and controlling the technology: towards a self-critical antenatal care?

An earlier chapter (chapter 6) of this book noted the rise in the 1950s of

The Captured Womb

a perinatal epidemiology which embodied the first systematic commitment to the scientific evaluation of antenatal care. Although there has
still been no randomized controlled trial of antenatal care, the impetus
to evaluate has been maintained, and has borne fruit in several ways.

In 1980 Marion Hall, a consultant obstetrician in Aberdeen, carried
out, together with her colleagues, a critical retrospective analysis of the
'productivity' of routine antenatal care. Looking at the case records of
the 1907 women in Aberdeen who delivered babies in 1975, and for
whom complete records were available, Hall and her co-workers
examined the extent to which certain items of a woman's medical or
obstetric history were actually picked up at the hospital booking visit,
and they also noted the capacity of subsequent visits to diagnose accurately three important antenatal conditions: intrauterine growth retardation (IUGR), fetal malpresentation, and pre-eclampsia. The results
would have disappointed the keen antenatalists of the 1920s and 1930s
who saw antenatal care as perfect preventive medicine. Many relevant
obstetric and medical factors recorded on the case-notes by the midwives at the booking visit were not perceived or acted upon by the
obstetricians. For instance, 23 per cent of serious medical conditions
(e.g. diabetes, epilepsy) recorded by midwives were not noted by
obstetricians. Moreover, the problem with the idea of risk-prediction
(see pp. 220–1) is that many obstetric risks appear to be unpredictable. In
the Aberdeen study, half the women who experienced perinatal death
had no antenatal risk factors at all. For IUGR, only 44 per cent of cases
were identified before delivery. Moreover, for every such condition
correctly diagnosed, there were 2.5 'false positives'; 205 fetuses were
falsely accused of being growth retarded, as against the 83 who were
correctly accused. For breech presentation the record was better, and 88
per cent of breech fetuses were detected antenatally. As to the detection
and prevention of pre-eclampsia, that great hope of the early antenatalists, 30 per cent of women suffering from this condition first had
symptoms in labour or post-natally, and therefore could not be expected
to have been identified at their antenatal visits. Table 12.1 gives some
information about antenatal diagnoses of pre-eclampsia and transient
hypertension (temporarily raised blood pressure which then settles).
The figures in the second column amount to false positives, so once
again the number of women incorrectly diagnosed as having pre-
eclampsia is about the same as those rightly identified as having this
condition. Additionally, less than 1 per cent of cases of pre-eclampsia
were diagnosed before 34 weeks of pregnancy, so routine antenatal care
to detect pre-eclampsia before this time would seem, perhaps, to be

Table 12.1 The antenatal diagnosis of pre-eclampsia and transient hypertension in Aberdeen in 1975

Stage of pregnancy	*Ultimately pre-eclampsia*		*Transient hypertension*	
	%	(No.)	%	(No.)
6–20 weeks	13	(26)	10	(25)
20–30 weeks	9	(17)	10	(25)
30 weeks and above	79	(157)	80	(206)
Total	100	(200)	100	(256)

source: Hall, Marion *An Appraisal of Outpatient Antenatal Care* 1980, p. 25. With permission of the author.

hardly worth doing (even after 38 weeks the detection rate was only 2 per cent) (Hall, 1980; Hall, et al., 1980; Chng, et al., 1980).

The moral of these figures is mixed. On the one hand, every woman who has a 'real' complication diagnosed by antenatal care and subsequently successfully treated is a justification for the invention and propagation of antenatal care. Yet, on the other hand, the productivity of antenatal care is almost certainly less than many people (clinicians and non-clinicians) believe it to be. The crucial question is whether its productivity, taken in conjunction with its social and economic costs, is sufficiently high to legitimate the continued existence of antenatal care as a mass screening programme.

When the antenatalists of the 1930s concluded that antenatal care did not always work as well as people had hoped, principally because expectations for its achievements had been too high in the first place, they probably would have been alarmed to learn that half a century later this message would still not be appreciated. The Aberdeen research has led to a revamped antenatal scheme being introduced in Aberdeen (five visits for normal multigravidae, more use of midwives and peripheral community clinics), and has had some impact on antenatal care practice elsewhere. The Report of the RCOG Working Party on Antenatal and Intrapartum Care in 1982 suggested five antenatal visits for normal low-risk women. The Report said that only by reducing attendance could the necessary social and organizational improvements demanded by the 'consumer' in the running of antenatal clinics be carried out. These recommendations echoed other 'innovations' in which antenatal care has, in the last few years, been moved more towards a community locale, and transformed, at least partially, into a GP and user-sensitive exercise. In the vicinity of St Thomas's Hospital in London, consultant obstetricians started going out (one on his bicycle) to antenatal sessions at a local general practice, instead of asking the women to go to the hospital.[1]

In Glasgow in the late 1970s a community antenatal clinic was set up in one of the most socially and economically deprived areas of the city, and a randomized controlled trial was then organized to compare community clinic care with routine antenatal care in the Glasgow Royal Maternity Hospital. The study aptly demonstrated that a community-based antenatal service benefits mothers by reducing waiting and travelling time and increasing satisfaction among a segment of the population that can least afford the social and economic costs of ante-natal care (Reid and McIlwaine, 1980). In the community clinic, women made significantly fewer visits than women in the hospital group, and more than half saw only one or two doctors antenatally, while a mere 3 per cent of women attending the hospital clinic achieved this degree of continuity of care. There were no appreciable differences in obstetric outcome between the two groups, although a low birthweight rate of 13 per cent in the hospital group and one of 8 per cent in the community clinic group suggested a potential difference in favour of community care (Reid, et al., 1983).

A rather more mixed recent development was the experiment by a group of hospital obstetricians in Cardiff to monitor fetal hearts electro-nically, via the public telephone network. This had the advantage that women stayed in their homes, but the disadvantage that some of the telephones produced a disturbing noise (and some women do not have telephones) (Dalton, et al., 1983).

It is, of course, a real challenge to integrate the appropriate use of antenatal technologies such as alphafetoprotein screening and ultrasound with a contracted and more user-sensitive format for antenatal care. The phrase 'appropriate technology' is now widely heard, both in the peri-natal field and more generally (Guidotti, 1983). It refers to the restric-tion of scientifically evaluated technologies to those population groups most likely to benefit from them. Uncontrolled routine use of unevalu-ated, possibly ineffective and/or hazardous technologies is not appropriate practice in the antenatal field or anywhere else.

In the late 1960s and early 1970s, the politics of technology in society

---

1. Bicycle-riding by consultants is no real revolution, since in the past many, especially in rural areas, must have engaged in it; the point is, rather, that doing it in the 1970s and 80s is significantly out-of-tune with mainstream antenatal practice, in which taking specialist antenatal care out into the community would be an unthinkable anachronism.

generally began to crystallize as an ethical, biological and financial issue:

long-established assumptions about the social benefits to be obtained from scientific and technological advance were called into question. Uncontrolled technology came to be associated with a variety of contemporary problems, among them hazards to health and safety . . . conflicts between amenity and commerce; mismatches between innovation and social need. Moreover, the number of obstacles to the democratic participation of ordinary people in decision-making increased in the face of technical experts and powerful industrial and government bureaucracies (Boyle, et al., 1977, p. xi).

From 1908, when the only problem thought by the British Royal Commission on the Motor Car to be associated with the invention of motor cars was dust on untarred roads, we have come a long way. Medical technology, including antenatal technology, is not exempt from the strictures of this new socio-political consciousness.

Technologies do not simply emerge or exist; they frequently imply a transformation in social relations by acquiring identities of their own. What the machine says is not only different (often) from what the patient says, but the machine, which supposedly operates according to 'unvarying automatic procedures' producing 'uniformly trustworthy evidence' is simply more liable than the patient to be trusted by those reared on science with its endemically mechanical worldview (Reiser, 1978). A central problem of technology everywhere is its overloading by commercial interests and the vested interests of particular professional groups. In obstetrics, the power of technology is partly fuelled by the professional power of obstetricians and partly by the manufacturers of technology, who owe their livelihood to its continued use. Scientific evidence as to the effectiveness of this or that technical procedure is not the main criterion used either by the technology manufacturers, or by obstetricians, in deciding how to treat their patients. If it were, there would be very little treatment going on, since the proportion of procedures thus evaluated is small, and the proportion whose effectiveness has been demonstrated even smaller (Enkin and Chalmers, 1982). When we look at the process of medical innovation more generally, we see that, aside from drug therapies, quality control in the introduction of new techniques is assured mainly by informal peer review within the medical community. Indeed, the right to innovate in whatever manner the individual clinician considers appropriate, is traditionally defended as endemic to clinical freedom (Richards, 1975). Peer review is a notably inconsistent and unreliable method of quality control, depending more on friendship networks, status-perceptions and plain patronage than on a stable evaluation of scientific principles (Peters and Ceci, 1982). In one study of the use of a new drug among American physicians, the most 'scientifically-orientated' doctors were the most eager adopters of a new drug, whose claims of superiority over its older competitors were not proven. Many physicians started to use the new drug because they knew other physicians who were doing so, or because physician-friends with whom they played golf told them about the drug. Only by mapping these informal relations between doctors could the process of drug innovation be understood; the notion of individual scientific appraisal of the drug's benefits and hazards did not provide an adequate explanation (Coleman, et al., 1966).

As David Banta (1983) has observed, the minimum requirements of a system for assessing medical technologies have not yet been implemented in any country of the world. Perhaps they will be so in the next decade, and, if they are, the impact on antenatal care could well be profound. Yet there is a real tension here: between those whose awareness of the potential social effects of technology prompts them to argue for its social control, and those professionals who 'own' the technical competence in question and whose very professionalism depends now, and in the future, on continuing exclusively to determine how the technology is used. At root, therefore, the evaluation of technology must call into question the standing of professionals in our society. The evaluation of antenatal technologies is not a separate question from the question of the ethics and satisfactoriness of present provider–user relations: it is the same question. Whether or not antenatal care will, indeed, become more self-critical in the future unavoidably depends on whether or not there is a shift in the balance of power between its providers and its users. The future assertiveness of the consumer movement is a key unknown. For, as in marriage there is no reason why chauvinist, power-seeking husbands should alter their habits unless the women with whom they live enjoin them to do so, so there is no reason why obstetricians should abrogate their power unless pregnant women and their advocates press home the message that a future dilution of power is an absolute ethical, social and practical necessity.

A golden age of fetal movement counts?

If we turn our heads and survey the future landscape of antenatal care from its other window, we see a composition of different developments. It would be facile to say that these somehow represent a return to a golden age before the rise of modern antenatal care. If there was such an age it took a far greater toll of maternal and infant deaths than any humane society could possibly be prepared to countenance. Nonetheless, there is a note of 'rediscovering the wheel' about some of these alternative developments.

Pregnant women have always possessed their own knowledge about the vitality of their fetuses. From the interior uterine movements of the fetus, women gain a sense of fetal character and wellbeing. It is, of course, exactly this useful intimate knowledge that obstetricians over the decades have pursued in the development of their own various modes of getting to know the fetus. These new modes are the modern medical-professional's response to Playfair's nineteenth-century injunction, that obstetricians must listen to mothers' accounts of the strength of fetal movements and induce labour on this basis.

From the mid-1970s, maternal fetal movement counting began to emerge as a 'simple low-technology test' superior to other methods for assessing fetal wellbeing which 'could become the basis of a new format of antenatal care' (Grant and Mohide, 1982, p. 41). In 1973 Sadovsky and his co-workers in Israel had demonstrated that mothers asked to note fetal movements were able to describe 87 per cent of those recorded by an electromagnetic device strapped to the abdomen, and that maternally-perceived reduction of fetal movements predated fetal death by a long enough interval to permit appropriate intervention (Sadovsky, et al., 1973; Sadovsky and Yaffe, 1973). In 1976 Pearson and Weaver in Cardiff showed that a low maternal fetal movement count was associated with fetal asphixia and death even when other clinical indices, such as urinary oestrogen levels, appeared to be normal. In 1980 an important trial of this 'new' technique was done in Copenhagen which showed an apparently dramatic reduction in antenatal fetal deaths among mothers who were asked to count their babies' movements (Neldam, 1980; see Grant and Mohide, 1982, for a discussion). In asking mothers systematically to count fetal movements, obstetricians are, of course, demanding that maternal experience be translated into technical obstetrical language. Nevertheless, this systematization of patient experience does represent an authentically new direction for contemporary antenatal care. Other ways of capitalizing on pregnant women's own bodily expertise are also emerging. One example is the rediscovery of an ancient stimulus for inducing labour — massage of the nipples (Elliott and Flaherty, 1983).

In the same landscape of a more user-sensitive antenatal care, we may also note a move to return the patient to her social environment, and to include some social causes of poor antenatal health as falling within, rather than outside, the brief of clinical antenatal surveillance. Such 'social' factors as diet had certainly been seen as important in the early days of antenatal care, but their visibility declined with the accelerated growth of a more technical type of care: the 1935 edition of F. J. Browne's germinal *Antenatal and Postnatal Care*, contained 20 pages on the subject of diet which had been eclipsed to four by the 1970 edition. Dietary interventions to promote good pregnancy outcome were popular throughout the 1930s and 1940s and even into the 1950s, when an Australian attack on carbohydrate-eating was described in the *Lancet* (Hamlin, 1952) as a necessary, and almost sufficient, strategy to eliminate pre-eclampsia and eclampsia from the national and international antenatal scene.

In 1901 an editorial on 'Diet in Pregnancy' in the *British Medical Journal* said that the scientific study of maternal and fetal nutrition was shrouded in fog, but a 'freshening breeze of . . . investigation' was at last causing the mists to roll away (*British Medical Journal*, 19 October 1901, p. 1187). This view of unravelling mists was perhaps over-optimistic. But in the last 10 years, assessment of dietary status and dietary interventions in pregnancy has succeeded in taking on a generally more rigorous and persuasive character (RCOG, 1983a). Of course the interventions themselves are not new: chapter 6 gave an example of the fashion for these in the 1940s, and the impact of maternal diet on pregnancy outcome was constantly stressed in the early official reports on the state of maternity care. Some of the findings of the more recent studies are internally contradictory as to the exact effect of diet on maternal and fetal health, but their consensus is undoubtedly that nutrition is a significant influence on antenatal health. The nutritional hypothesis is also under the spotlight with regard to specific causes of death and illness, especially neural tube defects (spina bifida and anencephaly). Work by Smithells and his colleagues (1981) suggests that such defects could be caused by vitamin deficiency, and thus prevented by vitamin supplementation. A randomized controlled trial of this proposal has met with resistance from the consumer groups who believe the case for vitamins already proven. Diet is something everyone is an expert on, and the idea that malformed fetuses can be prevented by a healthy diet is an idea with a long history and a commonsense appeal. While some of antenatal care's users, and some of its purveyors, are articulating a recharged interest in dietary forms of antenatal care, the issue is marked by confrontation rather than co-operation between them (AIMS Newsletter, Autumn 1983, p. 5), thereby illustrating one most basic point about the structured hierarchies of power embedded in the provision and use of antenatal care.

Nutrition is the lynchpin of another new and seemingly social innovation in antenatal care: that exercise variously called 'prepregancy', 'preconceptional' or 'preconceptual' care. (The third of these terms is increasingly favoured although it is the least sensible, since pregnancy begins with a conception and not with a concept.) The essence of preconceptional care is attention to women's health before pregnancy. The conceptus must be received into an already healthy environment instead of merely prodding its mother, once pregnant, to make herself more healthy. Standard preconceptional advice and treatment includes medical examination of both prospective parents, admonitions to give up oral contraception well before pregnancy and to relinquish the pleasures and hazards of alcohol, smoking and 'junk foods'. Genetic counselling may be done and also complex biochemical investigations of a woman's health status using bits of her nails, hair, etc. Some preconceptional clinics have sprung up in NHS hospitals, but in the main they take the shape of private industry. 'Foresight' (The Association for the Promotion of Preconceptual Care) was started in 1979 as a registered charity with a formidable list of eight medical advisers. By late 1982 its newsletter was going out to 5,000 people, the organization had 18 'Foresight Clinics' in operation around the country, and was participating in a range of international preconceptional care initiatives, including the first European Seminar on Hair Analysis in Amsterdam. A *Foresight Wholefood Cookbook* for building health families was in production, and a raffle was being held to raise £10,000 as a down payment on a hair analysis machine to be housed at Aston University.

In the same way that the early demands for antenatal care came not from doctors but from the lay public, so the main initial moves towards preconceptional care have been made by lay voluntary groups active in the maternity field, both in Britain and other countries. In early 1983 a 'joint statement' on 'Prepregnancy Care in Britain' was issued by the Maternity Alliance and the National Council for Voluntary Organizations' Health and Handicap Group. This contended that:

(1) In the future a comprehensive prepregnancy care service could reduce baby deaths and handicap just as antenatal and delivery care does today.

(2) Routine prepregnancy care should be introduced into the existing statutory services.

(3) A publicity campaign to alert parents-to-be and professionals of the value of good health before conception should be undertaken by statutory and voluntary initiatives (Maternity Alliance and National Council, 1983, p. 10).

If we compare these sentiments with those expressed during the early days of antenatal care, we cannot fail to be impressed by the parallels. In both the clarion call for antenatal care and that for preconceptional care there is the same urgency of absolute faith in the potential of the new practice to prevent illness and save lives, the same demand for its routine statutory introduction and the same specification of the overarching need for publicity to convince the world that the right answer has arrived. And in a very similar way the practitioners of maternity care have, and are, joining the bandwagon of the new advocacy and adding the new precepts to the care they already provide. Even the stately RCOG in its 1982 Report on Antenatal Care was prepared to recommend the soliciting of medical advice by women intending to become pregnant.

The cultural dilemma of antenatal care

In this new paradigm of preconceptional care we see illuminated the central dilemma of antenatal care throughout its history. Everyone's commonsense dictates that antenatal care is a good idea. For, if women are to bear healthy babies and retain their own health in the process, care must be taken to ensure that this happens. It is not sufficient to trust Nature — significantly dubbed *Mother* Nature precisely for her unreliability in this regard? Natural processes are wasteful of human life and humans have invented the resources to do something about this wastefulness. Nobody doubts the honourable motivations of most obstetricians to act in the best interests of their pregnant patients.

That is one side of the dilemma. The other side is what happens when care is taken to protect the health of mothers and children within the particular socio-political context of a profoundly class- and gender-divided culture, one, moreover, in which the power of professionals to shape people's lives has increasingly escalated to become one central mark of life in the twentieth century. In these circumstances the wombs of women — whether already pregnant or not — are containers to be captured by the ideologies and practices of those who, to put it most simply, do not believe that women are able to take care of themselves.

Antenatal care, in all its various formats, has evolved within a society, not only class- and gender-divided, but also split down the middle by an unhappy dislocation between two modes of existence, each of which is actually an integral part of the human experience. Fritjof Capra in *The Turning Point* (1982, p. 39) identifies the split as between 'rational knowledge over intuitive wisdom, science over religion, competition over co-operation, exploitation of natural resources over conservation' — and men over women. In Capra's view unless this fissure is healed the very survival of our culture is in question. Perhaps it may be seen as far-fetched to locate the present and future dilemmas of antenatal care within such a broad paradigm crisis: yet the science-fiction scenarios of artificial reproduction even now being played out in our hospital labor-atories are hardly less far-fetched in their potential for 'future shock', in their capacity to revolutionize the biological bedrock of the industrial world. The capturing of women's wombs is the domination of the physicalist and masculinist scientific paradigm, the ultimate logic, not purely of the medicalization of life, but of a Cartesian world-view, in which the behaviour of bodies can be explained and controlled indepen-dently of minds. Unless we relinquish this dangerously simplistic world-view, the world is not likely to change very much — and neither is antenatal care.

Appendix I
Statistics

Alison Macfarlane

This appendix uses available statistics to illustrate the background of the historical changes in maternity care discussed in the text. All the graphs refer to England and Wales, but some indication is given of the data available for Scotland and Ireland.

Such nationally aggregated data often mask local variations. Most of the publications referred to here include data for areas within each country, but a major source of local data before 1974 is the annual reports which Medical Officers of Health were required by law to produce. Since 1974, some Health Authorities in England and Wales, Health Boards in Scotland and Health and Social Services Boards in Northern Ireland have published local data.

Constructing series of historical data is somewhat contentious exercise. Even if a data series appears to cover a long time span, the way the statistics themselves are compiled and interpreted will inevitably have changed. Often, however, there are more explicit changes in the data which are collected. Both the data and these problems are discussed more fully in *Birth Counts: statistics of pregnancy and childbirth* (Macfarlane and Mugford, 1984).

Births and deaths

Figures A.1 to A.5 in this Appendix are derived from the civil registration of births and deaths. The registration of live births and deaths dates back to 1837 in England and Wales, 1855 in Scotland and 1864 in Ireland. Stillbirths did not have to be registered until 1927 in England and Wales, 1939 in Scotland and 1961 in Northern Ireland, and they are still not registered in the Irish Republic. These data appear in the annual publications of the Registrars General for England and Wales, Scotland and Northern Ireland. The term 'perinatal mortality' (defined as the number of stillbirths and deaths in the first week of life per thousand live and still births) was not used until the early 1950s, when the series in figure A.3 was constructed retrospectively.

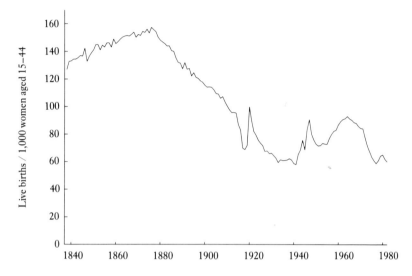

Figure A.1 Fertility rates, England and Wales, 1838–1982
source: OPCS Birth statistics, Series FM1

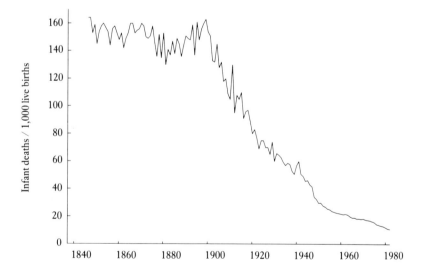

Figure A.2 Infant mortality rates, England and Wales, 1846–1982
source: OPCS Mortality statistics

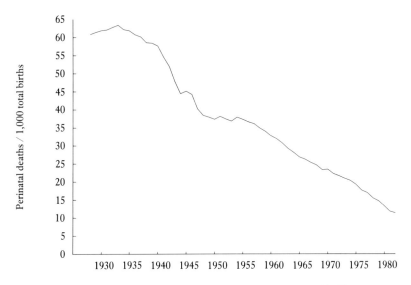

Figure A.3 Perinatal mortality rates, England and Wales, 1928–82
source: OPCS Mortality statistics, Series DH3

Although the registration of live births was started in England and Wales in 1837, it was not made compulsory until 1874, and the babies who died shortly after birth were particularly likely not to be registered. This means that the fertility and infant mortality rates for the mid-nineteenth century, included in figures A.1 and A2, are likely to be considerably underestimated.

While death registration was probably fairly complete by this period, deaths due to pregnancy and childbirth were considerably under-reported until the General Register Office introduced its system of medical enquiries in 1881 (General Register Office, 1883). Figure A.4 shows 'true maternal' deaths, that is those attributed directly to the effects of pregnancy and childbirth. There is a further category of 'associated deaths' which are deaths of women known to be pregnant but whose deaths were attributed to other causes.

Distinguishing between these two categories is clearly a subjective process and the definitions were changed on a number of occasions when the International Classification of Diseases (ICD) was revised (Ministry of Health, 1937, Taylor and Dauncey, 1954). For example, deaths attributed to 'criminal abortion' were moved from the 'violent deaths' section to 'true maternal deaths' in the fifth revision of the ICD, which came into use in England and Wales in 1940.

Appendix I

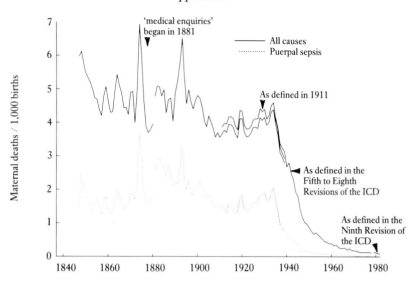

Figure A.4 Maternal mortality rates, England and Wales, 1847–1982
source: OPCS Mortality statistics

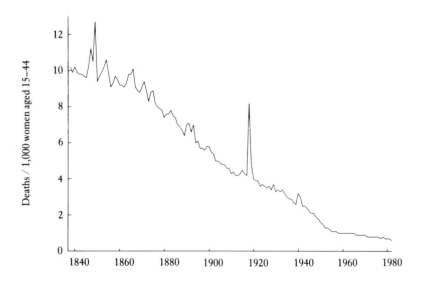

Figure A.5 Death rates from all causes in women aged 15–44, England and Wales, 1838–1982
source: OPCS Mortality statistics

In the nineteenth century the main subdivision within the category of maternal deaths was into 'accidents of childbirth' and 'puerperal sepsis' which was also known as 'metria'. Further subdivisions became more usual around the turn of the century and these were changed at successive revisions of the ICD. Puerperal sepsis remained a relatively stable category and deaths attributed to it are shown in figure A.4, where it can be seen that peaks in maternal mortality in the late nineteenth century were associated with peaks in deaths from puerperal sepsis. On the other hand, the peak in mortality in 1918–19, shown in figure A5 was associated with the influenza epidemic of 1918.

Place of delivery

Births registered in England and Wales have been routinely analysed by place of delivery since 1954 and the data are plotted in figure A.6. This also includes data from special analyses published in the Registrar General's Statistical Reviews for 1927, 1932 and 1937.

No data are available on a national scale about the numbers of births either in voluntary lying-in hospitals or about births in workhouses and poor law infirmaries before the First World War, but the *Minority*

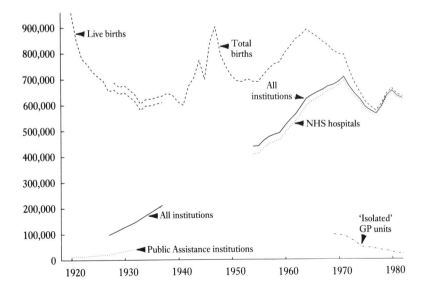

Figure A.6 Numbers of births in hospitals and other institutions, England and Wales, 1920–82
source: OPCS Birth statistics

Report of the Poor Law Commission of 1909 estimated that about 11,000 children were born in workhouses in England and Wales in 1907 (Webb and Webb, 1909). There are local data in individual hospital reports and reports of Medical Officers of Health (some of these are drawn on in the text).

Numbers of women admitted to certain types of institutions with maternity beds were tabulated from 1931 and 1939 in the annual reports of the Ministry of Health and the Welsh Board of Health. These used different categories from the Registrar General, included only women whose care was funded by local authorities and did not distinguish between antenatal and delivery admissions. Similar data were published in the annual reports of the Scottish Department of Health. Recent data about place of delivery in Scotland and Northern Ireland are published in *Scottish Health Statistics* and *Health and Personal Social Services Statistics for Northern Ireland*.

Table A.1 Numbers of maternity beds in hospitals and related institutions for the physically ill, England 1861–1938

	Voluntary		Public	
	Number of hospitals	*Number of beds*	*Number of hospitals*	*Number of beds*
1861	12	139		
1891	16	210		
1911	8	311		
1921	14	462	199	2463
1938	235	3587	1/6	6442

source: R. Pinker *English Hospital Statistics 1861–1938*. With permission of the author.

Data about hospital beds from 1861 to 1938 compiled from a variety of sources (Pinker, 1966) are shown in table A.1. The fact that there appear to have been no maternity beds in public hospitals before World War I suggests that the lying-in wards of Poor Law institutions were not counted. In addition, this source is not consistent with the annual reports of the Ministry of Health, which together with the Welsh Board of Health published the numbers of beds in municipal and voluntary maternity homes from 1920 to 1938. In 1931, the numbers of maternity beds in hospitals and public assistance institutions which had been transferred to local authorities under the Local Government Act of 1929 were added in. Similar data were published from 1931 to 1938 in the annual reports of the Scottish Department of Health. Statistics about arrangements during the Second World War were published in these reports and drawn together in Richard Titmuss's *Problems of social policy* (1950).

After 1948, the numbers of maternity beds in NHS hospitals were published in the annual reports of the Ministry of Health, the Welsh Board of Health and the Scottish Home and Health Department. More recently they have been published in the volumes of *Health and Personal Social Services Statistics* for England, Wales and Northern Ireland and in Scottish Health Statistics. Numbers of maternity beds from 1920–39 and since 1939 are plotted in figure A.7 with breaks to indicate changes in the basis for data collection.

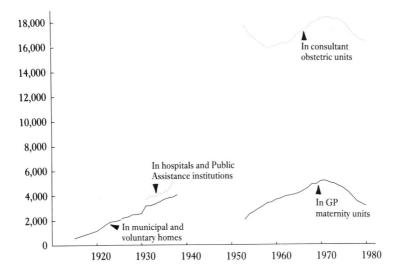

Figure A.7 Numbers of maternity beds, England and Wales, 1915–80
source: Ministry of Health, DHSS and Welsh Office

Antenatal care

The official reports mentioned in the preceding paragraphs also contain data about clinics. The rise through the 1920s and 1930s in the numbers of maternal and child welfare clinics and antenatal clinics is shown in figure A.8. The statistics collected in the early years of the NHS relate to the number of sessions held rather than the number of clinics, so they cannot be compared with earlier data.

Figure A.9 shows the numbers of women attending antenatal clinics and, for reference, the numbers of live and stillbirths. As some women

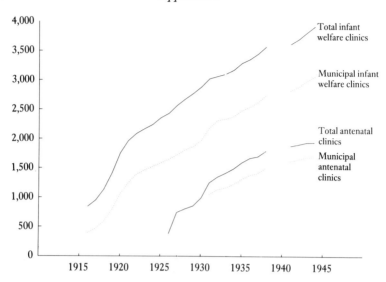

Figure A.8 Numbers of infant welfare and antenatal clinics, England and Wales, 1916–44
source: Local Government Board and Ministry of Health

attended more than one type of clinic there is likely to be some double counting. While data for hospital clinics for 1949 onwards are based on numbers of new outpatients, these data were not compiled for community clinics before 1949 or after 1961. For this reason, the somewhat less well defined 'number of women attending' has been plotted in figure A.9.

Collection of data about community antenatal clinics stopped after 1978, but statistics are still collected about attendances at NHS mothercraft and relaxation classes and are shown in figure A.10. these do not include those run by voluntary bodies, mainly the National Childbirth Trust.

Staff providing care

Also shown in figure A.10 are first visits to expectant mothers by health visitors during the 1930s. The Ministry of Health's Annual Report for 1938 remarked that the decline in these visits in that year was a consequence of the Midwives Act of 1936 which gave midwives greater responsibility for this task.

In the 1920s and 1930s a considerable proportion of health visitors' time was spent on what was broadly described as maternal and child

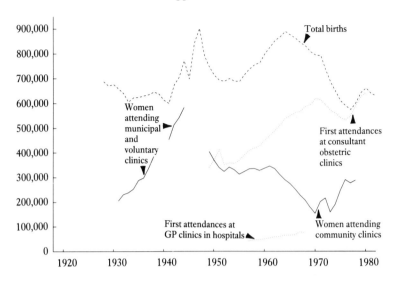

Figure A.9 Numbers of women attending various types of antenatal clinics, England and Wales, 1931–80
source: Ministry of Health, DHSS and Welsh Office

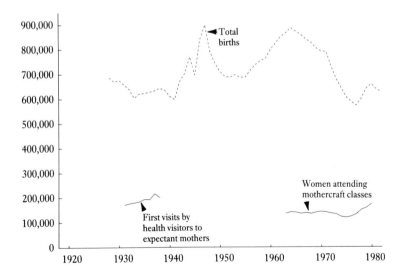

Figure A.10 Numbers of women receiving other types of antenatal care, England and Wales, 1931–80
source: Ministry of Health, DHSS and Welsh Office

welfare, but some women combined the role of health visitor, midwife and district nurse. The Ministry of Health reports for the inter-war years give the 'whole-time equivalent' number of women devoted to health visiting each year and this is plotted in figure A.11. These data need to be interpreted with care as the length of the working week is not stated. It is also difficult to compare them with data for post-war years when working hours decreased and the proportion of health visitors' time devoted to maternal and child health was smaller (Dunnell and Dobbs, 1982).

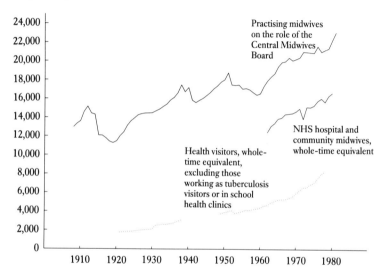

Figure A.11 Numbers of midwives and health visitors, England and
Wales, 1908–81
source: Central Midwives Board, Ministry of Health, DHSS and Welsh Office

Figure A.11 includes data from the Central Midwives Board about the numbers of midwives practising and, for more recent years, DHSS and Welsh Office data about whole time equivalent midwifery staff. In the interwar years, midwives worked much longer hours and domiciliary midwives were almost always on call. Since the start of the NHS, midwives' hours have decreased, the most recent occasion being in 1980, so the data have to be interpreted in the light of this. *Health and Personal Services Statistics* for England and for Wales classify midwives as either 'hospital' or 'community', but since the 1974 reorganization many midwives employed from hospitals work in the community as well.

Figure A.12, based on published and unpublished data from the LHS 27/3 returns, illustrates the decreasing numbers of deliveries done by community midwives over the past 20 years. The corresponding changes in the involvement of GPs is illustrated by data derived from their claims to Family Practitioner Committees for item-for-service payments for providing different types of maternity care (figure A.13).

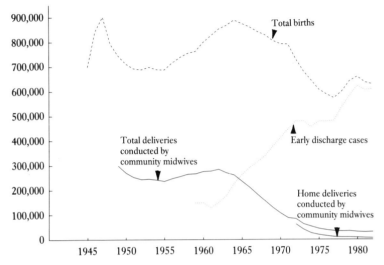

Figure A.12 Numbers of deliveries and early discharge cases attended by domiciliary/community midwives, England and Wales, 1949–82
source: Ministry of Health, DHSS and Welsh Office

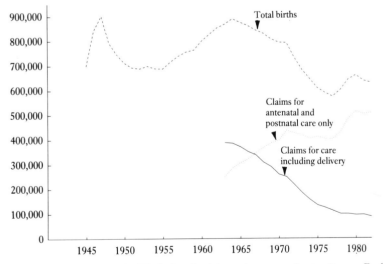

Figure A.13 Numbers of claims by GPs for fees for giving various types of maternity care, England and Wales 1963–82
source: Ministry of Health, DHSS and Welsh Office

No data were published about numbers of obstetricians before the setting up of the NHS. Figure A.14 shows the numbers of consultants since 1948, while table A.2 shows the distribution by gender of members and fellows of the Royal College of Obstetricians and Gynaecologists alive in 1983.

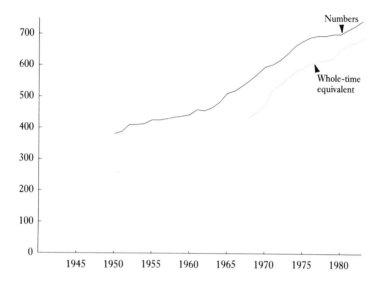

Figure A.14 Numbers of consultants in obstetrics and gynaecology working in the National Health Service, England and Wales, 1950–83
source: Ministry of Health, DHSS and Welsh Office

Table A.2 Members and fellows of the Royal College of Obstetricians and Gynaecologists alive in 1983 and practising in the United Kingdom, the Republic of Ireland and the armed forces

| Year of election | Fellows | | | | Members | | | |
	Male	Female	Total	Per cent Female	Male	Female	Total	Per cent Female
1929–49	29	5	34	14.7	24	32	56	57.1
1950–59	75	18	96	18.8	25	32	57	56.1
1960–69	270	40	310	12.9	88	89	177	50.3
1970–79	319	74	393	18.8	671	229	900	25.5
1980–83	208	29	237	12.2	429	184	613	30.0
Total	904	166	1070	15.5	1237	566	1803	31.4

source: Royal College of Obstetricians and Gynaecologists
The preponderance of women members in the older age groups reflects not only the higher death rate among men, but men's greater chances of rising to become fellows.

There are other data, not presented here, which relate to antenatal care. In particular, the Maternity Hospital In-Patient Enquiry gives estimates of numbers of antenatal stays in hospital. As successive stays by the same woman are not linked, they cannot be used to estimate the number of women who are admitted to hospital antenatally.

Although the data which are relevant to antenatal care are limited in many ways, and in particular reflect the organisation rather than the quality of care, they nevertheless give some idea of the major trends in practice which have taken place since the beginning of the century and changes in the outcome of pregnancy since the mid-nineteenth century. At the time of writing, data collection systems recommended for use in England by the Steering Group on Health Services Information are being pilot tested. If implemented, they may answer some of the criticisms which have been levelled at the data currently available.

Appendix I: *Data sources*

Vital Statistics

Annual Reports of the Registrar General for England and Wales for the years 1837–1920

Registrar General's Statistical Reviews for England and Wales for the years 1921–73

OPCS Birth statistics, Series FM1 } 1974 onwards
OPCS Mortality statistics, Series DH1–5 }

Annual Reports of the Registrar General for Scotland, 1855 onwards

Annual Reports of births, marriages and deaths in Northern Ireland, 1922 onwards

Irish Free State, Reports of the Registrar General, 1922–35

Irish Republic, Reports of the Registrar General, 1936–57

Irish Republic, Vital Statistics, 1958 onwards

Annual Reports of the Registrar General, Isle of Man, 1880 onwards (also includes health services statistics)

Health Services Statistics

Annual Reports of the Ministry of Health and the Welsh Board of Health, 1919–67

Annual Reports of the Chief Medical officer of the Department of Health and Social Security, 1968 onwards

NHS Hospital and Specialist Service Statistics, 1949–53

Ministry of Health Digest of Health Service Statistics, 1954–71

Health and Personal Social Services Statistics for England and Wales, 1972

Health and Personal Social Services Statistics for England 1973–78, 1982

Health and Personal Social Services Statistics for Wales, 1974 onwards

Annual Reports of the Scottish Board of Health, 1919–28

Annual Reports of the Scottish Department of Health, 1929–61

Annual Reports of the Scottish Home and Health Department, 1962 onwards

Scottish Health Statistics, 1968 onwards

Health and Personal Social Services Statistics for Northern Ireland, 1974 onwards

Annual Reports of the Medical Officers of Health for the States of Jersey and Guernsey (also contain vital statistics)

Appendix II

*The efforts of an obstetrician in cosmic time:
an interview with Dugald Baird,
23 May 1980*

Dugald Baird qualified in medicine in 1922, the year before the death of
J. W. Ballantyne. He worked with nearly all the famous names in the
early years of antenatal care — R. W. Johnstone, Eardley Holland,
Munro Kerr (to whom he attributes responsibility for his own life-long
commitment to obstetrics), and he worked in Scotland where, as we
have seen, the British movement for capturing the womb really began.
Dugald Baird has pioneered many important and controversial ideas and
practices in his lifetime: from epidemiology for obstetricians, to abortion
on demand, from induction of labour for postmaturity, to a genuinely
uncompetitive partnership between clinicians and social scientists with a
shared interest in finding out what is good, and making things better, for
mothers and babies. In the 1940s and 1950s he and his redoubtable
wife, May, gave the impression of running the city of Aberdeen —
where Baird went shortly before the Second World War as Regius
Professor of Midwifery — between them. In 1948 in her capacity as
convenor of the Aberdeen Public Health Committee and Chairman of
the North-East Scotland Regional Hospital Board, May was appointed a
member of the Steering Committee for the national working party
inquiry into the reasons for the shortage of midwives. My father,
Richard Titmuss, was a member of the working party which was, as far
as he was concerned, but an episode in a long collaboration and friendship with the Bairds.

   After my father's death in 1973, papers relating to this collaboration
came into my possession. These included a spirited correspondence
between Dugald and my father on the subject of what antenatal care
could hope to achieve. The correspondence related to the *Maternity in
Great Britain* Survey carried out in 1946. Baird was not directly involved,
but my father was on the Joint Committee of the Royal College of

Obstetricians and Gynaecologists and the Population Investigation Committee (representing the latter) which carried out, and analysed the results of, the Survey. Baird and Titmuss were concerned with the particular issue of an interpretation made by James Douglas, Director of the Committee, to the effect that a small number of antenatal attendances was responsible for premature births; or, to put it another way, that sufficient antenatal attendances could prevent premature birth. Talking about the social class III, IV and V women with a high incidence of premarital conceptions and a high prematurity rate, Baird wrote to Douglas in June 1949 in the following terms:

> The point is, would they have a low prematurity rate if they could be persuaded to attend regularly? You quote a reduction of from 28.7 to 24.6 per cent of the babies weighing 6½lbs or less in a working class group where there had been 9 antenatal attendances and no paid work for the last 5 months of pregnancy — not a very significant change . . . Over 50 per cent of the premature had 'adequate antenatal care' and yet were premature. How could 9 visits to a crowded antenatal clinic with waits of up to 3 hours on hard benches + examination of urine + blood pressure estimations + abdominal palpation + a general exhortation to drink milk, orange juice, etc., prevent prematurity? This is, you will agree, the position at many clinics.

The letter continued by discussing social class differences in birthweight by place of delivery, and ended by saying:

> Everyone who studies social class differences in reproductive performance knows that the causes are complex and interwoven, but the fact remains that social class IV and V contain a larger proportion of small stunted women in a poor state of health, who produce small and less robust babies than those in classes I and II. This is probably the effect of a generation or two of unhealthy living. It seems clear that the most important single factor is poor diet. How much of this poor standard of living is related to the lack of intelligence of the mother, faulty home environment, poor education, or poverty, is an interesting study.
>   Any antenatal clinic which can change all this in 9 sessions is doing wonderful work.

I was five years old at the time of this correspondence. Some 25 years later I found myself in the grip of a powerful interest in the functioning of the maternity services, which I could hardly suppose to be genetic in origin. To mark my personal debt to Dugald Baird's influence on my own professional socialization, therefore, and because of his own enormous contribution to the welfare of women and children in this country, and because otherwise some of these stories might simply disappear in the black hole of cosmic time, I am including as an appendix to the history of antenatal care (about which I was trying to interview Dugald that day in the spring of 1980) some of his own observations on life as an obstetrician.[1]

Becoming an obstetrician/gynaecologist/epidemiologist

Two years after graduation I had held a variety of house appointments, all of which were unpaid. It was then suggested to me that I apply for a post of resident registrar which was being created by Professor Munro Kerr in his department of gynaecology in the Glasgow Royal Infirmary. This may well have been the first paid post (£250 per annum) in Scotland. The Professor happened to have seen me play in an international rugby trial and is alleged to have said that 'if he turned out to be as good an obstetrician and gynaecologist as he was a footballer then they had made a good appointment.' When Munro Kerr found that I also played golf we were soon on the Old Prestwick course at Troon. It was, at that time, one of the champion courses and I was so excited with the prospect of playing on this famous course that on that occasion I managed to do the first nine holes in 37 strokes. After a decade of exciting and strenuous work, in which physical strength was an undoubted asset, I found myself in the Chair of Obstetrics and Gynaecology in Aberdeen.

My maternal grand-father was well-known breeder of Clydesdale horses. By the time I was fourteen I was quite an expert on sex and reproduction. Mares received better attention in 1914 than some women today. Note was taken of their weight increase, diet and exercise. I became quite an expert in clinical assessment of the quality of young growing horses. I recollect that one famous horse had to be taken 'off the road' because it had too many abortions — this was rather earlier than similar questions were raised in relation to human reproduction.

In the human, much use has been made of the husband's social class as a measure of the quality of environment and its relationship to reproductive efficiency. This information is easy to obtain, but is rather indirect and less efficient than an interview by a person with the necess-

---

1. I have edited the interview, and present sections of it here under headings.

ary knowledge — not unlike the skilled farmer's method of assessing health and efficiency in animals. In one study all primigravidae attending the antenatal outpatient department in Aberdeen had their health and physique assessed at their first visit. In due course it was found that those assessed A, the top group, had a small incidence (3 per cent) of low birthweight babies compared with 16 per cent in group D, those with the poorest health and physique. Reproductive efficiency is also affected by age, and the aristocracy has always acted on this. The young are reared in an environment which allows them to grow to their genetically determined height and to start reproduction at an age (twenty to twenty-five) when fertility is at its height. There is no postponement of pregnancy so that an honours degree can be finished or promotion in a career secured. The production of an heir is the first priority. In these circumstances labour is easy and the perinatal mortality rate very low.

By contrast I remember being shocked many years ago by the case of a woman sent in labour from Peterhead, about 30 miles away from Aberdeen. After many hours of labour the baby's head was still high in the pelvis and there was obvious serious disproportion. She had six previous pregnancies, the first two resulting in stillbirths after long labours, the next a breech presentation with neonatal death, and subsequently 3 live births. Despite this past experience and increasing age a home confinement had been planned.

One of my first acts after coming to Aberdeen in 1936 was to consult Professor Tom Smith (now Sir Thomas) the Professor of Scots Law on the legal position relating to therapeutic abortion in Scotland. He made it clear that the authorities would not allow a case to be brought against a doctor unless there was substantial evidence of criminal intent. A doctor was free to use his own judgement as in all other medical situations. I was prepared to act on this statement and started to study the place of therapeutic abortion in society. After 10 years a meeting of all general practitioners whose patients had had an abortion was called. They were asked to give an assessment of the immediate and long-term results of the operation in their patients. This they did meticulously and their opinions were uniformly favourable.

Communicating with the patient

I once had a request from the sister in charge of a large maternity unit in Glasgow to see a staff nurse for whom she had the highest regard. She was in her early thirties and her life revolved between her work as a midwife and the care of a mother who was bedridden with rheumatic arthritis. The mother died and for the first time in years the daughter could have a holiday. She went to Norway to learn to ski but her education did not stop there and she arrived back in Glasgow very depressed and quite dehydrated. I said 'well you've thought about all the pros and cons and you're a bright girl. There are three alternatives, which do you want?'

'Oh I'm afraid an abortion would be the best for me.'

'All right we'll do it tomorrow.'

'So you'll do what I want?'

'Of course you're the one who's pregnant and I know you've spent a lot of time thinking about it and you still want it done.' So we did it. The next day she was weeping, and I said 'I'm coming tomorrow to have a long talk to you about the whole matter, because you have got to get it straight.' The first question I asked was 'Was he nice to you? Did you enjoy it?'

'Oh' she said, quite calmly, 'I must say it was very nice'.

'Well, you're very lucky, a lot of women have never had that experience. So you are a privileged person in some ways. You are a very attractive woman and I feel sure that Glasgow men will not leave you alone for very long and you are now better equipped to deal with the situations as they arise.' The sister in charge wrote me a letter some time later saying she could not thank me enough because the nurse had completely settled down and was relaxed and happy again. Things could have gone badly wrong she said, because the nurse had a very strict religious upbringing.

I said to one woman, 'thank you very much for telling me about your sex life.'

'Oh, Professor, I'd have told you anything.'

'Oh, why is that?'

'Well, I was lying in the antenatal twenty years ago, and you came in with a couple of students, and you said to one of them "now will you palpate Mrs Smith's abdomen"' — she had the words right, you see — 'and he put his hands on me, and they were cold and I jumped, so you took the students away and you said "now, young man, just let this be a good lesson to you, *never* examine a patient with cold hands."' So because of that she'd tell me anything about her sex life!

A woman came to me with sex problems, and I said, 'What are you like with other men?'

'Oh, how do you know?' she said. Well, I didn't know, but I could apologize if I was wrong, couldn't I?'

I said to another woman, 'you've only had three children, all you wanted, how did you manage it?'

'Well, I've a very good husband, he doesnae bother me very much Professor.'

'Oh, what do you do?'

'Well, you see, he goes to football on Saturday and on Saturday night I just hand him a condom and that's that.'

I said, 'how do you get the condoms?'

'Well', she said, 'you see, I've an understanding with the chemist. I go in and ask him for coughdrops and I hand him the money and he hands over the "coughdrops" and there's no questions asked or anything. If the shop's full of people it doesnae matter.'

Patients like to know more about what is going on in hospital. My impression was that a talk on the mechanism of labour to a small group was more effective as a preparation for labour than relaxation exercises. The fellow who designed the mechanism of labour must have been a very clever chap.

On one occasion there was a difference of opinion as to whether an anaesthetic was necessary for the procedure of rupture of the membranes to induce labour. The patients agreed that an anaesthetic would not be given unless they particularly requested it. Afterwards they were asked to comment on their experience and feeling. Meantime the sisters and staff nurses had graded the skill and personal qualities of the obstetricians, seniority notwithstanding. Gradings were submitted in strict confidence to the senior consultant anaesthetist who was held in the highest regard by all. In the event it was clear that the higher the grading of the doctor by the nursing staff the more certain the patient was that an anaesthetic was unnecessary. To this day only the anaesthetist knows the details.

Important debates and historical moments

Since the end of the last war there has been a great expansion in the field of preventive medicine, sociology, epidemiology and nutrition. Unfortunately, for many reasons, the relationship between clinicians and professionals in these other disciplines has not always been satisfactory. In the field of reproduction the obstetrician has an advantage, because the clinical application of scientific advances in knowledge and the benefits can be seen more quickly than those resulting from advances in preventive medicine. Attempts to improve maternal reproductive efficiency may mean a wait of almost 20 years till a new generation has grown to maturity. Non-medical research workers may be jealous of the 'power' of the doctor and may think his manner dictatorial, on the other hand they do not, and might not care to, have his responsibility. The doctor may say that sociological research has discovered little that the competent clinician does not already know.

The time is now ripe for more attention to be paid to the emotional needs of mothers in relation to childbirth, a subject which, until now, tended to be pushed aside in the face of all the technical advances and the methods of finding out about how our bodies work. The net reproduction rate today is 0.823 and is unlikely to rise in Europe in the foreseeable future. This has diminished the problems of women in one way but other problems have emerged, for example those arising from the long-term use of oral contraceptives and the stress of facing up to the difficulties in establishing their rightful place in society. Meanwhile sex problems for the male stay as simple as they have always been, but what is required is a more careful look at their general role as husbands in modern society.

Having been a patient on several occasions recently and having been almost 'written off' on one occasion many years ago, I have been able to see very clearly the qualities necessary for the 'good' doctor and nurse. In 1928 I had septicaemia and a temperature of between 102 and 104F for four months but after a transfusion with fresh blood donated by two house physicians (an unusual procedure in those days) my temperature started to fall immediately. This helps to explain why Leonard Colebrook rang me up from Queen Charlotte's hospital one day in 1936 and said 'Dugald, you must come to London, I have something I want to show you.'

'Oh', I said, 'do I have to come?'

'Yes', he said, 'You'll enjoy it once you get here.' So I travelled to London and to the isolation block at Charlotte's. They showed me the temperature charts of many women who had had septicaemia due to the dreaded haemolytic streptococcus and were successfully treated with 'Prontosil Rubrum'. In many cases the temperature was normal in 48 hours. Between my personal experience of septicaemia and the realization that this was the beginning of the end of maternal mortality, this was one of the most memorable periods of my life.

Another important moment for me was the reading of Richard Titmuss's book on social conditions and infant mortality (*Birth, Poverty and Wealth*, 1943). I was able, with some difficulty to run him to earth in a large government building during the war years. He stimulated me to take an intelligent interest in the effect of the environment in which we are reared and its relationship to our subsequent health and thinking. He also had an important influence in the staffing of the Obstetric Medicine Research Unit (MRC) in Aberdeen which broke much new ground in the field of obstetrics. His quiet manner concealed great determination and courage. I wish more sociologists today would use the simple English which he used so effectively.

God and golf in cosmic time

Munro Kerr was ninety when I went to see him in Canterbury and he said, 'Dugald, do you believe in a hereafter?'

And I said 'well I haven't really thought about it, I'm not at that stage yet. You should know more about that than I do'.

He said, 'Well, I'd like to go out on the first tee at Killermont, put a ball down, hit a real beauty down the first fairway and then drop.'

I was brought up in a good religious home. With my father and younger brother I walked four miles (two miles there and two miles back) to Church on Sunday mornings, two miles to Sunday school in the afternoon and sometimes we had a reading of chapters of the bible at night. In due course I had a visit from the minister wanting me to join the Church. He was too much of a fundamentalist for me and I said 'About God, well, you know, man has been in existence for two million years and I believe it's now nearer four million years, surely he has left it very late coming about 2,000 years ago to send his son to look after his flock? What happened in the long years between?' It was disappointing to find that he had no answer to give to the question. My mother, a farmer's daughter, was very angry with me for speaking to the minister like that, but my father, a science master at my school, said 'leave the boy alone, we've all to work out these problems for ourselves.'

People said to me on retirement 'what would you like to be remembered for?'

I might say 'well, if you don't mind it's rather a silly question. My children will remember me, but after that I'll be a long time dead'.

They then said 'well, could I phrase it differently. What have you had most pleasure in doing?'

I say, 'that's more sensible. But in cosmic time, what can you do? The only thing you can do is to keep from being bored. Life's more interesting if you exert yourself, and do things, and you can hope that you're making the world, at the end of the day, a little more attractive for the people who are coming along.'

Bibliography

Abel-Smith, B. (1964) *The Hospitals 1800–1948* London, Heinemann.
Ahlfeld, F. (1905) *Mschr. Geburtsch-Gynäk.*, 21, p. 143.
Allan, P. and Jolley, M. (eds.) (1982) *Nursing, Midwifery and Health Visiting Since 1900* London, Faber and Faber.
Allbutt, T. C. (1897) 'Albuminuria in Pregnancy' *Lancet* 27 February, pp. 579–82.
Allen, E. and Doisy, E. A. (1923) 'An Ovarian Hormone; preliminary report on its location, extraction and partial purification, and action on test animals' *J. Amer. Med. Assoc.* 54, pp. 819–21.
Alter, B.P. (1981) 'Prenatal Diagnosis of Haemoglobinopathies: a status report' *Lancet* 21 November, pp. 1152–5.
Althusser, L. (1971) 'Ideology and Ideological State Apparatuses' in Althusser, L. (ed.) *Lenin and Philosophy and Other Essays* London, New Left Books.
Alvarez, H. and Caldeyro, R. B. (1950) 'Contractility of the Human Uterus Recorded by New Methods' *Surg. Gynec. and Obst.* 91, p. 1.
Anderson, A. and Turnbull, A. (1982) 'Effect of Oestrogens, Progestogens and Betamimetics in Pregnancy' in Enkin and Chalmers (eds.).
Arms, S. (1975) *Immaculate Deception* New York, Bantam Books.
Arney, W. R. (1982) *Power and the Profession of Obstetrics* London, University of Chicago Press.
Aschheim, S. and Zondek, B. (1928) 'Schwangerschafts diagnose aus dem Harn (Durch Hormonnachweis)' *Klin. Wchschr.* 7, p. 8.
Association for Improvements in the Maternity Services (1976) Discussion Paper for Meeting with the DHSS, 5 March (unpublished).
Audral, G. (1843) *Essai d'Hématologue Pathologique* Brussels, Societé Encyclopédique des Sciences Médicales.

Bailey, K. V. (1926) 'Medicinal Induction of Labour' *Lancet* 6 February, pp. 282–84.
Baines, C. (forthcoming) 'A History of the Induction of Labour'.
Baird, D. (1960) 'The Evolution of Modern Obstetrics' *Lancet* 10 September, pp. 557–64.
Baird, D., Thomson, A. M. and Duncan, E. H. L. (1953) 'The Causes and Prevention of Stillbirths and First Week Deaths. II Evidence from Aberdeen Clinical Records' *J. Obstet. Gynae. Brit. Emp.* 60, pp. 17–30.
Bakketeig, L. S. and Bergsjø, P. (1977) 'Transportfødsel i Norge' *Saertrykk av Tidsskrift for Den Norske Laegeforening* 17–18, pp. 923–70.
Bakketeig, L. S., Eik-Nes, S. H., Jacobsen, G., Ulstein, M. K., Brodtkorb, C. J., Balstad, P., Eriksen, B. C., Jörgensen, N. P. (1984) 'Randomized controlled trial of ultrasonic screening in pregnancy' *Lancet* 28 July, pp. 207–10.
Ballantyne, J. W. (1901a) 'A Plea for a Pro-Maternity Hospital' *British Medical Journal* 6 April, pp. 813–4.
Ballantyne, J. W. (1901b) 'A Visit to the Wards of the Pro-Maternity Hospital' *The American Journal of Obstetrics and Diseases of Women* May, no. 5, pp. 593–7.
Ballantyne, J. W. (1902) and (1904) *Manual of Ante-Natal Pathology and Hygiene* I *The Foetus*

(1902) II *The Embryo* (1904) Edinburgh, William Green and Sons.

Ballantyne, J. W. (1904) *Essentials of Obstetrics* Edinburgh, William Green and Sons.

Ballantyne, J. W. (1906–7) 'Inaugural Address on the Future of Obstetrics' *Trans. Edin. Obst. Soc.* 32, pp. 3–28.

Ballantyne, J. W. (1907–8) 'Hospital Treatment of Morbid Pregnancies' *Obst. Trans. Edin.*, 33, pp. 2–61.

Ballantyne, J. W. (1914) *Expectant Motherhood: its supervision and hygiene* London, Cassell and Co.

Bang, J. (1980) 'Strategy for Safety Studies and the Place of Epidemiology' in Kurjak (ed.) (1980b).

Banta, H. D. (1983) 'National Level Experience in the Evaluation of Technologies'. Paper presented at National Seminar and International Consultation in Perinatal Surveillance and Care Beijing, China, 31 October–5 November.

Barnes, A. C. (1975) 'Foreword' in Gruenwald, P. (ed.).

Beard, R. (1977) 'Changes in Obstetrics: an interview with Professor Richard Beard' *British Medical Journal* 23 July, pp. 251–3.

Beard, R. and Campbell, S. (1977) 'The Current Status of Fetal Heart Rate Monitoring and Ultrasound in Obstetrics' *Proceedings of a Scientific Meeting at the R.C.O.G.*, London.

Beech, B. (1981) 'The Work of the Association for Improvements in the Maternity Services' Paper presented to 4th Human Relations in Obstetrics Seminar, University of Glasgow, 13 September 1981, unpublished.

Benison, S. (1971) 'Oral History: a personal view' in Clarke, E. (ed.) *Modern Methods in the History of Medicine* London, Athlone Press.

Bennett, M. J. and Campbell, S. (eds.) (1980) *Real-Time Ultrasound in Obstetrics* Oxford, Blackwell Scientific Publications.

Beral, V. and Colwell, L. (1980) 'Randomized Trial of High Doses of Stilboestrol and Ethisterone in Pregnancy: long-term follow-up of mothers' *British Medical Journal* 281, pp. 1098–1101.

Bergsjø, P., Bakke, T., Salanonsen, L. A., Støa, K. F. and Thorsen, T. (1973) 'Urinary Oestriol in Pregnancy, Daily Fluctuation and Correlation with Fetal Growth' *J. Obstet. Gynae. Brit. Comm.* 80, pp. 305–10.

Berkeley, C. (1929) 'Maternal Morbidity: with special reference to abortions' Fifth English-speaking Conference on Maternal and Child Welfare. Report of Proceedings, National Association for the Prevention of Infantile Mortality.

Bishop, E. H. (1964) 'Pelvic Scoring for Elective Induction' *Obstet. Gynec.* 24, pp. 266–268.

Bjerkedal, T. and Bakketeig, L. S. (1972) *Medical Registration of Births in Norway 1967–8. Some Descriptive and Analytical Reports.* Institute of Hygiene and Social Medicine, University of Bergen.

Blair Bell, W. (1909) 'The Pituitary Body' *British Medical Journal* 4 December, pp. 1609–13.

Blair Bell, W. (1931) 'Maternal Disablement' *Lancet* 30 May, pp. 1171–7.

Blom, I. (1980) *Barne-begrensning — synd eller sunn fornuft* Oslo, Universitetsforlaget.

Blondel, B., Saurel-Cubizolles, M. J. and Kaminski, M. (1982) 'Impact of the French System of Statutory Visits on Antenatal Care' *Journal of Epidemiology and Community Health* 36, pp. 183–6.

Blondel, J. (1727) *The Strength of Imagination in Pregnant Women Examined: And the Opinion that Marks and Deformities in Children arise from thence, Demonstrated to be a Vulgar Error* London, J. Peele.

Blundell, J. (1834) *The Principles and Practice of Obstetricy* London, E. Cox.

Board of Education (1911) *Annual Report for 1910* London, HMSO.

Board of Education (1914) *Annual Report for 1913* London, HMSO.

Board of Education (1915) *Annual Report for 1914* London, HMSO.

Boddy, K. and Mantell, C. D. (1972) 'Observations of Fetal Breathing Movements Transmitted Through Maternal Abdominal Wall' *Lancet*, 2, pp. 1219–20.

Boddy, K. and Robinson, J. S. (1971) 'External Method for Detection of Fetal Breathing in Utero' *Lancet* 2, pp. 231–3.

Bode, O. (1931) 'Das Elektrohysterogramm' *Arch. Gynaec.* 146, p. 123.

Boissonnas, R. A., St. Guttmann, Jacquemond, P.-A. and Waller, J.-P. (1955) Une Nouvelle Synthèse de D'Oxytocine' *Helvetica Chimica Acta* XXXVIII, no. 179, pp. 1491–1501.

Borglin, N. E. (1962) 'Intranasal Administration of Oxytocin for Induction and Stimulation of Labour' *Acta Obst. and Gyn. Scand.* 41, pp. 238–53.

Bots, R. S. G. M., Nijhuis, J. G., Martin, C. B. and Prechtl, H. F. R. (1981) 'Human Fetal Eye Movements: detection in utero by ultrasonography' *Early Human Development* 5, pp. 87–94.
Bourne, G. (1975) *Pregnancy* London, Pan Books.
Boyd, E., Abdulla, U., Donald, I., Fleming, J. E. E., Hall, A. J. and Ferguson-Smith, M. A. (1971) 'Chromosome Breakage in Ultrasound' *British Medical Journal* 2, pp. 501–2.
Boyle, G., Elliott, D. and Roy, R. (1977) *The Politics of Technology* New York, Longman.
Braxton-Hicks, J. (1872) 'On the Contractions of the Uterus Throughout Pregnancy' *Transactions of the London Obstetrical Society*.
British Medical Association (1935) 'Memorandum Regarding a National Maternity Service'. Supplement to the *British Medical Journal* 7 December, pp. 245–8.
Brock, D. J. H. and Sutcliffe, R. G. (1972) 'Alphafetoprotein in the Antenatal Diagnosis of Anencephaly and Spina Bifida' *Lancet* 2, pp. 197–99.
Brook, D. (1976) *Naturebirth* Harmondsworth, Penguin.
Browne, A. D. H. (1969) 'Optical Amnioscopy' in Huntingford, et al. (eds.).
Browne, F. J. (1931) 'The Health of the Woman Citizen as Potential and Actual Mother' *Journal of State Medicine* XXXIX, pp. 688–702.
Browne, F. J. (1932) 'Antenatal Care and Maternity Mortality' *Lancet* 2 July, pp. 1–4.
Browne, F. J. (1934) 'Are We Satisfied with the Results of Ante-Natal Care?' *British Medical Journal* 4 August, pp. 194–7.
Browne, F. J. (1935) *Antenatal and Postnatal Care* London, J. and A. Churchill. New editions 1937, 1939, 1942, 1944, 1946, 1951, 1955 (authors Browne, F. J. and Browne, J. C. McC.), 1960, 1970, 1978 (authors Browne, F. J., Browne, J. C. McC. and Dixon, G.).
Browne, J. C. McC. and Veall, N. (1953) 'The Maternal Placental Blood Flow in Normotensive and Hypertensive Women' *J. Obstet. Gynae. Brit. Emp.* 60, pp. 142–7.
Budin, P. (1897) 'Photographie par les Rayon X D'un Bassin de Naegelé' *L'Obstetrique* 2.
Bull, T. (1837) *Hints to Mothers for the Management of Health During the Period of Pregnancy and in the Lying-in Room* London, Longmans, Orme, Brown, Green and Longmans.
Burke, F. J. (1935) 'Amniography' *J. Obstet. Gynae. Brit. Emp.* Vol. 42, pp. 1096–1106.
Burns, Rt. Hon. J. (1906) 'President's Inaugural Address' in National Conference on Infantile Mortality *Report of the Proceedings of the National Conference on Infantile Mortality* Caxton Hall, Westminster, 13–14 June 1906, London, P. S. King and Son.
Buster, J. E., Bustillo, M., Thorneycroft, I. H., Simon, J. A., Boyers, S. P., Marshall, J. R., Louw, J. A., Seed, R. W., Seed, R. G. (1983) 'Non-surgical Transfer of In Vivo Fertilised Donated Ova to 5 Infertile Women: report of 2 pregnancies' (letter) *Lancet* 23 July, pp. 223–4.
Butler, N. R. and Alberman, E. D. (1969) *Perinatal Problems* Edinburgh, E. and S. Livingstone.
Butler, N. R. and Bonham, D. (1963) *Perinatal Mortality* Edinburgh, E. and S. Livingstone.

Campbell, J. (1917) *Report on the Physical Welfare of Mothers and Children Vol. 2* Carnegie United Kingdom Trust, Liverpool, C. Tinling and Co.
Campbell, J. A. (1977) 'Antenatal Radiation Hazards' in Campbell, J. A. (ed.) *Obstetrical Diagnosis by Radiographic, Ultrasonic, and Nuclear Methods* Baltimore, Williams and Wilkins.
Campbell, R., Davies, I. M. and MacFarlane, A. (1982) 'Perinatal Mortality and Place of Delivery' *Population Trends* 28, Summer, pp. 9–12.
Campbell, S. (1968) 'An Improved Method of Fetal Cephalometry by Ultrasound' *J. Obstet. Gynae. Brit. Comm.* 75, pp. 568–76.
Campbell, S. and Little, D. J. (1980) 'Clinical Potential of Real-Time Ultrasound' in Bennett and Campbell (eds.).
Campbell, S., Reading, A. E., Cox, D. N., Sledmere, C. M., Mooney, R., Chudleigh, P., Beedle, J. and Ruddick, H. (1982) 'Ultrasound Scanning in Pregnancy: the short-term psychological effects of early real-time scans' *Journal of Psychosomatic Obstetrics and Gynaecology* 1–2, pp. 57–61.
Campion, S. (1950) *National Baby* London, Ernest Benn.
Cannings, R. B. (1922) *The City of London Maternity Hospital: a short history* London, J. S. Forsaith and Son.
Capra, F. (1983) *The Turning Point* New York, Bantam Books.
Carmichael, J. H. E. and Berry, R. J. (1976) 'Diagnostic X-rays in Late Pregnancy and in the Neonate' *Lancet* 1, pp. 351–2.
Cartwright, A. (1979) *The Dignity of Labour? A study of childbearing and induction* London, Tavistock.

Cates, J. (1915) 'A Working Scheme in Ante-natal Hygiene' in National Association for the Prevention of Infantile Mortality *Mothercraft Part II* London, The National League for Physical Education and Improvement.

Central Health Services Council (Standing Maternity and Midwifery Advisory Committee) (1961) *Human Relations in Obstetrics* London, HMSO.

Central Midwives Board (1937) *Report on the Work of the C.M.B. for the Year ended 31 March 1937* London, HMSO.

Central Office of Information (1944) *Women at Work* London, Central Office of Information.

Chalmers, I. (1979) 'Maternal Mortality' (letter) *British Medical Journal* 17 November, p. 1294.

Chalmers, I. and Richards, M. (1977) 'Intervention and Causal Inference in Obstetric Practice' in Chard and Richards (eds.).

Chamberlain, G. (1975) 'Antenatal Education' *Midwife, Health Visitor and Community Nurse*, 11, pp. 289–92.

Chamberlain, G. (1976) 'The Usefulness of Antenatal Care' in Turnbull and Woodford (eds.).

Chamberlain, G., Howlett, B., Philipp, E. and Masters, K. (1978) *British Births 1970* 2 *Obstetric Care* London, Heinemann.

Chard, T. and Richards, M. (eds.) (1977) *Benefits and Hazards of the New Obstetrics* London, Spastics International Medical Publications.

Chavasse, P. H. (1832) *Advice to a Wife on the Management of her Own Health* London (8th edition 1911).

Chief Medical Officer *Annual Report of the Chief Medical Officer of the Ministry of Health* for 1933, published 1934; for 1936, published 1937; for 1946, published 1947; for 1952, published 1953; for 1954, published 1955; for 1958, published 1959; for 1963, published 1964. London, HMSO.

Chilowsky, C. and Langevin, M. P. (1916) 'Procédés et Appareil Pour Production de Signaux Sous-marins Dingés et Pour la Localization á Distance d'Obstacles Sous-marins' *French Patent No. 502913.*

Chng, P. K., Hall, M. H. and MacGillivray, I. (1980) 'An Audit of Antenatal Care: the value of the first antenatal visit' *British Medical Journal* 1 November, pp. 1184–6.

Cianfrani, T. (1960) *A Short History of Obstetrics and Gynecology* Springfield, Illinois, C. C. Thomas.

Clarke, J. (1806) (2nd edition) *Practical Essays on the Management of Pregnancy and Labour* London, J. Johnson.

Clark-Kennedy, A. E. (1955) 'Medicine in Relation to Society' *British Medical Journal* 1, pp. 619–23.

Cole, G. D. H. and Postgate, R. (1961) *The Common People 1746–1946* London, Methuen.

Colebrook, L. and Kenny, M. (1936a) 'Treatment of Human Puerperal Infections in Mice with Prontosil' *Lancet* 6 June, pp. 1279–90.

Colebrook, L. and Kenny, M. (1936b) 'Treatment with Prontosil of Puerperal Infections' *Lancet* 5 December, pp. 1319–26.

Coleman, J. S., Katz, E. and Menzel, H. (1966) *Medical Innovations a diffusion study* New York, Bobbs-Merrill.

Collip, J. B. (1930) 'Further Observations on an Ovary Stimulating Hormone of the Placenta' *Can. Med. Assoc. J.* 22, p. 761.

Collver, A., Have, R. T. and Speare, M. C. (1967) 'Factors Influencing the Use of Maternal Health Services' *Social Science and Medicine* 1, pp. 293–308.

Cookson, I. (1954) 'Domiciliary Obstetrics' *British Medical Journal* 10 April, pp. 841–7.

Cookson, I. (1967) 'The Past and Future of Maternity Services' *Journal of the College of General Practitioners* 13, pp. 143–62.

Cranbrook Committee (1959) *Report of the Maternity Services Committee*, London, HMSO.

Crawford, R. (1980) 'Healthism and the Medicalization of Everyday Life' *International Journal of Health Services* 10, 3, pp. 365–88.

Cremer, M. (1906) 'Ueber die Direkte Ableitung der Aktionsströme des Menschlichen Merzens Vom Oesophagus und über das Elektrokardiogramm des Fötus' *München med. Wchnschr.* 53, p. 811

Crew, F. A. E. (1930) 'Pregnancy Diagnosis Station — Report on First Year's Working' *British Medical Journal* 5 April, pp. 662–664.

Curry, A. S. and Hewitt, J. V. (1974) *Biochemistry of Women: clinical concepts* Cleveland, Ohio, CRC Press.

Dale, H. (1906) 'On Some Physiological Actions of Ergot' *Journal of Physiology* 34, pp. 163–206.

Dalton, K. J., Dawson, A. J. and Gough, N. A. J. (1983) 'Long Distance Telemetry of Fetal Heart Rate from Patients' Homes using Public Telephone Network' *British Medical Journal* 14 May, p. 1545.

Davies, A. C., Chalmers, I. and Fahmy, D. R. (1977) 'Predicting Fetal Death' (letter) *British Medical Journal* 12 February p. 443.

Davies, C. (n.d.) '"Little Credit and Less Cash": the maternity and child welfare doctors of the interwar years' Unpublished paper, University of Warwick.

Davies, M. L. (1915) *Maternity: letters from working women* London, G. Bell and Sons. Reprinted 1978, Virago.

Davin, A. (1978) 'Imperialism and Motherhood' *History Workshop* Spring, 5, pp. 9–65.

Denman, T. (1794) *An Introduction to the Practice of Midwifery* London, Johnson. Fifth edition 1821.

Department of Health for Scotland (1935) *Report on Maternal Mortality and Morbidity in Scotland* Edinburgh, HMSO.

Department of Health and Social Security (1977) *Reducing the Risk: safer pregnancy and childbirth* London, HMSO.

Department of Health and Social Security (1982) *Report on Confidential Enquiries into Maternal Deaths in England and Wales 1976–8* London, HMSO.

Departmental Committee on Maternal Mortality and Morbidity (1930) *Interim Report*, London, HMSO.

Departmental Committee on Maternal Mortality and Morbidity (1932) *Final Report* London, HMSO.

Devore, G. R. and Hobbins, J. C. (1980) 'The Use of Ultrasound in Fetoscopy' in Bennett and Campbell (eds.).

Devries, R. G. (1981) 'Birth and Death: social construction at the poles of existence' *Social Forces* 59, 4, pp. 1074–93.

Dewsbury, A. R. (1980) 'What the Fetus Feels' (letter) *British Medical Journal* 16 February, p. 481.

Dick-Read, G. (1942) *Childbirth Without Fear* London, Heinemann.

Diczfalusy, E. and Mancuso, S. (1969) 'Oestrogen Metabolism in Pregnancy' in Klopper and Diczfalusy (eds.).

Dilling, W. and Gemmell, A. (1929) 'A Preliminary Investigation of Foetal Deaths Following Quinine Induction' *J. Obstet. Gynae. Brit. Emp.* 36, pp. 352–66.

Dillon, T. F., Douglas, R. G. and Du Vigneaud, V. (1962) 'Further Observations on Transbuccal Administration of Pitocin for Induction and Stimulation of Labor' *Obstetrics and Gynecology* 20, pp. 434–41.

Dilman, V. M. (1977) 'Metabolic Immunodepression Which Increases the Risk of Cancer' *Lancet* 10 December, pp. 1207–9.

Domagk, G. (1935) *Deutsche med. Wchnschr.* 61, 15 February, p. 250.

Donald, I. (1965) 'Diagnostic Uses of Sonar in Obstetrics and Gynaecology' *J. Obstet. Gynae. Brit. Comm.* 72, pp. 907–19.

Donald, I. (1967) 'Ultrasonics in Obstetrics and Gynaecology' *British Journal of Radiology* 40, pp. 604–11.

Donald, I. (1968) 'Ultrasonics in Obstetrics' *British Medical Bulletin* 24, 1, pp. 71–5.

Donald, I. (1969) 'On Launching a New Diagnostic Science' *American Journal of Obstetrics and Gynecology* 1 March, pp. 609–28.

Donald, I. (1974a) 'New Problems in Sonar Diagnosis in Obstetrics and Gynaecology' *American Journal of Obstetrics and Gynecology* 118, 3, 1 February, pp. 299–309.

Donald, I. (1974b) 'Sonar: what it can and cannot do in obstetrics' *Scottish Medical Journal* 19, 5 September, pp. 203–10.

Donald, I. (1976) 'The Biological Effects of Ultrasound' in Donald, I. and Levi, S. *Present and Future of Diagnostic Ultrasound* New York, John Wiley.

Donald, I. (1979) *Practical Obstetric Problems* London, Lloyd-Luke.

Donald, I. (1980) 'Sonar — its Present Status in Medicine' in Kurjak (ed.) (1980a).

Donald, I. and Abdulla, U. (1968) 'Placentography by Sonar' *J. Obstet. Gynae. Brit. Comm.* 75, October, pp. 992–1006.

Donald, I., MacVicar, J. and Brown, T. G. (1958) 'Investigation of Abdominal Masses by Pulsed Ultrasound' *Lancet*, I, p. 1188.

Donnison, J. (1977) *Midwives and Medical Men* London, Heinemann.

Dorland, W. A. N. and Hubeny, M. J. (1926) *The X ray in Embryology and Obstetrics* London, Henry Kimpton.

Douglas, C. A. (1955) 'Trends in the Risks of Childbearing and in the Mortalities of Infancy During the last 30 Years' *J. Obstet. Gynae. Brit. Emp.* 62, pp. 216–31.

Duncan, E. H. L., Baird, D., and Thomson, A. M. (1952) 'The Causes and Prevention of Stillbirths and First Week Deaths Part I: the evidence of vital statistics' *J. Obstet. Gynae. Brit. Emp.* 59, pp. 183–96.

Duncan, J. M. (1868) *Researches in Obstetrics* New York, W. Wood and Co.

Duncan, J. M. (1870) *On the Mortality of Childbed and Maternity Hospitals* Edinburgh, Adam and Charles Black.

Dunnell, K. and Dobbs, J. (1982) *Nurses Working in the Community*, O.P.C.S. Social Survey Report 551141, London, HMSO.

Durandy, A., Griscelli, C., Dumez, Y., Oury, J. F., Henrion, R., Briard, M. L., and Frezal, J. (1982) 'Antenatal Diagnosis of Severe Combined Immuno-deficiency from Fetal Cord Blood' (letter) *Lancet* 10 April, pp. 852–3.

Dussik, K. T., Dussik, F. and Why, L. (1947) 'Aufdem wege zur hyperphonographie des Gehurhes' *Wien. Med. Wochenschr.* 97, pp. 425–429.

Dyhouse, C. (1978) 'Working-class Mothers and Infant Mortality in England 1895–1914' *Journal of Social History* 12, Winter, pp. 248–67.

Eastman, N. J. (1938) 'The Induction of Labor' *Americal Journal of Obstetrics and Gynecology* 35, pp. 721–9.

Eccles, A. (1982) *Obstetrics and Gynaecology in Tudor and Stuart England* London, Croom Helm.

Eden, T. W. (1929) 'An Address on the National Inquiry into the Causes of Our High Maternal Mortality Rate' *British Medical Journal* 20 July, pp. 81–5.

Eden, T. W. (1933) 'Midwifery in the Home' *British Medical Journal* 11 March, pp. 399–403.

Elliott, J. P. and Flaherty, J. F. (1983) 'The Use of Breast Stimulation to Ripen the Cervix in Term Pregnancies' *American Journal of Obstetrics and Gynecology* 1 March, pp. 553–6.

Emanuel, J. (1982) The Politics of Maternity in Manchester (1919–1939): a study from within a continuing campaign. Unpublished M. Sc. Dissertation, University of Manchester.

Embrey, M. P. and Yates, M. J. (1964) 'A Tocographic Study of the Effects of Sparteine Sulphate on Uterine Contractility' *J. Obstet. Gynae. Brit. Comm.* Vol. 71, pp. 33–6.

Engelmann, G. J. (1883) *Labor Among Primitive Peoples.* St Louis, J. H. Chambers and Co.

Engström, L. (1959) 'Induction of Labour Around Fulterm Especially by means of Synthetic Oxytocin in Intravenous Drip' *Acta Obstetrica et Gynecologica Scandinavia* XXXVIII Supplement 3.

Enkin, M. and Chalmers, I. (eds.) (1982) *Effectiveness and Satisfaction in Antenatal Care* London, Spastics International Medical Publications.

Fairbairn, J. S. (1927) 'Observations on the Maternal Mortality in the Midwifery Service of the Queen Victoria's Jubilee Institute' *British Medical Journal* 8 January, pp. 47–50.

Farr, A. D. (1979) 'Blood Group Serology — the first 4 Decades (1900–1939)' *Medical History* 23, pp. 215–26.

Farr, W. (1885) *Vital Statistics* London, Edward Stanford.

Farrant, W. (1980) 'Stress after Amniocentesis for High Serum Alphafetoprotein Concentrations' (letter) *British Medical Journal* 20 September, p. 452.

Faulk, W. P., Stevens, P. J., Burgos, H., Matthews, R., Bennett, J. P. and Hsi, B.-L. (1980) 'Human Amnion as an Adjunct in Wound Healing' *Lancet* 31 May, pp. 1156–8

Fawdry, R. D. S. (1982) Printed Items Relevant to History Taking. Unpublished Paper.

Feminist Self-Insemination Group (1980) *Self-Insemination* London.

Ferguson, J. H. (1912) 'Some Twentieth Century Problems in Relation to Marriage and Childbirth' *Trans. Edin. Obstet. Soc.* Vol. 38, pp. 3–39.

Ferguson, S. M. and Fitzgerald, H. (1954) *Studies in the Social Services* London, HMSO.

Fields, H., Greene, J. W. and Smith, K. (1965) *Induction of Labor* New York, Macmillan.

Figlio, K. (1977) 'The Historiography of Scientific Medicine: an invitation to the human sciences' *Comparative Studies in Society and History*, 19, 3, pp. 262–86.

Fitzgerald, W. J. (1958) 'Evolution of the Use of Ergot in Obstetrics' *New York State Medical Journal* 15 December, pp. 4081–3.

Forber, Lady (Lane-Claypon, J.) (1936) 'The Position of Midwives in Independent Practice' *The Medical Officer* 14 March, p. 107.

Forster, F. M. C. (1967) *Progress in Obstetrics and Gynaecology in Australia* Sydney, John Sands Ltd.

Foucault, M. (1977) *Discipline and Punish: the birth of the prison* London, Allen Lane.

Fox, D. (1834) *The Signs, Disorders and Management of Pregnancy: the Treatment to be Adopted during and after Confinement: and the Management and Disorders of Childbirth* Derby, Henry Mozley and Sons.

Foy, H., Kondi, A., Parker, A.M., Stanley, R. and Venning, C.D. (1970) 'The α-fetoprotein Test in Pregnant Women on Oral Contraceptives, Newborn Babies and Pyridoxine-deprived Baboons' *Lancet*, I, pp. 1336–7.

Francis, J. G., Turnbull, A. C. and Thomas, F. F. (1970) 'Automatic Oxytocin Infusion Equipment for Induction of Labour' *J. Obstet. Gynae. Brit. Comm.* Vol. 77, pp. 594–602.

Francome, C. and Huntingford, P. J. (1980) 'Birth by Caesarean Section in the United States of America and in Britain' *Journal of Biosocial Science* 12, pp. 353–62.

Freidson, E. (1972) *Profession of Medicine* New York, Dodd, Mead and Co.

Fullerton, L. S. P., Davidson, H. W., Howie, J. W., Croll, J. M., Orr, J. B. and Godden, W. (1933) 'Observations in Nutrition in Relation to Anaemia' *British Medical Journal*, 22 April, pp. 685–89.

Galbraith, J. K. (1974) *Economics and the Public Purpose* London, Andre Deutsch.

Garcia, J. (1982) 'Women's Views of Antenatal Care' in Enkin and Chalmers (eds.).

Garrow, J. S. and Douglas, C. P. (1968) 'A Rapid Method for Assessing Intrauterine Growth by Radioactive Selenomethionine Uptake' *J. Obstet. Gynae. Brit. Comm.* Vol. 75, pp. 1034–9.

Gau, G. S., Bhundia, J., Napier, K. and Ryder, T. A. (1983) 'The Worm that Wasn't' (letter) *Lancet* 21 May, pp. 1160–1.

Gellhorn, G. (1927) 'Can Quinine Kill the Fetus in Utero?' *American Journal of Obstetrics and Gynecology* 13, pp. 779–82.

General Register Office (1883) *Forty-fourth Annual Report of the Registrar General.* London, HMSO.

Gibberd, G. F. (1929a) 'A Contribution to the Study of the Maternal Death Rate' *Lancet* 14 September, pp. 535–8.

Gibberd, G. F. (1929b) 'The Results of Induction of Labour with Animal Bladders' *British Medical Journal* 5 October, pp. 617–8.

Gilbert, B. G. (1966) *The Evolution of National Insurance in Great Britain* London, Michael Joseph.

Gill, D. G. (1971) 'The British National Health Service: professional determinants of administrative structure' *International Journal of Health Services* 1, 4, pp. 342–53.

Gill, D. G. (1980) *The British National Health Service: a sociologist's perspective* United States Department of Health and Human Services NHS Pub. No. 80–2054.

Gillett, J. (1976) 'A Report on the Survey on Preparation for Childbirth within the Catchment of Copthorne Maternity Unit, Shrewsbury, December 1972–June 1973, *International Journal of Nursing Studies* 13.

Gluck, L., Kulovich, M. V., Borer, R. C., Brenner, P. H., Anderson, G. G., and Spellacy, W. N. (1971) 'Diagnosis of the Respiratory Distress Syndrome by Amniocentesis' *American Journal of Obstetrics and Gynecology* 109, pp. 440–5.

Godber, G. (1963) 'The Effect of Specialisation on Maternity Services' *Lancet* 18 May, pp. 1061–66.

Goldthorpe, W. O. and Richman, J. (1974) 'Maternal Attitudes to Unintended Home Confinement' *Practitioner* 212, pp. 845–853.

Graham, H. (1950) *Eternal Eve* London, T. Brun.

Graham, H. (1978) 'Problems in Antenatal Care' DHSS/Child Poverty Action Group Conference, Reaching the Consumer of the Antenatal and Child Health Services.

Graham, H. and McKee, L. (1979) *The First Months of Motherhood Volume I: Summary Report* London, Health Education Council, unpublished report.

Grant, A. and Chalmers, I. (forthcoming) 'Epidemiology in Obstetrics and Gynaecology' in MacDonald, R. R. (ed.) *Scientific Basis of Obstetrics and Gynaecology* (3rd Edition) Edinburgh, Churchill Livingstone.

Grant, A., Chalmers, I. and Enkin, M. (1982) 'Physical Interventions Intended to Prolong Pregnancy and Increase Fetal Growth' in Enkin and Chalmers (eds.).

Grant, A. and Mohide, P. (1982) 'Screening and Diagnostic Tests in Antenatal Care' in Enkin and Chalmers (eds.).

Granville, A. B. (1819) *A Report of the Practice of Midwifery at the Westminster and General Dispensary During 1818* London, Burgess and Hill.

Greene, J. W., Duhring, J. L. and Smith, K. (1965) 'Placental Function Tests' *American Journal of Obstetrics and Gynecology* 92, 7, pp. 1030–58.

Grigg, J. (1789) *Advice to the Female Sex in General, Particularly those in a State of Pregnancy and Lying-In* Bath, S. Hazard.

Gruenwald, P. (1975) 'Introduction' in Gruenwald (ed.).

Gruenwald, P. (ed.) (1975) *The Placenta and Its Maternal Supply Line* Lancaster, Medical and Technical Publishing Co.

Guidotti, R. (1983) 'Appropriate Perinatal Technology' Paper presented at National Seminar and International Consultation on Perinatal Surveillance and Care, Beijing, China, 31 October–5 November.

Guillebaud Committee (1956) *Report of the Committee of Enquiry Into The Cost of the National Health Service* London, HMSO.

Gustavii, B. (1983) 'First-Trimester Chromosomal Analysis of Chorionic Villi Obtained by Direct Vision Technique' *Lancet* 27 August, pp. 507–8.

Haire, D. (1972) *The Cultural Warping of Childbirth* International Childbirth Education Association.

Halban, J. (1905) Die Innere Secretion von Ovarium und Placenta und ihre Bedentung für die Funktion der Milchdrüse *Arch. Gynäk.* 75, p. 353.

Hall, M. H. (1980) An Appraisal of Outpatient Antenatal Care Aberdeen, unpublished Paper.

Hall, M. H., Chng, P. K. and MacGillivray, I. (1980) 'Is Routine Antenatal Care Worthwhile?' *Lancet* 12 July, pp. 78–80.

Hamilton, A. (1781) *Treatise on Midwifery* London, J. Murray.

Hamlin, R. H. J. (1952) 'The Prevention of Eclampsia and Pre-eclampsia' *Lancet* 12 January, pp. 64–8

Hammacher, K. (1969) 'The Clinical Significance of Cardiotocography' in Huntingford, et al. (eds.).

Hammacher, K., Hüter, K. A., Bokelmann, J. and Werners, P. H. (1968) 'Foetal Heart Frequency and Perinatal Condition of the Foetus and Newborn' *Gynaecologia* 166, pp. 349–60.

Hanmer, J. (1980) 'Reproductive Engineering: the final solution?' *New Society* 24 July, pp. 163–4.

Harrison, B. (1981) 'Women's Health and the Women's Movement in Britain 1840–1940' in Webster, C. (ed.) *Biology, Medicine and Society 1840–1940* Cambridge, Cambridge University Press.

Hassani, S. N. (1978) *Ultrasound in Gynaecology and Obstetrics* New York, Springer Verlag.

Haultain, W. F. T. and Chalmers Fahmy, E. (1929) *Antenatal Care: a practical handbook of antenatal care and of the abnormalities associated with pregnancy* Edinburgh, E. and S. Livingstone.

Hellman, L. M., Morton, G. W., Tolles, W. E. and Fillisti, L. P. (1963) 'A Computer Analysis of the Atrophine Test for Placental Function' *American Journal of Obstetrics and Gynecology* 85, pp. 610–618.

Henriksen, E. (1941) 'Pregnancy Tests of the Past and Present' *West. J. Surg. Obstet. Gynec.* 49, pp. 567–75.

Henrion, R., Oury, J. F., Aubry, J. P. and Aubry, M. C. (1980) 'Prenatal Diagnosis of Ectrodactyl' (letter) *Lancet* 9 August, p. 319.

Hess, J. H. (1917) 'The Diagnosis of the Age of the Fetus by the Use of Roentgenograms' *American Journal of Diseases of Children* 14, 6, pp., 397–423.

Heward, J. A. and Clarke, M. (1976) 'Communications to an Antenatal Clinic' *British Medical Journal* 15 May, pp. 1202–4.

Hilson, D., Bruce, R. L. and Sims, D. G. (1978) 'Successful Pregnancy Following In-Vitro Fertilization' (letter) *Lancet* 26 August, p. 473.

Hirst, B. C. (1900) *A Textbook of Obstetrics* London, W. B. Saunders.

Hitschmann, F. and Adler, L. (1908) Der Ban der Uterusschleimhaut des Geschlechtsreifen

M

Weibes Mit Besonderer Berucksichtigung der Menstruation *Monatsschr. Geburtsch. u. Gynäk.*, 27, 1.

Hobel, C. J. (1978) 'Risk Assessment in Perinatal Medicine' *Obstetrics and Gynecology* 21, pp. 287–95.

Hofbauer, J. (1955) 'Forty Years of Postpituitary Extract in Obstetrics' *American Journal of Obstetrics and Gynecology* 69, pp. 822–5.

Holland, E. (1935) 'Maternal Mortality' *Lancet* 27 April, pp. 973–6.

Holmes, H. B. Hoskins, B. B. and Gross, M. (eds.) (1981) *The Custom-Made Child?* Clifton, New Jersey, Humana Press.

Holton, J. B. (1976) 'Assessment of Fetal Lung Maturity and Prediction of Respiratory Distress Syndrome' in Turnbull and Woodford (eds.).

Hon, E. H. (1961) *A Manual of Pregnancy Testing* London, J. and A. Churchill.

Honigsbaum, F. (1979) *The Division in British Medicine* London, Kogan Page.

Hope, E. W. (1917) *Report on the Physical Welfare of Mothers and Children Volume I* Carnegie United Kingdom Trust, Liverpool, C. Tinling and Co.

Houd, S. and Oakley, A. (1983) Alternative Perinatal Services in the European Region and North America: a pilot survey. World Health Organization, Copenhagen, unpublished paper.

Howard, H. I. (1962) 'Obstetrics in General Practice: A Five-Year Survey. Part I General Outline' *The Practitioner* 188, pp. 239–42, and 'Part II Detailed Analysis' *The Practitioner* 188, pp. 383–93.

Howie, P. W. (1977) 'Induction of Labour' in Chard and Richards (eds.).

Howry, D. H. and Bliss, W. R. (1952) 'Ultrasonic Visualization of Soft Tissue Structures of the Body' *J. Lab. Clin. Med.* 40, pp. 579–92.

Hoyer, L. W., Lindsten, J., Blomback, M., Hagenfeldt, L., Cordesins, E. M., Stromberg, P. and Gustavii, B. (1979) 'Prenatal Evaluation of Fetus at Risk for Severe von Willebrand's Disease' (letter) *Lancet* 28 July pp. 191–2.

Hubert, J. (1974) 'Belief and Reality: social factors in pregnancy and childbirth' in Richards, M. P. M. (ed.) *The Integration of a Child Into a Social World* Cambridge, Cambridge University Press.

Huntington, J. L. (1913) 'Relation of the Hospital to the Hygiene of Pregnancy' *Boston Medical and Surgical Journal* 21, pp. 763–5.

Huntingford, P. J., Beard, R. W., Hytten, F. E. and Scopes, J. W. (eds.) (1971) *Perinatal Medicine* Proceedings of the Second European Congress, London, Basel, Karger.

Huntingford, P. H., Hüter, K. A. and Saling, E. (eds.) (1969) *Perinatal Medicine* Proceedings of the First European Congress, Berlin, London, Academic Press.

Hutchinson, D. L. (1967) 'Amniotic Fluid' in Marcus and Marcus (eds.).

Hytten, F. E. (1976) 'Metabolic Adaptations of Pregnancy' in Turnbull and Woodford (eds.).

Illich, I. (1975) *Medical Nemesis* London, Calder and Boyars.

Illsley, R. (1956) 'The Duration of Antenatal Care' *The Medical Officer* 24 August, pp. 107–11.

Interdepartmental Committee on the Physical Deterioration of the Population (1904) *Report* London, HMSO.

Jameson, J. E. and Handfield-Jones, R. P. C. (1954) 'Obstetrics and the General Practitioner' *Lancet* 27 March, pp. 665–9.

Jefferys, M. (1978) 'The Consumer's View' DHSS/Child Poverty Action Group Conference on Reaching the Consumer in the Antenatal and Child Health Services.

Jellett, H. (1899) *A Short Practice of Midwifery* (2nd edition) London, J. and A. Churchill.

Johnstone, R. W. (1913) *A Textbook of Midwifery* London, Adam and Charles Black.

Johnstone, R. W. (1947) 'Ballantyne's Ghost' *Trans. Edin. Obstet. Soc.* 54, pp. 1–13.

Johnstone, R. W. (1950) 'Fifty Years of Midwifery' *British Medical Journal* 7 January, pp. 12–15.

Joint Committee of the Royal College of Obstetricians and Gynaecologists and the Population Investigation Committee (1948) *Maternity in Great Britain*, Oxford, Oxford University Press.

Kaback, M. M. (1976) 'Introduction' in Kaback and Valenti (eds.).

Kaback, M. M. and Valenti, C. (eds.) (1976) *Intrauterine Fetal Visualization: a multidisciplinary approach* Amsterdam, Excerpta Medica.

Karim, S. M. M., Trussell, R. R., Hillier, K. and Patel, R. C. (1969) 'Induction of Labour with Prostaglandin F2x' *J. Obstet. Gynae. Brit. Comm.* 76, 9. pp. 769–82.

Karim, S. M. M., Trussell, R. R., Patel, R. C. and Hillier, K. (1968) 'Response of Pregnant Human Uterus to Prostaglandin — F_{2a} — Induction of Labour' *British Medical Journal* 4, pp. 621–3.

Kerr, J. M. (1933) *Maternal Mortality and Morbidity: a study of their problems* Edinburgh, E. and S. Livingstone.

Kerr, J. M. (1956) *Operative Obstetrics* (6th edition by J. Chassar Moir) London, Baillière, Tindall and Cox.

Kerr, J. M., Johnstone, R. W. and Phillips, M. H. (eds.) (1954) *Historical Review of British Obstetrics and Gynaecology 1800–1950* Edinburgh, E. and S. Livingstone.

Kerr, J. M. and MacLennan, H. R. (1932) 'An Investigation into the Mortality in Maternity Hospitals' *Lancet* 19 March, pp. 633–7.

Kerr, M. (1975) 'Problems and Perspectives in Reproductive Medicine' Inaugural Lecture, University of Edinburgh, 25 November.

Kerr, M. (1980) 'The Influence of Information on Perinatal Practice' in Chalmers, I. and McIlwaine, G. (eds.) *Perinatal Audit and Surveillance* Proceedings of the Eighth Study Group of the Royal College of Obstetricians and Gynaecologists, London.

Kirke, P. (1975) 'The Consumer's View of the Management of Labour' in Beard, R., Brudenell, M., Dunn, P. and Fairweather, D. (eds.) *The Management of Labour* Proceedings of the 3rd Study Group of the Royal College of Obstetricians and Gynaecologists, London.

Kitzinger, S. (1962) *The Experience of Childbirth* London, Gollancz.

Klopper, A. (1969) 'The Assessment of Placental Function in Clinical Practice' in Klopper and Diczfalusy (eds.).

Klopper, A. and Diczfalusy, E. (eds.) (1969) *Foetus and Placenta* Oxford, Blackwells Scientific Publications.

Klopper, A. and Farr, V. (n.d.) 'Proceedings of the International Symposium on the Treatment of Foetal Risks'. University of Vienna Medical School, Department of Obstetrics and Gynaecology.

Knaus, H. H. (1926) 'The Action of Pituitary Extract Administered by the Alimentary Canal' *British Medical Journal* 6 February, pp. 234–5.

Kopelevich, Y. X. (n.d.) 'Towards a History of the Problem of the Effect of the Mother's Organism on the Fetus', (in Russian).

Kossoff, G. (1980) 'Look Into the Future of Diagnostic Ultrasound' in Kurjak (ed.) (1980b).

Koster, H. and Perrotta, L. (1943) 'Elective Painless Rapid Childbirth Anticipating Labor' *Ex. Med. Surg.* I, pp. 143–7.

Kubli, F. (1971) 'Measurement of Placental Function' in Huntingford, et al. (eds.).

Kuensberg, C. (1980) 'Personal View' *British Medical Journal* 25 October, p. 1138.

Kuenssberg, E. V. and Sklaroff, S. A. (1958) 'General-Practice Midwifery' *The Practitioner* 180, pp. 717–28.

Kurjak, A. (ed.) (1978) *Recent Advances in Ultrasound Diagnosis* International Congress Series 436, Amsterdam, Excerpta Medica.

Kurjak, A. (1980a) *Progress in Medical Ultrasound* Volume I Amsterdam, Excerpta Medica.

Kurjak, A. (ed.) (1980b) *Recent Advances in Ultrasound Diagnosis* International Congress Series 498 Amsterdam, Excerpta Medica.

Lambert, P. (1976) 'Perinatal Mortality: social and environmental factors' *Population Trends* 4, Summer, pp. 4–8.

Landsteiner, K. and Wiener, A. S. (1940) 'An Agglutinable Factor in Human Blood Recognized by Immune Sera for Rhesus Blood *Proc. Soc. Exp. Biol. Med.* 43, p. 223.

Lane-Claypon, J. (1920) *The Child Welfare Movement* London, G. Bell.

Langevin, M.P. (1928) Les Oudes Ultrasonores *Revue Général de l'Electricité* 23, p. 626.

Lash, A. F. and Lash, S. R. (1950) 'Habitual Abortion: the incompetent internal os of the cervix' *American Journal of Obstetrics and Gynecology* 59, pp. 68–74.

Law, R. G. (1980) *Ultrasound in Clinical Obstetrics* Bristol, John Wright and Sons.

Leboyer, F. (1977) *Birth Without Violence* London, Fontana.

Leishmam, W. (1873) *A System of Midwifery* Glasgow, James Maclehose.

Lejumeau de Kedaradec, J. A. (1822) *Mémoire sur l'Auscultation Appliqué a l'Étude de la Grossesse* Paris, Méquignon-Marvis.

Lesinski, J. S. (1975) 'High Risk Concept in Maternity Care' *International Journal of Gynaecol. Obstet.* 13, pp. 65–73.

Letchworth, A. T. and Chard, T., (1972) 'Placental Lactogen Levels as a Screening Test for Fetal Distress and Neonatal Asphyxia' *Lancet* I, pp. 704–706.

Lewis, E. (1982) 'Attendance for Antenatal Care' *British Medical Journal* 1, p. 788.

Lewis, J. (1975) 'Beyond Suffrage: English feminism in the 1920s' *Maryland Historian* 7, Spring, pp. 1–17.

Lewis, J. (1980) *The Politics of Motherhood* London, Croom Helm.

Lewis, J. (1983) 'Dealing with Dependency: State practices and social realities, 1870–1945' in Lewis, J. (ed.) *Women's Welfare, Women's Rights* London, Croom Helm.

Lewis, J. and Davies, C. (1982) 'Sociological Models and Historical Scholarship'. Paper given to British Sociological Association Medical Sociology group and Society for the Social History of Medicine Annual Conference, University of Durham, 24–6 September.

Lewis, P. J., De Swiet, M., Boylan, P. and Bulpitt, C. J. (1980) 'How Obstetricians in the United Kingdom Manage Preterm Labour' *British Journal of Obstetrics and Gynaecology* 87, pp. 574–77.

Lewis, T. L. T. (1964) *Progress in Clinical Obstetrics and Gynaecology* London, J. and A. Churchill (2nd edition).

Leybourne-White, G. and White, K. (1945) *Children for Britain* London, Pilot Press.

Liley, A. W. (1976) 'Experiences with Uterine and Fetal Instrumentation' in Kaback and Valenti (eds.).

Lilford, R. J. and Chard, T. (1981) 'Microcomputers in Antenatal Care: a feasibility study on the booking interview' *British Medical Journal* 22 August, pp. 533–9.

Llewellyn-Jones, D. (1969) *Fundamentals of Obstetrics and Gynaecology Volume I Obstetrics* London, Faber and Faber.

Local Government Board (1910) *Thirty Ninth Annual Report for 1909–10. Supplement on Infant and Child Mortality*; (1913) *Report for 1912*; (1914) *Report for 1913*; (1915a) *Report for 1914–15, Supplement*; (1915b) *Memorandum on Health Visiting and on Maternity and Child Welfare Centres*, by the Medical Officer of the Board; (1917) *Report for 1915–16*; (1918) *Report for 1917–18*: London, HMSO.

Lofland, J. (1976) 'Open and Concealed Dramaturgic Strategies: the case of state execution' in Lofland, L. (ed.) *Toward a Sociology of Death and Dying* Beverly Hills, Sage.

Logan, D. (1934) 'The General Practitioner and Midwifery' *Lancet* 17 November, pp. 1141–3.

Logan, R. F. L., Pasker, P. and Klein, R. (1971) 'Patients as Consumers' *British Journal of Hospital Medicine* January, pp. 29–34.

London County Council (1918) *Annual Report of the County Medical Officer for London for 1917*, London, P. S. King and Co.

Lueck, J., Brewer, J. I., Aladjem, S. and Novotny, M. (1983) 'Observation of an Organism Found in Patients with Gestational Trophoblastic Disease and in Patients with Toxaemia of Pregnancy' *American Journal of Obstetrics and Gynecology* 145, pp. 15–26.

Lumley, J. (1983) 'Antepartum Fetal Heart Rate Tests and Induction of Labour' in Young (ed.).

Lumley, J. and Astbury, J. (1980) *Birth Rites, Birth Rights* Melbourne, Sphere Books.

Lynch, M. A. (1975) 'Ill-health and Child Abuse' *Lancet* 16 August, pp. 317–19.

McCleary, G. F. (1904) 'The Infant's Milk Depot: its history and function' *The Journal of Hygiene* July, pp. 329–68.

McCleary, G. F. (1905) *Infantile Mortality and Infants' Milk Depots* London, P. S. King and Son.

McCleary, G. F. (1933) *The Early History of the Infant Welfare Movement* London, H. K. Lewis.

McCleary, G. F. (1935) *The Maternity and Child Welfare Movement* London, P. S. King and Son.

McCleary, G. F. (1945) *Race Suicide* London, Allen and Unwin.

McDonald, I. A. (1957) 'Suture of the Cervix for Inevitable Miscarriage' *J. Obstet. Gynae. Brit. Emp.* Vol. 64. pp. 346–50.

MacFarlane, A. (1978) 'Variations in Number of Births and Perinatal Mortality by Day of the Week in England and Wales' *British Medical Journal* 2, pp. 1670–3.

MacFarlane, A. (1979) 'Perinatal Mortality' (letter) *Lancet* 4 August, pp. 255–6.

MacFarlane, A. and Mugford, M. (1984) *Birth Counts: statistics of pregnancy and childbirth* London, HMSO.

MacGregor, A. (1967) *Public Health in Glasgow 1905–46* Edinburgh, E. and S. Livingstone.

McGregor, R. M. and Martin, L. V. H. (1961) 'Obstetrics in General Practice' *Journal of the College of General Practitioners* 4, pp. 542–51.

McIlwaine, G. (1980) Oral Evidence given to the Social Services Committee (Short Report, 1980).

MacIntyre, S. (1977) 'The Management of Childbirth: a review of sociological research issues' *Social Science and Medicine* 11, pp. 477–84.

MacIntyre, S. (1981) 'Expectations and Experiences of First Pregnancy' Occasional Paper no. 5. University of Aberdeen, Institute of Medical Sociology.

Macintosh, J. C. and Davey, D. A. (1970) 'Preliminary Communications: chromosome aberrations induced by an ultrasonic fetal pulse detector' *British Medical Journal* 4, pp. 92–3.

MacKenzie, W. L. (1917) *Scottish Mothers and Children*. East Port, Dunfermline, The Carnegie United Kingdom Trust.

McKinlay, J. B. (1970) 'A Brief Description of a Study on the Utilization of Maternity and Child Welfare Services by the Lower Working Class Subculture' *Social Science and Medicine* 4, pp. 551–6.

McKinlay, J. B. (1979) 'Epidemiological and Political Determinants of Social Policies Regarding the Public Health' *Social Science and Medicine* 13A, pp. 541–58.

McKinlay, J. B. (1981) 'From "Promising Report" to "Standard Procedure": seven stages in the career of a medical innovation' *Milbank Memorial Fund Quarterly* 59, 3, pp. 374–411.

McLachlan, G. and Shegog, R. (eds.) (1970) *In the Beginning: studies of the maternity services* Oxford, Oxford University Press.

McNally, F. (1979) *Women for Hire* London, Macmillan.

MacVicar, J. and Donald, I. (1963) 'Sonar in the Diagnosis of Early Pregnancy and its Complications' *J. Obstet. Gynae. Brit. Comm.* 70, pp. 387–95.

Mandelstam, D. A. (1971) 'The Value of Antenatal Preparation: a statistical survey' *Midwife and Health Visitor* 7, pp. 217–24.

Marcus, S. L. and Marcus, C. C. (eds.) (1967) *Advances in Obstetrics and Gynecology Volume I* Baltimore, Williams and Wilkins.

Mass Observation (1945) *Britain and Her Birth Rate* London, John Murray.

Maternity Alliance and National Council for Voluntary Organizations Health and Handicap Group (1983) Prepregnancy Care: a joint statement *Socialism and Health* March/April, p. 10.

Mathie, J. G. and Dawson, B. H. (1959) 'Effect of Castor Oil, Soap Enema and Hot Bath on the Pregnant Human Uterus Near Term' *British Medical Journal* I, pp. 1162–1165.

Maurice, Major-General Sir J. F. (1903) 'National Health, A Soldier's Study' *Contemporary Review* January, pp. 41–56.

Mead, M. (1974) *Los Angeles Times* 5 February part 4, p. 6.

Mead, M. and Newton, N. (1967) 'Cultural Patterning of Perinatal Behaviour' in Richardson and Guttmacher (eds.).

Mechling, J. (1975) 'Advice to Historians on Advice to Mothers' *Journal of Social History* 9, 1–2, pp. 44–63.

Medical Research Committee (1917) *The Mortalities of Birth, Infancy and Childhood* London, HMSO.

Medical Research Committee (1926) *Child Life Investigations: a clinical and pathological study of 1673 cases of dead-births and neo-natal deaths* (by Holland, E. and Lane-Claypon, J.) London, HMSO.

Medical Research Council (1978) Working Party. 'An Assessment of the Hazards of Amniocentesis' *British Journal of Obstetrics and Gynaecology* Supplement 2, p. 85.

Melchior, J. (1969) 'Comments on Fetal Heart Rate Monitoring' in Huntingford, et al. (eds.).

Merrington, W. R. (1976) *University College Hospital and Its Medical School: a history* London, Heinemann.

Metropolitan Borough of Battersea (1905) *Annual Report of the Council for the Year ended 31 March 1905*.

'Miles' (Maurice, Major-General Sir J. F.) (1902) 'Where to Get Men' *Contemporary Review* January, pp. 78–86.

Miller, J. A. and Marini, A. (1958) 'Cardiac Activity in Apneic Five Hundred Eighty Gram Human Fetus' *Journal of the American Medical Association* 167, pp. 976–82.

Miller, J. H. (1978) '"Temple and Sewer": childbirth, prudery and Victoria Regina' in Wohl, A. S. (ed.) *The Victorian Family* London, Croom Helm.

Ministry of Health (1922) *Report on the Causation of Foetal Death* (by Holland, E.) Reports on Public Health and Medical Subjects No. 7, London HMSO.

Ministry of Health (1923a) *Notes on the Arrangements for Teaching Obstetrics and Gynaecology in the Medical Schools* (by Campbell, J. M.) Reports on Public Health and Medical Subjects No. 15, London, HMSO.

Ministry of Health (1923b) *The Training of Midwives* (by Campbell, J. M.) Reports on Public Health and Medical Subjects No. 21, London, HMSO.

Ministry of Health (1924) *Maternal Mortality* (by Campbell, J.M.) Reports on Public Health and Medical Subjects No. 25, London, HMSO.

Ministry of Health (1927) *The Protection of Motherhood* (by Campbell, J. M.) Reports on Public Health and Medical Subjects No. 48, London, HMSO.

Ministry of Health (1929a) *Infant Mortality* (by Campbell, J. M.) Reports on Public Health and Medical Subjects No. 55, London, HMSO.

Ministry of Health (1929b) *Report of the Departmental Committee on the Training and Employment of Midwives* London, HMSO.

Ministry of Health (1932) *High Maternal Mortality in Certain Areas* (by Campbell, J. M., Cameron, I. D. and Jones, D. M.) Reports on Public Health and Medical Subjects No. 68, London, HMSO.

Ministry of Health (1937) *Report on an Investigation into Maternal Mortality* London, HMSO.

Ministry of Health (1949) *Report of the Working Party on Midwives* London, HMSO.

Montgomery, W. F. (1856) *An Exposition of the Signs and Symptoms of Pregnancy* London, Longman, Brown, Green, Longmans and Roberts (first edition 1838).

Moore, S. G. (1928) 'The Relative Value of Intensive Methods Employed for the Reduction of Infant Mortality' in National Association for Maternal and Child Welfare *Annual Conference Reports 1924–31.*

Morris, J. N. and Heady, J. A. (1955) 'Social and Biological Factors in Infant Mortality: V mortality in relation to the father's occupation 1911–1950' *Lancet* 12 March, pp. 554–9.

Morris, N. (1960) 'Human Relations in Obstetrics' *Lancet* 23 April, pp. 913–5.

Morton, D. G. (1933) 'Induction of Labor by Means of Artificial Rupture of Membranes 'Castor Oil and Quinine and Nasal Pituitrin' *American Journal of Obstetrics and Gynecology* 26, pp. 323–29.

Murphy, D. P. (1947) *Uterine Contractility in Pregnancy* Philadelphia, Lippincott.

Murray, G. C. P. (1858) 'Diagnosis of the Fetus in Utero by Means of External Palpation' *Lancet* 13 March, pp. 262–3.

Myers, R. E. (1979) 'Maternal Anxiety and Fetal Death' in Zichella, L. and Pancheri, P. (eds.) *Psychoendocrinology in Reproduction* Elsevier, Holland, North-Holland Biomedical Press.

Nabors, G. C. (1958) 'Castor Oil as an Adjunct to Induction of Labor: critical reevaluation' *American Journal of Obstetrics and Gynecology* 75, pp. 36–8.

National League for Health, Maternity and Child Welfare (1915) *Report*, London.

Navarro, V. (1976) *Medicine Under Capitalism* New York, Prodist.

Neilson, J. P. and Whitfield, C. R. (1981) 'Ultrasound in Obstetrics' (letter) *Lancet* 11 July, p. 94.

Neldam, S. (1980) 'Fetal Movements as an Indicator of Fetal Wellbeing' *Lancet* 7 June, pp. 1222–4.

Newcombe, R. G. and Chalmers, I. (1981) 'Assessing the Risk of Preterm Labour' in Elder, M. G. and Hendricks, C. H. (eds.) *Preterm Labour* London, Butterworth.

Newman, G. (1906) *Infant Mortality: a social problem* London, Methuen.

Newman, G. (1930) *Health and Social Evolution* London, Allen and Unwin.

Niswander, K. R., Patterson, R. J. and Randall, C. L. (1960) 'Elective Induction of Labor' *American Journal of Obstetrics and Gynecology* 79, 4, pp. 797–80.

Niven, J. (1906) 'The Teaching in Schools of Elementary Hygiene in Reference to the Rearing of Infants' in *Report of the Proceedings of the National Conference on Infantile Mortality*, London.

Nixon, W. C. W. and Smyth, C. N. (1959) 'Old and New Methods for Induction of Labor and of Premature Labor' *American Journal of Obstetrics and Gynecology* 77, pp. 393–405.

Oakley, A. Unpublished data, Transition to Motherhood Project, Bedford College, University of London, 1974–9.

Oakley, A. (1980) *Women Confined* Oxford, Martin Robertson.

Oakley, A., Macfarlane, A. and Chalmers, I. (1982) 'Social Class, Stress and Reproduction' in Rees, A. R. and Purcell, H. (eds.) *Disease and the Environment* Chichester, Sussex, John Wiley.

Obata, I. (1912) 'Die Knoehenkerne des Fötalen Menschlichen Beckens' *Zeitschr. f. Geb. u. Gynäk. Bd.* LXXII, pp. 533–74.

O'Brien, M. and Smith, C. (1981) 'Women's Experiences of Antenatal Care' *Practitioner* 225, pp. 123–5.

O'Brien, P. (1963) 'The General-Practitioner Obstetrician' *Lancet* 14 September, pp. 568–73.

O'Driscoll, K. and Meagher, D. (1980) *Active Management of Labour* London, W. B. Saunders.

Office of Population Censuses and Surveys (1982) *Birth Statistics 1980* London, HMSO.

Oppenheimer, J. M. (1968) 'Some Historical Relationships between Teratology and Experimental Embryology' *Bull. Hist. Med.* 42, pp. 145–159.

Ounsted, C., Roberts, J., Gordon, M. and Milligan, B. (1982) 'Fourth Goal of Perinatal Medicine' *British Medical Journal* 20 March, pp. 879–82.

Owen, G. M. (1982) 'Health Visiting' in Allan and Jolley (eds.).

Oxley, W. H. F., Phillips, M. H. and Young, J. (1935) 'Maternal Mortality in Rochdale: an achievement in a black area' *British Medical Journal* 16 February, pp. 304–7.

Page, E. W. (1943) 'Response of Human Pregnant Uterus to Pitocin Tannate in Oil' *Proc. Soc. Exp. Biol.* 2, pp. 195–7.

Palmer, D. (n.d.) 'The Departmental Committee on Maternal Mortality (1928–32): the Ministry of Health's attempt to tackle a persistent public health problem'. Unpublished paper, Department of Sociology, University of Warwick.

Paneth, N., Kiely, J., Stein, Z. and Susser, M. (1981) 'The Incidence of Cerebral Palsy: which way are we going?' *Dev. Med. Child. Neurol.* 23, pp. 111–2.

Pankhurst, S. (1930) *Save the Mothers* London, Knopf.

Parkes, A. S. (1966) 'The Rise of Reproductive Endocrinology 1926–40' *J. Endocrin.* 34, pp. xx–xxiv.

Parsons, W. D. and Perkins, E. R. (1980) 'Why Don't Women Attend for Antenatal Care?' Leverhulme Health Education Project, University of Nottingham, Occasional Paper No. 23.

Patterson, J. H. (1961) 'G.P.s' Clinical Authority' *British Medical Journal* 2, Supplement, pp. 172–3.

Pearson, J. F. and Weaver, J. B. (1976) 'Fetal Activity and Fetal Wellbeing: an evaluation' *British Medical Journal* 29 May, pp. 1305–7.

Pedersen, J. F. (1980) 'Ultrasound Evidence of Sexual Difference in Fetal Size in First Trimester' *British Medical Journal* 8 November, p. 1253.

Peel Committee (1970) (Standing Maternity and Midwifery Advisory Committee) *Domiciliary Midwifery and Maternity Bed Needs* London, HMSO.

Perkins, E. R. (1980) 'The Pattern of Women's Attendance at Antenatal Classes: is this good enough?' *Health Education Journal* 39, 1, pp. 3–9.

Peters, D. P. and Ceci, S. J. (1982) 'Peer-review Practices of Psychological Journals: the fate of published articles submitted again' *The Behavioural and Brain Sciences* 5, pp. 187–255.

Pfaundler, M. (1936) 'Studien über Frühtod, Geschlechtsvarhältnis und Selection' *Ztsch. Kinderheilk* 57, pp. 185–227.

Philipp, E. (1975) *Childlessness* London, Arrow.

Pinard, A. (1889) *Traité de Palper Abdominal au Point de Vue Obstétrical, et de la Version par Manoeuvres externes* Paris, 2nd edition.

Pinker, R. (1966) *English Hospital Statistics 1861–1938* London, Heinemann.

Playfair, W. S. (1898) *A Treatise on the Science and Practice of Midwifery* London, Smith Elder (first edition 1876).

Playfair, P. L. (1941) 'Uroselectan B as a Method of Inducing Labour' *Journal of Obstetrics and Gynaecology* 48, pp. 41–59.

Plentl, A. A. and Friedman, E. A. (1963) 'Sparteine Sulfate: a clinical evaluation of its use for the induction of labour' *American Journal of Obstetrics and Gynecology* 85, pp. 200–8.

Podleschka, K. (1932) 'Die Cystotokographie, eine Methode zur Registrierung des Weheneffektes auf den Uterusausführungsgang' *Arch. Gynäk.* 152, p. 159.

Political and Economic Planning (1937) *Report on the British Health Services* London.

Political and Economic Planning (1946) *A Complete Maternity Service* Broadsheet No. 244, 31 January.

Porritt, N. (1934) *The Menace and Geography of Eclampsia in England and Wales* Humphrey Milford, Oxford University Press.

Potts, M. (1980) 'Antenatal, anti-natal' *Guardian* 10 March.

Poullet, J. (1880) 'Du Tocographe. Application de la Methode Graphique aux Accouchements' *Arch. de Tocologie* 7, pp. 65–80.

Pusch, D. and Schmidt, E. (1983) Prenatal Care in European Countries. Unpublished Report, World Health Organization.

Queen Charlotte's Textbook of Obstetrics (1970) by J. S. Tomkinson, London, J. and A. Churchill.

Quilligan, E. J. and Freeman, R. K. (1969) 'The Status of Fetal Monitoring in Decision-Making and in Patient Management' in Reid, D. E. and Barton, T. C. (eds.) *Controversy in Obstetrics and Gynecology* W. B. Saunders.

Radcliffe, W. (1967) *Milestones in Midwifery* Bristol, John Wright and Sons.

Rasor, P. A. (1981) 'Gurkha Obstetrics and Perinatal Mortality in the New Territories: Hong Kong *Journal of the Royal Army Medical Corps* 127, pp. 26–30.

Reading, A. E., Campbell, S., Cox, D. N. and Sledmere, C. M. (1982) 'Health Beliefs and Health Care Behaviour in Pregnancy' *Psychological Medicine* 12, pp. 379–83.

Redman, C. (1982) 'Management of Pre-Eclampsia' in Enkin and Chalmers (eds.).

Redman, T. F. and Walker, S. C. B. (1954) 'Evolution of Hospitals and Local Authority Antenatal Care under the N.H.S. Act' *British Medical Journal* 3 July, pp. 41–3.

Reece, L. N. (1935) 'The Estimation of Foetal Maternity by a New Method of X-ray Cephalometry: its bearing on clinical midwifery' *Proc. Roy. Soc. Med.* 18 January, pp. 489–504.

Rees, H. G. St. M. (1961) 'A Domiciliary Obstetric Practice 1948–58' *Journal of the College of General Practitioners* 4, pp. 47–71.

Registrar-General (1929) *Statistical Review for 1927* London, HMSO.

Registrar-General (1935) *Statistical Review for 1932* London, HMSO.

Reid, M. E., Gutteridge, S. and McIlwaine, G. M. (1983) A Comparison of the Delivery of Antenatal Care between a Hospital and a Peripheral Clinic. Social Paediatric and Obstetric Research Unit, Glasgow, Report submitted to Health Services Research Committee, Scottish Home and Health Department.

Reid, M.E. and McIlwaine, G. M. (1980) 'Consumer Opinion of a Hospital Antenatal Clinic' *Social Science and Medicine* 14A, pp. 363–8.

Reid, R. (1978) *Marie Curie* London, Paladin.

Reilly, W. J. (1979) 'Personal View' *British Medical Journal* 21 April, p. 1077.

Reiser, S. J. (1978) *Medicine and the Reign of Technology* Cambridge, Cambridge University Press.

Reynolds, S. R. M., Harris, J. S. and Kaiser, I. H. (1954) *Clinical Measurement of Uterine Forces in Pregnancy and Labor* Springfield, Illinois, C. C. Thomas.

Rhodes, P. (1977) *Doctor John Leake's Hospital. A History of the General Lying-In Hospital 1765–1971* London, Davis-Poynter.

Rhys-Williams, Lady (1936) 'Malnutrition as a Cause of Maternal Mortality' *Public Health* 50, October, pp. 11–19.

Riley, E. M. D. (1977) 'What Do Women Want? The question of choice in the conduct of labour' in Chard and Richards (eds.).

Richards, M. P. M. (1975) 'Innovation in Medical Practice: obstetricians and the induction of labour in Britain' *Social Science and Medicine* 9, pp. 595–602.

Richards, M. P. M. (1980) 'Is Neonatal Special Care Overused?' *Birth and the Family Journal* 7, 4, pp. 225–7.

Richardson, S. A. and Guttmacher, A. F. (eds.) (1967) *Childbearing — Its Social and Psychological Aspects* Baltimore, Williams and Wilkins.

Riddell, J. R. (1907) 'Measurement of Pelvic Diameters by the Roentgen Rays' *British Medical Journal* 14 September, pp. 636–7.

Riley, M. (1968) *Brought to Bed* New York, A. S. Barnes.

Roberts, A. B., Little, D. J., Cooper, D. and Campbell, S. (1980) 'Fetal Activity in Normal and Growth-Retarded Fetuses' in Bennett and Campbell (eds.).

Robinson, D. (1973) *Patients, Practitioners and Medical Care* London, Heinemann.

Robinson, S., Golden, J. and Bradley, S. (1982) 'The Role of the Midwife in the Provision of Antenatal Care' in Enkin and Chalmers (eds.).

Rodeck, C. H., Patrick, A. D., Pembrey, M. E., Tzannatos, C. and Whitfield, A. E. (1982) 'Fetal Liver Biopsy for Prenatal Diagnosis of Ornithine Carbamyl Transferase Deficiency' *Lancet* 27 August, pp. 297–9.

Rosebery, Earl of (1900) *The Times* 17 November.

Rosen, A. (1974) *Rise Up, Women!* London, Routledge and Kegan Paul.

Ross, J. S. (1952) *The National Health Service in Great Britain: an historical and descriptive study* London, Oxford University Press.

Rowland, B. (ed.) (1981) *Medieval Woman's Guide to Health* London, Croom Helm.

Rowntree, S. (1937) *The Human Needs of Labour* London, Longmans, Green and Co.

Royal College of Obstetricians and Gynaecologists (1944) *Report on A National Maternity Service* London, RCOG.

Royal College of Obstetricians and Gynaecologists (1982a) *Report of the RCOG Working Party on Antenatal and Intrapartum Care* London, RCOG.

Royal College of Obstetricians and Gynaecologists (1982b) *Report of the Working Party on Further Specialization Within Obstetrics and Gynaecology* London, RCOG.

Royal College of Obstetricians and Gynaecologists (1983a) *Nutrition in Pregnancy: proceedings of the 10th study group of the RCOG* London, RCOG.

Royal College of Obstetricians and Gynaecologists (1983b) *Report of the RCOG Ethics Committee on in vitro Fertilization and Embryo Replacement or Transfer* London, RCOG.

Royal College of Obstetricians and Gynaecologists (1984) *Prenatal Diagnosis; proceedings of the 11th study group of the RCOG* London, RCOG.

Royal College of Obstetricians and Gynaecologists and Royal College of General Practitioners (1981) *Report on Training for Obstetrics and Gynaecology for GPs by a Joint Working Party of the RCOG and RCGP* London.

Royal Commission on the Population (1945) *Statement* London, HMSO.

Royal Commission on the Population (1949) *Report* London, HMSO.

Rubovits, F. E., Cooperman, N. R. and Lash, A. F. (1953) 'Habitual Abortion: a radiographic technique to demonstrate the incompetent internal os of the cervix' *American Journal of Obstetrics and Gynecology* 66, pp. 269–80.

Russell, A. W. (1912) *Prophylaxis in Obstetrics and Other Papers on Obstetrical and Gynaecological Subjects* Glasgow, James Maclehose and Sons.

Russell, C. S. (1956) 'Home Confinement' *Lancet* 12 May, pp. 681–3.

Russell, H. (1971) *J. W. Ballantyne 1861–1923* Edinburgh, Royal College of Physicians.

Ruzek, S. B. (1979) *The Women's Health Movement* New York, Praeger.

Sadovsky, E., Polishuk, W. Z., Mahler, Y., Malkin, A. (1973) 'Correlation between Electromagnetic Recording and Maternal Assessment of Fetal Movement' *Lancet* 26 May, pp. 1141–3.

Sadovsky, E. and Yaffe, H. (1973) 'Daily Fetal Movement Recording and Fetal Prognosis' *Obstet. Gynecol.* 41, pp. 845–50.

Saint-Hilaire, E.-G. (1822) *Philosophie Anatomique: des monstruosités humaines* Paris, Rignoux.

Saleeby, C. W. (1915) 'The Problem of the Future' in National League for Physical Education and Improvement *Mothercraft. A course of lectures delivered under the auspices of the National Association for the Prevention of Infant Mortality* London.

Saling, E. (1962) 'Die Amnioskopie, ein Neus Verfahren sum Erkennen von Gefahrenznständen des Feten bei noch Stehender Fruchtblase *Geburtsch. u. Frauenheilk* 22, p. 830.

Saling, E. (1969) 'Opening Address' in Huntingford, Hüter and Saling (eds.).

Salmond, R. W. A. (1937) 'The Uses and Value of Radiology in Obstetrics' in Browne (1937).

Schatz, F. (1872) 'Beitrage zur Physiologischen Geburtskunde' *Arch. Gynäk.* 3, p. 58.

Scrimgeour, J. B. (1974) (eds.) 'Fetoscopy' in Motulsky, A. G. and Lenz, W. (eds.) *Birth Defects:*

proceedings of the 4th International conference International Congress Series No. 310, Amsterdam, Excerpta Medica.

Scully, D. (1980) *Men Who Control Women's Health* Boston, Houghton Mifflin.

Seaman, B. and Seaman, G. (1978) *Women and the Crisis in Sex Hormones* New York, Bantam.

Selwyn, H. J. (1982) 'Review of Obstetrical Risk Assessment Methods' in Institute of Medicine and National Research Council *Research Issues in the Assessment of Birth Settings* Washington, National Academy Press.

Shanks, S. C. (1950) 'Fifty Years of Radiology' *British Medical Journal* 7, 1, pp. 44–8.

Shaw, W. F. (1954) *Twenty Five Years: the story of the Royal College of Obstetricians and Gynaecologists 1929–54* London, J. and A. Churchill.

Shirodkar, V. N. (1953) 'Some Observations on Non-Malignant Conditions of the Cervix' *Journal of Obstetrics and Gynaecology of India*, 3, pp. 287–9.

Short Report (1980) (Second Report from the Social Services Committee) *Perinatal and Neonatal Mortality* London, HMSO.

Siddall, A. C. (1980) 'Bloodletting in American Obstetric Practice 1800–1945' *Bulletin of the History of Medicine* 54, pp. 101–10.

Simkin, P. (1983) 'Amniotomy' in Young, D. (ed.).

Simpson, H. and Walker, G. (1980) 'When do Pregnant Women Attend for Antenatal Care?' *British Medical Journal* 2, pp. 104–7.

Sleep, J., Grant, A., Garcia, J., Elbourne, D., Spencer, J. and Chalmers, I. (1983) 'The West Berkshire Perineal Management Trial' Paper presented at the 23rd British Congress of Obstetrics and Gynaecology, Birmingham, 13 July.

Smith, A. (1970) 'Progress in the 1960s and Problems for the 1970s' in McLachlan and Shegog (eds.).

Smith, F. B. (1979) *The People's Health 1830–1910* London, Croom Helm.

Smith, F. W., Adam, A. H. and Phillips, W. D. P. (1983) 'NMR Imaging in Pregnancy' *Lancet* I, pp. 61–2.

Smith, G. V. and Smith, O. W. (1933) 'Excessive Anterior-Pituitary-Like Hormone and Variations in Oestrin in the Toxemias of Late Pregnancy' *Proc. Soc. Exper. Biol. and Med.* 30, pp. 918–919.

Smithells, R. W., Shepherd, S., Schorah, C. J., Seller, M. J., Nevin, N. C., Harris, R., Read, A. P. and Fielding, D. W. (1981) 'Apparent Prevention of Neural Tube Defects by Vitamin Supplementation' *Arch. Dis. Childh.* 56, pp. 911–8.

Snowden, R. and Mitchell, G. D. (1983) *The Artificial Family* London, Unwin.

Solesh, G. I., Masterson, J. G., Hellman, L. M., (1961) 'Pelvic Arteriography in Obstetrics' *American Journal of Obstetrics and Gynecology* 81, pp. 57–66.

Sontag, S. (1977) *Illness as Metaphor* New York, Farrar, Straus and Giroux.

Spastics Society (1981) *Who's Holding the Baby Now?* London, Spastics Society.

Speidel, E. and Turner, H. H. (1924) 'The Roentgen Ray Diagnosis of Normal and Abnormal Pregnancies' *Amer. J. Obst. Gyn.* 7, pp. 697–702.

Spencer, H. R. (1901) 'The Dangers and Diagnosis of Breech Presentation and its Treatment by External Version Towards the End of Pregnancy' *British Medical Journal* 18 May, pp. 1192–6.

Spencer, H. R. (1927) *The History of British Midwifery from 1650–1800* John Bale, Sons and Danielsson Ltd.

Spring Rice, M. (1939) *Working Class Wives* London, Penguin (reprinted Virago 1981).

Stacey, M. (1976) 'The Health Service Consumer: a sociological misconception' in Stacey, M. (ed.) *The Sociology of the National Health Service* Monograph 22, University of Keele, Staffordshire.

Standing Medical Advisory Committee (1963) *The Field of Work of the Family Doctor* London, HMSO.

Standing Medical Advisory Committee (1979) *Report by the Working Party on Screening for Neural Tube Defects* London, HMSO.

Steinbacher, R. (1981) 'Futuristic Implications of Sex Preselection' in Holmes, et al.

Steptoe, P. C. and Edwards, R. G. (1978) 'Birth after the Implantation of a Human Embryo' *Lancet* 12 August, p. 366.

Stern, L., Lind, J. and Kaplan, B. (1961) 'Direct Human Foetal Electrocardiography (with studies of the effects of adrenaline, atrophine, clamping of the umbilical cord and placental separation of the foetal ECG)' *Biol. Neonat.* 3, p. 49.

Stevens, R. (1966) *Medical Practice in Modern England: the impact of specialization on state medicine* New Haven, Yale University Press.

Stewart, A. L., Reynolds, E. O. R. and Lipscombe, A. P. (1981) 'Outcome for Infants of VLBW: survey of world literature' *Lancet* 9 May, pp. 1038–41.

Stewart, A., Webb, J., Giles, D. and Hewitt, D. (1956) 'Malignant Disease in Childbood and Diagnostic Irradiation in Utero' *Lancet*, 2, p. 447.

Stilwell, J. A. (1979) 'Relative Costs of Home and Hospital Confinement' *British Medical Journal* 28 July, pp. 257–9.

Stone, M. L. (1979) 'Presidential Address' *American College of Obstetricians and Gynecologists Newsletter* 4 May.

Stratmeyer, M. E. (1980) 'Research in Ultrasound Bioeffects: a public health view' *Birth and the Family Journal* 7, 2, pp. 92–100.

Sturrock, J. (1958) 'Early Maternity Hospitals in Edinburgh' *British Journal of Obstetrics and Gynaecology* 65, pp. 122–31.

Sturrock, J. (1969) 'James Haig Ferguson and his Contribution to Obstetrics' William Meredith Fletcher Shaw Memorial Lecture, 41st Annual Report of the Royal College of Obstetricians and Gynaecologists, pp. 81–94.

Sutherland, I. (1949) *Stillbirths: their epidemiology and social significance* London, Oxford University Press.

Taylor, R. (1979) *Medicine Out of Control* Melbourne, Sun Books.

Taylor, S. (1944) *Battle for Health* London, Adprint Ltd.

Taylor, W. and Dauncey, M. (1954) 'Changing Patterns of Mortality in England and Wales' *Brit. J. Prev. Soc. Med.* 8, pp. 172–5.

Tew, M. (1977) 'Where to be born?' *New Society* 20 January, pp. 120–1.

Theobald, G. W. (1974) 'The Induction of Labour' in Hawkins, D. F. (ed.) *Obstetric Therapeutics* London, Baillière and Tindall.

Theobald, G. W., Kelsey, H. A. and Muirhead, J. M. B. (1956) 'The Pitocin Drip' *J. Obstet. Gynae. Brit. Emp.* 63, 5, pp. 641–62.

Thoms, H. (1935) *Classical Contributions to Obstetrics and Gynecology* Springfield, Illinois, C. C. Thomas.

Titmuss, R. M. (1943) *Birth, Poverty and Wealth* London, Hamish Hamilton.

Titmuss, R. M. (1950) *Problems of Social Policy* London, HMSO.

Titmuss, R. M. (1959) 'Health' in Ginsberg, M. (ed.) *Law and Opinion in the Twentieth Century* London, Steven and Sons.

Titmuss, R. M. and Abel-Smith, B. (1956) *The Cost of the National Health Service in England and Wales* National Institute of Economic and Social Research Occasional Papers, 18, Cambridge.

Titmuss, R. and Titmuss, K. (1942) *Parents' Revolt* London, Secker and Warburg.

Topping, A. (1936) 'Maternal Mortality and Public Opinion' *Public Health* 45, pp. 342–9.

Townsend, P. and Davidson, N. (1982) *Inequalities in Health* Harmondsworth, Penguin.

Trounson, A. and Conti, A. (1982) 'Research in Human In Vitro Fertilization and Embryo Transfer' *British Medical Journal* 24 July, pp. 244–8.

Tuckman, E. (1953) 'A General Practitioner Midwifery Service' *Medical World* 79, pp. 465–72.

Tulchinsky, D. (1974) 'Hormonal Changes in Pregnancy as Indicators of Fetoplacental Function' in Curry and Hewitt (eds.).

Turnbull, A. C. and Anderson, A. B. M. (1967) 'Induction of Labour' *J. Obstet. Gynae. Brit. Comm.* 7A, pp. 849–54.

Turnbull, A. C. and Anderson, A. B. M. (1968) 'Induction of Labour' *J. Obstet. Gynae. Brit. Comm.* 75, pp. 24–31.

Turnbull, A. C. and Woodford, F. P. (eds.) (1976) *Prevention of Handicap Through Antenatal Care* Amsterdam, Elsevier.

Tyler Smith, W. (1858) *A Manual of Obstetrics* London, John Churchill.

Underwood, E. A. (1957) 'William Conrad Röntgen (1845–1923) and the Early Development of Radiology' in Cope, Z. (ed.) *Sidelights on the History of Medicine* London, Butterworth.

Valenti, C. (1972) 'Endoamnioscopy and Fetal Biopsy: a new technique' *American Journal of Obstetrics and Gynecology* 114, pp. 561–4.

Van Dongen, L. G. R. (1956) 'Induction of Labour' *South African Medical Journal* 6 October, pp. 959–64.

Versluysen, M. (1981) 'Lying-in Hospitals in Eighteenth Century London' in Roberts, H. (ed.) *Women, Health and Reproduction* London, Routledge and Kegan Paul.

Vigneaud, V. Du, Ressler, C., Swan, J. M., Roberts, C. W. and Katsoyannis P. G. (1954) 'The Synthesis of Oxytocin' *J. Am. Chem. Soc.* 76, pp. 3115–21.

Visser, G. H. A., Goodman, J. D. S., Levine, D. H. and Davies, G. S. (1981) 'Micturition and the Heart Period Cycle in the Human Fetus' *British Journal of Obstetrics and Gynaecology* 88, pp. 803–5.

Vartan, C. K. (1962) 'Castor Oil for Induction of Labour' (letter) *British Medical Journal* 2, p. 1397.

Walters, W. and Singer, P. (1982) *Test-Tube Babies* Melbourne, Oxford University Press.

Webb, S. and Webb, B. (eds.) (1909) *The Break-up of the Poor Law, being part one of the Minority Report of the Poor Law Commission* London, Longmans, Green and Co.

Webb, S. and Webb, B. (1910) *The State and the Doctor* London, Longmans, Green and Co.

Wertz, R. W. and Wertz, D. C. (1977) *Lying-In: a history of childbirth in America* New York, the Free Press.

Westermark, F. (1893) 'Experimentelle Untersuchungen über die Wehentätigkeit des Menschlichen Uterus bie die Physiologischen Geburt. *Skandinav. Arch. f. Physiol.* 4, p. 331.

Westin, B. (1954) 'Hysteroscopy in Early Pregnancy' *Lancet* 2, p. 872.

Which? (1971) 'Maternity Services' June, pp. 164–71.

White, A. (1901) *Efficiency and Empire* London.

White, C. (1773) *A Treatise on the Management of Pregnant and Lying-in Women*, London.

Whitfield, C. R. (1969) 'The Significance of Methods for Monitoring the Fetal Heart' in Huntingford, et al (eds.).

Williams, J. W. (1903) *Obstetrics: a textbook for the use of students and practitioners* New York, D. Appleton and Co.

Williams, M. and Booth, H. D. (1974) *Antenatal Education: guidelines for teachers* Edinburgh, Churchill Livingstone.

Williamson, N. E. (1976) 'Sex Preferences, Sex Control and the Status of Women' *SIGNS: Journal of Women in Culture and Society* 1, pp. 847–62.

Williamson, R., Eskdale, J., Coleman, D. V., Niazi, M. Loeffler, F. E. and Modell, B. M. (1981) 'Direct Gene Analysis of Chorionic Villi: a possible technique for first-trimester antenatal diagnosis of haemoglobinopathies' *Lancet* 21 November, pp. 1125–9.

Willocks, J., Donald, I., Duggan, T. C. and Day, N. (1964) 'Foetal Cephalometry by Ultrasound' *J. Obstet. Gynae. Brit. Comm.* 71, pp. 11–20.

Windeyer, J. C. (1922) 'Pre-Maternity Work' *The Medical Journal of Australia* 16 September, pp. 325–7.

Winter, J. M. (1979) 'Infant Mortality, Maternal Mortality and Public Health in Britain in the 1980s' *The Journal of European Economic History* 8, 2, pp. 439–62.

Winter, J. M. (1981) 'Economic Instability and Infant Mortality in England and Wales 1920–50, in Winter, J. (ed.) *The Working Class in Modern British History* Cambridge, Cambridge University Press.

Wladimiroff, J. W. and Laar, J. (1980) 'Ultrasonic measurement of fetal body size: a randomised controlled trial' *Acta Obstet. Gynecol. Scand.* 59, pp. 177–9.

Wladimiroff, J. W., Leijs, R. and Smit, B. (1980) 'Human Fetal Stomach Profiles' in Kurjak (ed.) (1980b).

Woodbury, R. A., Hamilton, W. F. and Torpin, F. (1939) 'The Relationship between Abdominal, Uterine and Arterial Pressures During Labour' *American Journal of Physiology* 121, pp. 640–649.

Workers' Educational Association (n.d.) *The Future of the Family* London.

World Health Organization (1957) *Epidemiological and Vital Statistics Report* 57.

World Health Organization (1974) Scientific Group on Health Statistics *Methodology Related to Perinatal Events* WHO Document ICD/74.4, Geneva.

Wrigley, A. J. (1934) 'A Criticism of Ante-natal Work' *British Medical Journal* 19 May, pp. 891–4.

Young, D. (ed.) (1983) *Obstetrical Intervention and Technology in the 1980s* New York, the Haworth Press.

Young, J. H. (1964) *St Mary's Hospitals Manchester 1790–1963* Edinburgh, E. and S. Livingstone.

Yu, V. Y. H., Hewson, P. H. and Hollingsworth, E. (1979) 'Iatrogenic Hazards of Neonatal Intensive Care in Extremely Low Birthweight Infants' *Austr. Paediatr. J.* 15, pp. 233–7.

Zander, L. I., Watson, M., Taylor, R. W. and Morrell, D. C. (1978) 'Integration of General-Practitioner and Specialist Antenatal Care' *Journal of the Royal College of General Practitioners* August, pp. 455–8.

Zola, I. K. (1977) 'Healthism and Disabling Medicalization' in Illich, I., Zola, I. K., McKnight, J., Caplan, J. and Shaiken, H. *Disabling Professions* London, Marion Boyars.

Hospital and other archives, main sources

Bristol Lying-in Hospital (later Bristol Maternity Hospital): Reports for 1910–1946.

Bristol Royal Infirmary: Intern Maternity Book 1922, Admissions Book 1776–1781, Extern Midwifery Department Case Book 1912–3 and 1914–5.

Edinburgh Royal Maternity and Simpson Memorial Hospital: Directors' Minutes Books 1881, 1884, 1901; Reports by the Directors 1915–25; Annual Reports for 1929, 1938; Medical and Clinical Reports for 1934, 1937; House Committee Minutes 1915–1919.

Glasgow Royal Maternity and Women's Hospital (later Glasgow Royal Maternity Hospital): House Committee Minutes 1913–6; Miscellaneous Papers (held in Divisional Nursing Officer's Room); Minutes of Meetings 1913–48; Annual Reports 1858–76, 1908–47; Medical Reports 1929–51; G.R.M.H. and The Ross Hospital Clinical Reports 1960–2.

Reports of the Medical Officer of Health for Glasgow 1914–19, 1921–41, 1944, 1951, 1962, 1966, 1971.

Queen Charlotte's Lying-in Hospital (later Queen Charlotte's Hospital for Women): Case-book 1877; Clinical Reports 1907–14; Annual Clinical Reports 1915–72; Year Book 1973.

Reports of the Medical Officer of Health for Rochdale 1920, 1925, 1927–8.

Index